WE 707
GEN ✓
(NLM).

WE 707 GEN
£100.

D1422525

WE 707 GEN
£100.

Head and Neck Cancer
An Evidence-Based Team Approach

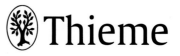

Head and Neck Cancer
An Evidence-Based Team Approach

Eric M. Genden, MD, FACS
Professor and Chairman of Otolaryngology–Head and Neck Surgery and Immunobiology
Director, Head and Neck Cancer Center
Mount Sinai Medical Center
New York, New York

Mark A. Varvares, MD
Chairman of Otolaryngology–Head and Neck Surgery
St. Louis University School of Medicine
Director, St. Louis University Cancer Center
St. Louis, Missouri

Thieme
New York • Stuttgart

Thieme Medical Publishers, Inc.
333 Seventh Ave.
New York, NY 10001

Consulting Editor: Esther Gumpert
Managing Editor: J. Owen Zurhellen IV
Vice President, Production and Electronic Publishing: Anne T. Vinnicombe
Production Editor: Heidi Pongratz, Maryland Composition
Vice President, International Sales and Marketing: Cornelia Schulze
Chief Financial Officer: Peter van Woerden
President: Brian D. Scanlan
Compositor: Compset Inc.
Printer: Everbest

Library of Congress Cataloging-in-Publication Data
Head and neck cancer : an evidence-based team approach / [edited by] Eric M. Genden, Mark A. Varvares.
   p. ; cm.
 Includes bibliographical references and index.
 ISBN 978-1-58890-636-6 1. Head—Cancer. 2. Neck—Cancer. 3. Evidence-based medicine. I. Genden, Eric M. II. Varvares, Mark A.
 [DNLM: 1. Head and Neck Neoplasms. 2. Evidence-Based Medicine. WE 707 H431726 2008]
 RC280.H4H3847 2008
 616.99'491—dc22

                                                                                    2007038559

Important note: Medical knowledge is ever-changing. As new research and clinical experience broaden our knowledge, changes in treatment and drug therapy may be required. The authors and editors of the material herein have consulted sources believed to be reliable in their efforts to provide information that is complete and in accord with the standards accepted at the time of publication. However, in view of the possibility of human error by the authors, editors, or publisher of the work herein or changes in medical knowledge, neither the authors, editors, nor publisher, nor any other party who has been involved in the preparation of this work, warrants that the information contained herein is in every respect accurate or complete, and they are not responsible for any errors or omissions or for the results obtained from use of such information. Readers are encouraged to confirm the information contained herein with other sources. For example, readers are advised to check the product information sheet included in the package of each drug they plan to administer to be certain that the information contained in this publication is accurate and that changes have not been made in the recommended dose or in the contraindications for administration. This recommendation is of particular importance in connection with new or infrequently used drugs.

Some of the product names, patents, and registered designs referred to in this book are in fact registered trademarks or proprietary names even though specific reference to this fact is not always made in the text. Therefore, the appearance of a name without designation as proprietary is not to be construed as a representation by the publisher that it is in the public domain.

Printed in China

5 4 3 2 1

ISBN: 978-1-58890-636-6

Dedication

To my loving wife and children for their support and understanding, to my mentors for their guidance, and to my patients for their trust.

  – *Eric M. Genden*

To all my teachers, colleagues, patients, and family members.

  – *Mark A. Varvares*

Contents

Foreword

The privilege of writing the foreword for a book is a mixed blessing. The privilege arises from recognition that, for some historical reason, you are viewed as someone who has a perspective from which to comment on the work or the ability to put the work in a context of its place among current and past publications. The burden of such an invitation is to cogently assess and summarize the significance of the book before it has stood the test of time. Unfortunately, the foreword cannot truly measure or reflect the impact of a work. One's humble efforts may include an assessment of the quality of the writing, the accuracy and utility of the author's efforts, and a judgment of how the work may be received. In this regard, it is my pleasure to introduce *Head and Neck Cancer: An Evidence-Based Team Approach*, edited by Eric M. Genden and Mark A. Varvares, as a welcome addition to our discipline's teaching literature.

This book presents a very concise and well-edited summary of traditional factors considered in the treatment and follow-up of patients with head and neck carcinoma. It is organized in a traditional fashion according to tumor site and includes the most recent evidence-based data and expert opinions that reflect current treatment approaches. Although a multidisciplinary team approach is emphasized throughout the text, each chapter tends to emphasize surgical treatment, reconstruction, and decision-making. It will provide a useful reference for residents and fellows in train-

ing and for nonsurgical oncologists who want to better understand the complexities of surgical decision-making. Relatively less emphasis is placed on controversy and complexity in decision-making and on complications of treatment.

A unique and welcome addition is the inclusion of actual case studies to each chapter. These provide useful examples that are immediate and practical applications of the principles presented in the text. The cases are well chosen to represent key issues.

With any new textbook, it is a challenge to be timely, yet timelessly remain grounded in principles that will withstand the rapid evolution of knowledge in cancer biology and treatment. This book meets that challenge. The inclusion of case studies is a step forward that foreshadows the eventual development of highly personalized future cancer treatment strategies. On the whole, this new contribution is a wonderful and easily digested review for the experienced clinician and a practical guide for the less experienced oncologist interested in head and neck cancer. Dr. Genden, Dr. Varvares, and the contributors have risen to the challenge and are to be congratulated.

Gregory T. Wolf, MD, FACS
Chairman of Otolaryngology
University of Michigan

Preface

The management of head and neck cancer has changed significantly over the past several years. The role of postoperative combined chemoradiation for advanced disease and the use of combined therapy for organ preservation have left many practitioners confused about the appropriate therapy for patients with tumors of the head and neck. Moreover, not all practitioners have access to a multidisciplinary tumor board for guidance. This book was written with the intent of providing surgeons and oncologists with an evidence-based guide to the contemporary management of head and neck cancer. Each chapter covers a specific cancer of a specific site, and is written by a team of physicians including a head and neck surgeon, a radiation oncologist, and a medical oncologist. The organization of the book provides the reader with a tumor board approach to tumors of the head and neck. The role of radiation—including the indications, contraindications, and common pitfalls—is discussed, as well as the indications for systemic chemotherapy and targeted therapy for patients with carcinoma of the upper aerodigestive track and thyroid gland.

The chapters are organized to provide the readership with a concise review of the anatomy, etiology, and options for management of head and neck cancer. Each chapter concludes with a series of patient cases that represent common clinical entities. The cases are discussed by the tumor board team in an effort to provide the reader with the benefit of a multidisciplinary approach to managing basic and complex cases.

This book incorporates the concepts and ingenuity of many surgeons and oncologists. It is our goal to simplify the often contradictory and confusing literature regarding the management of head and neck cancer.

Contributors

Peter E. Andersen, MD
Associate Professor of Otolaryngology
Director of Division of Head and Neck Oncology
Department of Otolaryngology–Head and Neck Surgery
Oregon Health and Science University
Portland, Oregon

Elise M. Brett, MD
Clinical Assistant Professor of Medicine
Division of Endocrinology
Mount Sinai School of Medicine
New York, New York

Houtan Chaboki, MD
Department of Otolaryngology
Mount Sinai School of Medicine
Mount Sinai Medical Center
New York, New York

Jonathan Clark, MBBS, BSc(Med), FRACS
Head and Neck Surgeon
Sydney Head and Neck Cancer Institute
Sydney Cancer Centre
Royal Prince Alfred Hospital
Newtown, Australia

Laura A. Dawson, MD, FRCPC
Associate Professor of Radiation Oncology
University of Toronto
Princess Margaret Hospital
Toronto, Ontario, Canada

Kenneth J. Dornfeld, MD, PhD
Assistant Professor of Radiation Oncology
University of Iowa
Iowa City, Iowa

Mark W. El-Deiry, MD
Assistant Professor of Otolaryngology–Head and Neck Surgery
University of South Florida
Moffitt Cancer Center
Tampa, Florida

Eric M. Genden, MD, FACS
Professor and Chairman of Otolaryngology–Head and Neck
    Surgery and Immunobiology
Director, Head and Neck Cancer Center
Mount Sinai Medical Center
New York, New York

David P. Goldstein, MD, FRCSC
Lecturer in Otolaryngology–Head and Neck Surgery
University of Toronto
Princess Margaret Hospital
Toronto, Ontario, Canada

Neil D. Gross, MD
Assistant Professor of Otolaryngology–Head and Neck Surgery
Oregon Health and Science University
Portland, Oregon

Patrick J. Gullane, MB, FRCSC, FACS
Professor and Chair of Otolaryngology–Head and Neck Surgery
University of Toronto
Otolaryngologist-in-Chief
Princess Margaret Hospital
Toronto, Ontario, Canada

Henry T. Hoffman, MD
Professor of Otolaryngology–Head and Neck Surgery
University of Iowa
Iowa City, Iowa

Jonathan C. Irish, MD, MSc, FRCSC, FACS
Professor of Otolaryngology–Head and Neck Surgery
University of Toronto
Princess Margaret Hospital
Toronto, Ontario, Canada

Adam S. Jacobson, MD
Assistant Professor of Otolaryngology–Head and Neck Surgery
Albert Einstein School of Medicine
New York, New York

Johnny Kao, MD
Assistant Professor of Radiation Oncology
Mount Sinai Medical Center
New York, New York

Merrill S. Kies, MD
Professor of Head and Neck Medical Oncology
University of Texas MD Anderson Cancer Center
Houston, Texas

William Lawson, MD
Professor and Vice Chairman of Otolaryngology
The Mount Sinai Medical Center
Mount Sinai School of Medicine
New York, New York

Brian A. Moore, MD, FRCSC
Clinical Assistant Professor of Otolaryngology
Tulane University
New Orleans, Louisiana
Chief of Otolaryngology
Eglin Air Force Base Hospital
Eglin Air Force Base, Florida

Michael J. Odell, MD
Assistant Professor of Otolaryngology–Head and Neck Surgery
St. Louis University School of Medicine
St. Louis, Missouri

Stuart H. Packer, MD
Associate Professor of Hematology/Oncology
Mount Sinai School of Medicine
New York, New York

Hans-Joachim Reimers, MD, PhD
Professor of Internal Medicine
Division of Hematology/Oncology
St. Louis University School of Medicine
St. Louis University Hospital
St. Louis, Missouri

David Rosenthal, MD
Professor of Radiation Oncology
University of Texas MD Anderson Cancer Center
Houston, Texas

Jonathan S. T. Sham, MBBS, MD, FRCR, FHRCR, FHKAM
Honorary Clinical Professor of Clinical Oncology
The University of Hong Kong
Queen Mary Hospital
Hong Kong, China

Lillian L. Siu, MD, FRCP(C)
Associate Professor of Medical Oncology and Hematology
University of Toronto
Princess Margaret Hospital
Toronto, Ontario, Canada

Peter M. Som, MD
Professor of Radiology, Otolaryngology, and Radiation Oncology
Mount Sinai School of Medicine
New York University
New York, New York

Douglas K. Trask, MD, PhD
Assistant Professor of Otolaryngology–Head and Neck Surgery
University of Iowa
Iowa City, Iowa

Mark A. Varvares, MD, FACS
Chairman of Otolaryngology–Head and Neck Surgery
St. Louis University School of Medicine
Director, St. Louis University Cancer Center
St. Louis, Missouri

Bruce J. Walz, MD
Professor of Radiation Oncology
St. Louis University School of Medicine
St. Louis, Missouri

Georges B. Wanna, MD
Chief Resident in Otolaryngology–Head and Neck Surgery
Mount Sinai Medical Center
New York, New York

Mark K. Wax, MD
Professor of Otolaryngology
Director of Microvascular Reconstructive Surgery
Program Director of Otolaryngology–Head and Neck Surgery
Oregon Health and Science University
Portland, Oregon

Randal S. Weber, MD
Professor and Chairman of Head and Neck Surgery
University of Texas MD Anderson Cancer Center
Houston, Texas

William I. Wei, MS, FRCS, FRCSE, FRACS(Hon), FACS, FHKAM(ORL)(SURG)
Li Shu Pui Professor of Surgery
Chair in Otorhinolaryngology
The University of Hong Kong
Queen Mary Hospital
Hong Kong, China

Richard Westreich, MD
Assistant Professor of Otolaryngology
SUNY-Downstate Medical Center
Brooklyn, New York

1

Carcinoma of the Oral Cavity

Eric M. Genden, Johnny Kao, and Stuart H. Packer

◆ Epidemiology

Carcinoma of the oral cavity is not uncommon. It comprises nearly 30% of all malignant tumors of the head and neck. Although the vast majority of these cancers are squamous cell carcinoma, sarcomas, and minor salivary gland tumors, a variety of dentigerous tumors may arise in the oral cavity. In North America, the most common risk factors for the development of carcinoma of the oral cavity include tobacco and alcohol use. Outside of North America, the chewing of beetle nut and of tobacco represent additional risks for the development of oral cancer. Beyond these risks, there is little evidence linking dietary factors or nutritional deficiencies to the development of oral cavity carcinoma.

◆ Etiology

The use of alcohol or of tobacco independently represents a risk for the development of oral cavity carcinoma, and the synergistic effect of these two risk factors has been well documented. It has been suggested that the use of alcohol suppresses DNA repair after exposure to nitrosamine compounds; however, the exact mechanism of the observed synergy remains poorly defined. There is significant literature to suggest a relationship between human papilloma virus and the development of squamous cell carcinoma of the cervix and tonsil; however, there has been little evidence of such an effect in the oral cavity.

Poor dental hygiene and chronic mechanical irritation have been associated with the development of carcinoma of the oral cavity. When the lateral aspect of the oral tongue is exposed to mechanical friction as a result of a sharp tooth edge or irritation of the oral cavity as a result of an ill-fitting denture, a cascade of events beginning with chronic irritation can lead to the development of squamous cell carcinoma. Ill-fitting dentures, poor dental hygiene, or chronic mechanical irritation have been linked to the development of oral cavity carcinoma; however, more recent evidence suggests a genetic factor may play a significant role in the development of carcinoma of the oral cavity. This is exemplified by a rise in the development of tongue cancer in nonsmoking young adults in the United States.

Since 1930, the prevalence of tongue cancer in young women has more than doubled. Such findings strongly suggest an environmental and/or a genetic predisposition to the development of carcinoma of the oral cavity may exist. Unlike other areas of the aerodigestive track, the oral cavity is accessible and easily examined. As a result, it is essential that screening be instituted in an effort to identify early cancers of the oral cavity. Although there are significant limitations to the current staging system of oral cavity carcinoma, it is clear that early identification, diagnosis, and management of oral cavity carcinomas result in an improved prognosis when compared with advanced disease.

◆ Development and Progression

Oral cavity carcinoma may develop as a result of one of two pathways (**Fig. 1–1**).[1] In some patients, there is a progressive systematic change in the oral cavity mucosa. Changes in the epithelium first result in hyperkeratosis, the development of parakeratosis, and eventually dyskeratosis. As the dyskeratotic cells invade, the lesion is considered a carcinoma in situ and eventually an invasive squamous cell carcinoma. However this is a common pathway for the development of invasive squamous cell carcinoma, not all patients undergo this well-defined progression. In fact, a significant number of patients develop an invasive squamous cell carcinoma without this well-defined progression.

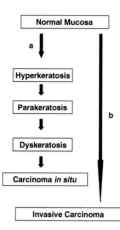

Figure 1–1 Pathway for the development of epithelial malignancy: (**A**) cellular evolution and (**B**) de novo development.

Patients who present with hyperkeratosis may develop leukoplakia represented as a white patch on the oral mucosa (**Fig. 1–2**). Commonly, this is a superficial lesion involving the oral cavity.[1] It has been estimated that leukoplakia will develop into an invasive squamous cell carcinoma in 4 to 6% of patients. A more ominous sign is the development of erythroplakia. Erythroplakia is represented as a red discoloration of the oral mucosa and has been associated with the development of invasive squamous cell carcinoma in as many as 30% of patients. Early identification of both leukoplakia and erythroplakia are essential in determining the risk of the development of invasive squamous cell carcinoma.

The oral cavity represents a unique aspect of the upper aerodigestive tract in that tumors of the oral cavity occur adjacent to the complex anatomy of the tongue, floor of the mouth, buccal mucosa, and mandible. Oral cavity carcinoma may present as a superficial lesion confined to the superior layers of the mucosa or the tumor may extend into the deep tissues invading the mandible, deep muscle, or

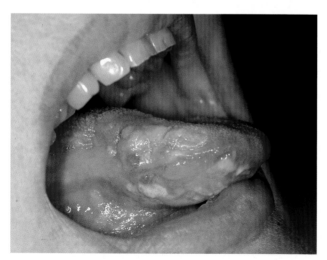

Figure 1–2 Presentation of leukoplakia. Leukoplakia may present as a dense confluent patch or a diffuse lesion involving any region of the upper aerodigestive system.

adjacent nerves. The adjacent mandible and neurovascular structures are at high risk even in early cancer of the oral cavity. Determining whether a tumor will invade and disseminate locally, regionally, or to distant sites is a function of the tumor biology and the specific histopathology. This is readily apparent in such tumors as adenoid cystic carcinoma. Although neurotropism is not a common characteristic in squamous cell carcinoma of the oral cavity, minor salivary gland tumors such as adenoid cystic carcinoma may extend into the underlying neurovascular structures involving the lingual, hypoglossal, or inferior alveolar nerves. Although local recurrence and neurotropic spread represent survival risks, adenoid cystic carcinoma most commonly spreads to distant sites such as the lung. In contrast, squamous cell carcinoma is less neurotropic but represents a high risk for local and regional spread. In squamous cell carcinoma, the specific histologic findings such as angioinvasion, lymphatic emboli, perineural spread, and poor host response are more reliable indicators of high-risk disease.[2] Therefore, the biologic behavior of a tumor is the result of both the tumor type and the histopathologic characteristics of the tumor.

◆ Anatomy of the Oral Cavity

The anterior border of the oral cavity is at the junction of the skin and vermillion border of the lip.[1] Posteriorly, the oral cavity is limited by the junction of the hard and soft palates superiorly and the circumvallate papilla inferiorly (**Fig. 1–3**). The anterior tonsillar pillars define the posterior lateral aspects of the oral cavity. The oral cavity is composed of the oral cavity gingiva, the lip, the hard palate, the oral tongue, the floor of the mouth, retromolar trigone, and buccal mucosa. In addition, the underlying mandible and maxilla are often included in the anatomy of the oral cavity. The oral cavity is composed of squamous cell epithelium populated by minor salivary glands. Although minor salivary glands can be demonstrated throughout the mucosa of the oral cavity, they are most concentrated within the hard and soft palates. For this reason, minor salivary gland tumors exist most commonly within these regions of the oral cavity.

In addition, the mandibular and maxillary alveoli are included in the oral cavity. The retromolar trigone, which is an area located in the posterior oral cavity posterior to the third molar, is a common site for carcinomas of the oral cavity. The overlying periosteum is particularly thin in the area of the retromolar trigone making invasion of the cortex common. The floor of the mouth extends from the inner margin of the lower alveolus to the ventral surface of the oral tongue. The structures of the floor of the mouth are supported by mylohyoid, geniohyoid, and genioglossus musculature. It is this muscular bed that separates the sublingual and submandibular spaces. The oral tongue located within the floor of the mouth is lined with squamous epithelium and fungiform, filiform, and circumvallate papilla. The complex movement of the tongue is generated by the intrinsic muscles responsible for swallowing and the articulation of speech. The blood supply of the oral cavity structures is provided by several branches of the external carotid artery including the facial and lingual arteries.

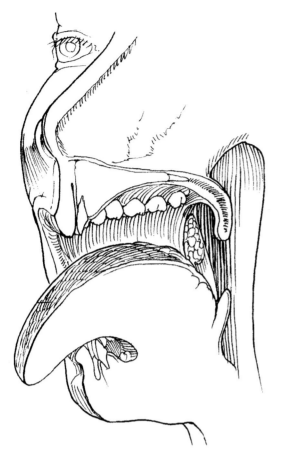

Figure 1–3 Anatomy of the oral cavity. The oral cavity includes the mucosa of the lips, buccal mucosa, floor of the mouth, alveolus, palate, and tongue extending posteriorly to the circumvallate papilla and anterior faucial arches.

The lymphatics of the oral cavity have been well characterized. Regional lymphatic channels extend from the oral cavity into the jugular digastric lymph nodes. Whereas lymphatic spread of primary oral cavity tumors commonly occurs in a predictable fashion, the rich lymphatic network of this complex area may result in skipped metastases. Additionally, the jugular digastric region serves as the first echelon of lymphatic drainage for most areas of the oral cavity; however, regions of the soft palate may drain to the retropharyngeal lymph nodes.

The complex processes of the oral cavity including speech, mastication, and deglutition are coordinated by the rich sensory and motor innervation. The second and third divisions of the trigeminal are largely responsible for the rich sensory innervation of the oral cavity. Taste and secretomotor functions of the glands within the oral cavity are provided by means of the caroticotympanic nerve, which travels along the lingual nerve to the submandibular gland. Motor control is provided by the facial nerve, the hypoglossal nerve, and the third division of the trigeminal nerve. The complex sensory muscular innervation of the oral cavity is essential for mastication, oral competency, and articulation of speech. For these reasons, it is essential that a thoughtful approach be taken when planning the management and reconstruction of an oral cavity malignancy.

◆ Staging and Prognostic Factors

The American Joint Committee on Cancer (AJCC) staging system serves as the primary tool for staging cancer of the oral cavity (**Table 1–1**). The AJCC staging system is based on surface dimensions.[3] Although staging of lip lesions is unchanged from the prior staging system, T4 lesions are now subdivided into superficially extensive (T4a) and deeply extensive (T4b). The latter denotes unresectable invasion of the masticator space, pterygoid plates, and/or skull base, and these lesions often may encase the carotid artery. The former suggests that the lesion is surgically resectable. Although the current staging system provides a useful system for reporting information, it is incomplete in its ability to predict prognosis. The survival and prognosis of a patient suffering from oral cavity carcinoma is a result of several important factors including patient comorbidity, performance status, nutritional status, and the patient's intact immune response. Although age itself is not a prognostic indicator, the comorbidities that are commonly associated with advanced age may represent a negative prognostic predictor.

There are a series of histopathologic features that may have significant impact on the prognosis of oral cavity carcinoma. The presence of perineural invasion, lymphocytic response, and depth of invasion are examples of histopathologic parameters that are not accounted for in the AJCC staging system. Additionally, extracapsular spread, which may be associated with a 50% reduction in survival, may have a significant impact on the prognosis of a patient with oral cavity carcinoma and regional disease.

Tumor thickness has been demonstrated to predict the risk of local recurrence and survival for oral tongue carcinoma.[4] The exact depth of invasion and correlation with survival is not clear; however, several studies have suggested that tumor thickness greater than 4.0 mm significantly increases the risk for cervical metastases and therefore has a negative impact on survival.[5] Other studies have suggested that 5.0 mm of tumor depth is associated with an increased rate of regional disease.[6] Currently, most surgical oncologists believe that tumor depth of 4.0 mm or greater is associated with an increased risk for regional metastases and as a result

Table 1–1 American Joint Committee on Cancer Staging System for Carcinoma of the Oral Cavity

T0	No evidence of tumor
Tis	Tumor in situ
T1	Lesions less than 2 cm
T2	Lesions 2 to 4 cm
T3	Lesions greater than 4 cm
T4(lip)	Tumor invades through the cortical bone, inferior alveolar nerve, floor of the mouth, or skin of the face.
T4a	Tumor invades adjacent structures (i.e., through cortical bone, into deep extrinsic muscle of the tongue).
T4b	Tumor invades the masticator space, pterygoid plates, or skull base and or encases the carotid artery.

Table 1–2 Factors That Influence the Presence of Occult Metastasis of the Neck

Tumor thickness >4 mm
Poorly differentiated tumors
Infiltrating-type invasion front
Presence of perineural invasion
Presence of angiolymphatic invasion
Lack of peritumor lymphocyte response
Islands of tumor >1 cm apart

recommend elective treatment of the N0 neck even in the absence of high-risk histopathologic features.

High-risk histopathologic features that influence the risk of local regional recurrence include angioinvasion, lymphatic emboli, and perineural invasion (**Table 1–2**). The most significant prognosticator in oral cancer, however, is the presence of extracapsular spread (ECS).[7,8] Because the presence of ECS has been identified as a poor prognostic indicator, patients with ECS are commonly treated with adjuvant therapy including radiation, systemic chemotherapy, or multimodality therapy. In spite of adjuvant therapy, one third of patients will still experience regional recurrence.[8]

The current AJCC staging system fails to include these factors and as a result does not appropriately reflect the impact of a given tumor on survival. Beyond these factors, there are several other important prognostic factors including lymph node fixation that are not included in the staging system. As a result, the computed tomography (CT) scan and physical examination may provide important information in determining the biologic behavior of a tumor.

◆ Presentation

The presentation of tumors of the oral cavity may vary depending upon the histology and the location of the tumor. Tumors may present as an ulcerative lesion (**Fig. 1–4A**), a raised exophytic lesion (**Fig. 1–4B**), or with irregular mucosa mass (**Fig. 1–4C**). Not uncommonly, ulcerative lesions may present as a subtle lesion on the surface; however, on further inspection and palpation, the lesion may extend deep into the soft tissue. For this reason, palpation is a key part of the exam. Similarly, tumors of the alveolus may present as an irregular patch of mucosa adjacent to a tooth socket. Peridental tumors may present as a limited lesion on the surface mucosa, yet they may extend deep into the tooth socket and

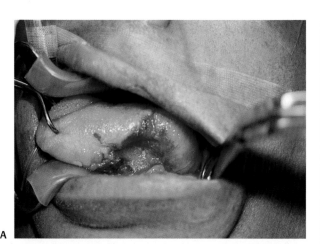

A

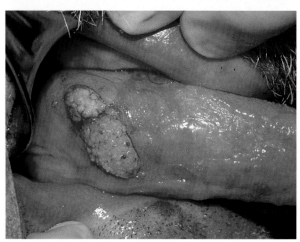

B

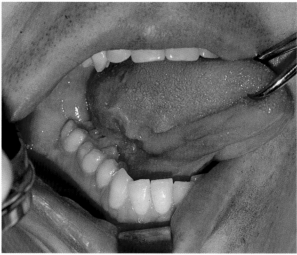

C

Figure 1–4 Variable presentations of oral cavity carcinoma. Carcinoma of the oral cavity may present as (**A**) an invasive ulcerative lesion, (**B**) an exophytic lesion, or (**C**) an irregular mucosal mass.

mandibular canal. In contrast, exophytic lesions may present as a papillomatous mass often described as a "cauliflower-like" growth. Although benign lesions may present in a similar fashion, bleeding or ulceration may suggest malignancy.

Malignancies of the oral cavity may present as painful lesions; however, presentation may be variable. Because tumors in this region are exposed to saliva, contamination and infection commonly lead to infection and pain. In contrast, if a malignant lesion erodes into sensory nerves (i.e., the lingual or alveolar nerves), the patient may present with anesthesia or hypesthesia of the lip or oral cavity. Finally, when a patient presents with complaints of trismus, invasion of the pterygoid space must be assumed until proved otherwise. Whereas infection and inflammation may also result in trismus, invasion of the pterygoid muscular may portend extensive invasion.

◆ Diagnosis and Workup

Local Disease

The diagnosis of an oral cavity carcinoma can be relatively straightforward. A complete history including use of alcohol, tobacco, and oral hygiene should be documented.

Because the oral cavity is readily accessible, changes in the mucosa are easily identified and evaluated. A surgical biopsy represents the most reliable method of diagnosis. More recently, brush biopsy has been used in the dental community as a screening tool. Several studies suggest that the sensitivity and specificity of this technique is unacceptably low.[9,10] Whereas the brush biopsy technique provides the cytologist with a sample of the surface of the lesion, surgical biopsy provides the pathologist with the tissue architecture necessary to make a definitive diagnosis of invasive carcinoma.

Noninvasive lesions, dysplasia, and carcinoma in situ require minimal workup with regard to evaluation; however, the diagnosis of invasive carcinoma mandates a thorough evaluation to assess the extent of tumor. Once a definitive diagnosis has been achieved, imaging is essential to gain an understanding of the stage of the tumor and presence of metastasis. Although extensive lesions may be heralded by trismus, otalgia, or hypesthesia, the lack of these signs does not exclude extensive invasion of the surrounding structures. CT[7] scan with contrast offers an initial assessment of soft tissue, bone, and mucosal involvement. The CT scan can be performed more quickly than a magnetic resonance imaging (MRI) scan and is performed in an "open" coil so that it is more easily tolerated by the patient. When performed with contrast, the CT scan can elucidate the mucosal extent of the tumor, the presence of bone invasion, and the presence of regional metastasis. If there is concern regarding the invasion of the deep soft tissue, muscle, or nerve, an MRI scan may prove more accurate. The MRI scan is ideal for the evaluation of soft tissue and, in some cases, nerve involvement. Enhancement of the lingual, alveolar, or trigeminal ganglion may suggest perineural involvement. The MRI scan is particularly helpful in evaluation of nonepidermoid carcinoma (i.e., adenoid cystic carcinoma) in which perineural invasion is not uncommon.

Mandibular Invasion

Plain radiography has been used extensively in the past for the diagnosis of extensive tumor invasion of the mandible; however, subtle changes associated with the cortex have been more difficult to identify. The introduction of the panoramic x-ray, CT, and MRI scans have increased the accuracy of preoperative imaging and staging. Significant debate still exists regarding the optimal modality or combination of modalities recommended for preoperative assessment. Although CT is a very accurate method for identifying gross bone invasion,[11] prior work has suggested that bone invasion may be missed in as many as 27% of patients with preoperative CT scans. The sensitivity of a CT scan for bone involvement of the retromolar trigone is ~50% with a negative predictive value of 60%; however, the positive predictive value is ~90%. It has been concluded that although the CT scan is accurate when bone erosion is clearly identified, its negative predictive value is unacceptably low and therefore an inaccurate indicator of bone invasion at the retromolar trigone. The CT scan renders an excellent view of both the soft tissue and bone of the mandible; however, it has several limitations, the most significant being artifacts caused by dental amalgams. Dental amalgams commonly create a shadow leading to artifact that can obscure invasion of the mandibular cortex. Additionally, the CT scan may misleadingly detect defects in the cortex secondary to irregular tooth sockets or periapical disease.

In light of these shortcomings, several investigators have reported on the use of a Dentascan. The Dentascan was introduced in the early 1980s to assist oral maxillofacial surgeons in planning for osseointegrated implants. The Dentascan images are derived by reformatting standard axial CT scans in two views: panelliptical and parasagittal. This reformatting permits assessment of the buccal and lingual cortices. The diagnostic accuracy of the Dentascan is accurate, yielding a sensitivity of 95% and a specificity of 79% with a positive predictive value of 87% and a negative predictive value of 92%. The Dentascan is an accurate method for preoperative evaluation of mandibular invasion in patients with squamous cell carcinoma of the oral cavity.

Whereas the CT scan and Dentascan may offer excellent methods for assessing bone, the MRI scan offers the advantage of imaging soft tissue and potentially the medullary bone space. Several studies have examined the use of MRI in assessing mandibular invasion, and it has been concluded that the MRI scan is superior for evaluating the medullary space of the mandible,[12] but inadequate for assessing mandibular invasion. Shaha[13] examined the value of various studies including panoramic x-rays, dental films, routine mandible films, bone scans, CT scans, and MRI and found that CT scanning was not very helpful mainly because of the presence of irregular dental sockets and artifacts. Many suggest that clinical evaluation is the most accurate in determining the presence of bone invasion and the optimal method of resection, marginal versus segmental.

Most centers consider the combination of a CT scan and a panoramic x-ray acceptable for preoperative imaging of the mandible and maxilla; however, the most accurate measure of bony invasion is determined clinically. Unless there is frank invasion of the bony cortex, periosteal stripping followed by frozen-section examination at the time of surgery is often the most reliable measure of bone invasion.

Regional Disease

MRI and CT are both effective in identifying regional disease; however, most centers prefer CT because it is well tolerated, highly sensitive, and less expensive than MRI. Both modalities are sensitive in identifying ECS. Identifying ECS is extremely important because of its impact on survival. Whereas tumor limited to the lymph node has been associated with survival rates ranging from 50 to 70%,[14] the presence of ECS diminished survival to 25 to 30% over 5 years. In the event that pathologic lymph nodes are identified, fine-needle aspiration (FNA) may be warranted. "Pathologic" lymph nodes are those nodes that demonstrate central necrosis, extracapsular spread, or are greater than 1 cm in diameter in levels I, III, IV, V, and VI or greater than 1.5 cm in the jugulodigastric region.[15] Identification of a pathologic node in the face of a known oral cavity malignancy does not always require assessment; however, in cases where there is an undetermined primary carcinoma or if there is a suspicious lymph node in an area outside the predicted nodal basin, FNA is warranted. When the lymph node is easily palpable, a fine-needle biopsy can be performed by palpation. In cases in which the lymph node is difficult to palpate, ultrasound-guided FNA is highly accurate.

Distant Disease

Distant metastatic disease is rare in epidermoid oral cavity carcinoma. It occurs in only 15% of patients who succumb to their disease. Distant metastatic disease rarely occurs without evidence of regional metastasis; however, when distant disease is discovered, survival is poor. In contrast, early-stage nonepidermoid carcinoma, in particular adenoid cystic carcinoma, may present with distant metastatic disease; however, patients can survive extended periods with distant disease.

Distant metastasis from epidermoid carcinoma may occur in the lung, bone, or liver. Although distant metastases rarely occur as a result of oral cavity carcinoma, when they do occur, histopathology often demonstrates aggressive patterns such as lymphatic, vascular, and/or perineural invasion. Additionally, we have found a strong association between peritumor lymphocytic infiltrate and survival.[2] Those patients whose tumors lack a peritumor infiltrate have a significantly increased risk of recurrence and death as a result of their disease. Although external beam radiation therapy has a positive impact on local regional recurrence, distant metastatic disease remains the most common cause of death from head and neck cancer. This has prompted several groups to incorporate systemic chemotherapy as a radiosensitizing agent and to limit distant metastasis.

The use of coregistered positron emission tomography (PET)[16] and CT scanning (PET-CT) has had an enormous impact on surveillance of local, regional, and distant sites.[16] The PET-CT scan has also proved useful for monitoring the response to therapy.[17,18] We find that the PET-CT scan is a reliable alternative to liver function studies, CT scan alone, and bone scanning for the evaluation of distant disease.

◆ Treatment

Tumors Involving the Tongue

Surgical Treatment

The overwhelming majority of cancers involving the oral cavity are squamous cell carcinoma; however, minor salivary gland tumors may also occur. Epidermoid cancer of the oral cavity may be treated with either radiation, surgery, or combined therapy. Although the goal is to achieve a cure, it is optimal to manage patients with single-modality therapy because it is associated with less treatment-related morbidity and, in many cases, an improvement in quality of life.

Early Disease Superficial carcinomas of the oral cavity can be treated with equivalent cure rates with either radiation therapy or surgical excision. Therefore, the choice of therapy is often based on factors such as patient preference, quality of life, cost, convenience, and patient compliance. Because surgical therapy can be achieved with minimal morbidity, surgery has become the gold standard for management of early cancers of the oral cavity. Although radiotherapy is equally effective for the treatment of early disease, the rates of long-term sequelae including xerostomia, dysphagia, and osteoradionecrosis are unacceptably high. Other advantages of surgical therapy include the cost of treatment. Surgical therapy requires a single intervention, whereas radiation therapy requires daily therapy in addition to catheter implants. Currently, radiation therapy is reserved for those patients who are unable to undergo surgery.

Advanced Disease Advanced disease of the oral cavity is best managed with multimodality therapy. Surgery coupled with preoperative or postoperative radiation therapy is often applied for advanced disease. The rationale for preoperative radiation is to decrease the tumor mass and therefore increase the "resectability" of the tumor; however, it is common practice to surgically resect the tumor based on the pre-radiation margins because it has been demonstrated that islands of viable tumor may persist in the initial peripheral margins. Additionally, preoperative radiation is associated with a higher rate of postoperative complications. For these reasons, most centers perform surgery followed by postoperative radiation.

Tumors involving the anterior two-thirds of the oral tongue can usually be managed through a transoral approach; however, more extensive tumors and tumors involving the posterior one-third of the tongue may require a lingual release.

Postoperative radiation therapy for the primary site is reserved for those cases in which the risk of recurrence is high. Defining the "high-risk" patient has been a topic of controversy; however, it is important to clarify that the indications for postoperative radiation therapy directed to the primary site are different from the indications for postoperative radiation directed at the neck. The goal of a surgical excision is to achieve a complete resection of the tumor with tumor-free margins. In cases where there are positive margins, a re-resection is recommended. In cases where a re-resection is performed and there is evidence of microscopic disease at the margins, radiation directed at the primary site should be considered. In cases where there is neck disease that is N2 or greater or the tumor pathology demonstrates aggressive surgical behavior (**Table 1–2**),[3] radiation therapy is warranted.

Radiation Therapy

Early disease that measures less than 1.5 mm thick on imaging may be treated with interstitial implantation using iridium-192 (^{192}Ir) to a dose of 60 to 65 Gy. Alternatively, an intraoral cone may be used to 40 Gy in 10 fractions. For lesions that invade deeper than 1.5 mm, radiation treatment should consist of external beam radiation to the gross tumor with at least 2-cm margins to 40 Gy with elective treatment of neck bilaterally (levels I to IV to 50 Gy) followed by ^{192}Ir interstitial implant to 35 to 40 Gy. For a well-lateralized lesion, treatment of the contralateral lower neck may be omitted. External beam radiotherapy alone results in suboptimal local control[19]; however, the appropriate use of brachytherapy can yield local control rates of 80 to 85% for T1 lesions and 65 to 80% for T2 lesions.[20,21]

Advanced disease is commonly managed surgically; however, when surgery would result in total glossectomy or severely impaired function, organ-preserving therapy with primary radiation should be considered in selected cases.

Radiation alone consists of 50 Gy to the gross tumor + 2-cm margin + bilateral levels 1 to 4 to 50 Gy followed by ^{192}Ir interstitial implant to 25 to 30 Gy. Local control rates of 45 to 65% for T3 and 0 to 10% for T4 are suboptimal.[21] Therefore, adding concomitant chemotherapy to radiation to improve local control is appropriate for these patients.

Acute complications of radiation therapy including mucositis and taste changes generally resolve within 3 months of completion of radiation. The degree of xerostomia is related to dose and volume of salivary glands irradiated. Severe late complications, such as mucosal ulceration or osteonecrosis, occur in ~10% of patients treated with definitive radiation and is related to tumor burden. Interestingly, one report from the University of Florida showed similar rates of late complications between surgery and radiation for T1 to T2 lesions. Primary radiation resulted in lower rates of late complications compared with surgery ± adjuvant radiation. The likelihood of complications can be reduced with attention to technique. For external beam irradiation, the tongue is depressed by an intraoral stent to allow blocking of the hard palate. Sparing a strip of submental skin may reduce the likelihood of late edema. For interstitial brachytherapy, to avoid bone complications, care should be given to insert packing into the floor of the mouth and to avoid placing catheters near the mandible.

Tumors Involving the Mandible

Surgical Treatment

Tumors invading the mandible can be managed either with a marginal resection or a segmental resection (**Fig. 1–5**). The decision regarding the optimal method of tumor resection is largely dependent on the degree of invasion. It has been

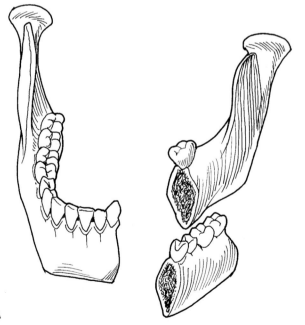

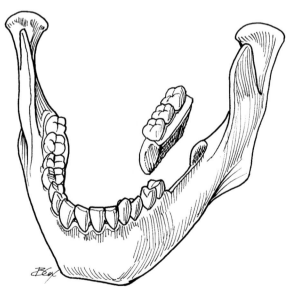

Figure 1–5 (**A**) Segmental resection. Tumors eroding the cortex and invading the mandibular canal require a segmental resection of the mandible. (**B**) Marginal resection. Tumors invading the superficial cortex of the mandible can be managed with a marginal resection of the mandible. The inferior 2-cm margin of the mandible must be preserved to provide strength to the mandible during mastication.

suggested that tumor invasion of the periosteum or cortical bone, without invasion of the medullary cortex, can be appropriately managed with a marginal resection. Tumors that erode into the medullary canal, however, require a segmental resection. It has been shown that once a tumor gains access to the medullary canal, tumor may travel through the canal via the neurovascular bundle. The inability to obtain frozen-section assessment of the mandible intraoperatively represents a management dilemma because decalcification of the mandible specimen requires 2 weeks.

The periosteum is relatively resistant to cancer invasion. With the exception of the tooth sockets, the periosteum acts as a dense barrier to the invasion of adjacent tumor. In spite of the protective periosteum, aggressive and long-standing tumors erode the periosteum and invade the adjacent mandible through a variety of pathways. Two distinct histologic patterns of tumor invasion have been identified. The first pattern is referred to as *infiltrative* and is characterized by finger-like projections of tumor, which advance independently and invade the cancellous spaces without the intervening connective tissue layer and with very little osteoclastic activity. The second pattern is referred to as *erosive*. In contrast with the infiltrative pattern, the erosive pattern is characterized by a broad front with a connective tissue layer and active osteoclast activity. The significance of the erosive and infiltrative patterns has been demonstrated in several reports, and it has been demonstrated that patient survival is significantly affected by the pattern of invasion. Wong et al found that the 3-year disease-free survival for infiltrative squamous cell carcinoma was 30%, whereas the 3-year disease-free survival for the erosive pattern was 73%.[22] It has been suggested that the pattern of invasion is a reflection of the biologic aggressiveness of the tumor and may impact the approach to ablative therapy. We commonly consult our pathologist regarding the pattern and use this information when considering the role of radiation therapy, chemotherapy, and posttreatment surveillance. Whereas most tumors that invade the mandible mandate postoperative external beam radiation, some have suggested that superficially invading tumors may not benefit from postoperative radiation. Given the aggressive behavior of the infiltrative pattern of invasion, we recommend postoperative radiation for all patients with this pattern of bone invasion.

Tumor within the oral cavity may invade the mandible and gain entrance into the mandibular canal through several routes. Not uncommonly, tumor will travel along the surface mucosa until it approaches the attached gingiva where the tumor cells may come into contact with the periosteum of the mandible. Tumor cells demonstrate a tendency to migrate into the dental sockets because this area represents a pathway of minimal resistance. In the edentulous patients, tumor cells will migrate onto the occlusal surface of the alveolus and enter the mandible through dental pits, which are cortical bone defects at the location of prior dentition. Less commonly, tumor may enter the mandible through mental or mandibular canals. Least commonly, adjacent tumor may erode through the cortical bone directly into the mandibular canal. As mentioned earlier, this is a rare mode of invasion.

Although the superficial invasion of the periosteum or cortical bone may be managed with a marginal mandibulectomy, once the tumor has eroded into the medullary cavity and mandibular canal, most advocate a segmental resection. Determining the presence of bone erosion and the extent of bone erosion represents an ongoing clinical dilemma. The poor predictability associated with preoperative imaging has led many to rely on preoperative clinical assessment as the primary method for determining the presence of mandibular invasion. Several groups have studied this issue and found that clinical evaluation of mandibular bone erosion is more sensitive than radiographic evaluation; however, radiographic assessment may be more specific and provide a higher reliability index.[23]

There are a few studies reviewing the impact of clinical assessment alone in determining the extent of mandibular invasion. This likely represents the difficulty in quantifying a clinical exam. Most agree, however, that clinical assessment for invasion is paramount. Several studies have evaluated the role of periosteal stripping as an indicator for tumor invasion of the mandible[24] and found that periosteal stripping at the time of resection represented an accurate predictor of the presence of mandibular invasion. We subscribe to this approach and find that without clear evidence of mandibular invasion, periosteal stripping followed by close inspection is an adequate approach. If there is evidence of cortical invasion, a marginal resection can be performed. If there is cortical invasion, the marginal resection can be converted to a segmental resection.

In conclusion, accurate preoperative assessment through the combination of clinical and radiologic examination is more accurate than using either modality alone. Intraoperative periosteal stripping at the time of resection represents an accurate predictor of the presence of mandibular invasion and may be the only reliable method of assessment.

Radiation Therapy

Radiation is seldom used for management of disease of the alveolus and retromolar trigone. When surgical therapy is not an option, T1 disease may be treated with external beam radiation, 50 Gy to primary tumor and lymph node basins IB to II followed by a 16-Gy boost to the primary tumor. For small T2 lesions, treatment consists of 50 Gy external beam radiation to primary tumor and lymph node basins I to III followed by an 18-Gy boost to the primary tumor. Local control is ~70 to 85%. Large T2 and T3 tumors may also be managed with radiation therapy. Recommended concomitant boost radiation consists of one treatment per day for the first 16 treatment days and two treatments for the final 12 treatment days. This strategy is designed to overcome accelerated repopulation of tumor cells during radiation. Local control is ~70 to 75%. T4 lesions with bone involvement are usually treated by surgery. An alternative treatment is concomitant chemotherapy and radiation, although there is a risk of bone exposure. The primary necks receive 50 Gy whereas the primary tumor receives 70 Gy with concomitant chemotherapy. Local control is ~35 to 60%.

Tumors of the Buccal Mucosa

Surgical Treatment

Buccal carcinoma comprises less than 10% of oral cavity carcinoma, and when it occurs, it commonly arises from a preexisting leukoplakia.[25,26] The principles of management of buccal carcinoma are no different than those of other subsites within the oral cavity. Surgical therapy is the preferred method of management. In early disease, surgical excision can usually be accomplished transorally. Tumors that invade the buccinator muscle and tumors that present with nodal disease or with poor prognostic features should be managed with postoperative radiation therapy. Negative surgical margins are paramount, and in an effort to achieve this goal, careful preoperative planning is essential to determine the extent of the tumor. An MRI scan is ideal for imaging of the buccal mucosa and soft tissue of the masticator space. Whereas early tumors of the buccal mucosa commonly present as an irregular mucosal mass, more than half of buccal tumors will present as deeply invasive tumors that may track along the parotid duct, masseter muscle, or into the palate. The proximity of the buccal mucosa to the parotid duct requires that the duct be traced retrograde and sampled to ensure a negative margin.

Deeply invasive lesions may break into the buccal fat pad. When this occurs, it is advisable to resect the entire fat pad because negative surgical margins in this area are difficult to confirm. The rich lymphatic network characteristic of the buccal region and the high rate of lymph node metastasis mandate that the neck be carefully evaluated and, in most cases, treated. Smaller tumor can usually be managed through a transoral approach; however, more advanced tumors may require a midline labiotomy incision (**Fig. 1–6**).

Radiation Therapy

Small tumors not involving the oral commissure are commonly treated surgically; however, radiation provides equivalent local control. Because buccal mucosal tumors are well lateralized, treatment consists of external beam radiation to a dose of 50 Gy to the primary tumor with a 2-cm margin. An external beam radiation boost is given to the primary tumor to achieve a final dose of 66 Gy for T1 and 70 Gy for T2 cancers. This can be accomplished with techniques that spare the contralateral parotid gland, such as a wedged photon pair or appositional mixed electron photon (4:1 ratio) portal. Alternatively, brachytherapy administered to a dose of 25 to 30 Gy can be employed as a boost. Local control is ~90% for T1 and 70% for T2. Advanced tumors are also usually treated surgically. Local control is ~70% for T3 and 50% for T4. Due to extension to midline structures, elective bilateral radiation to 50 Gy is generally indicated followed by a boost to the primary tumor to 70 Gy. Strong consideration of concomitant chemotherapy and radiation should be given to patients that present with T4 carcinoma. When a primary irradiation approach is selected, the primary tumor and uninvolved ipsi-

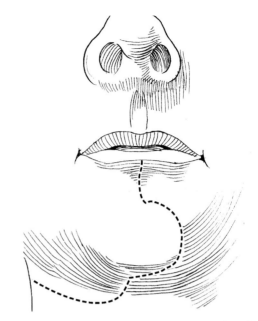

Figure 1–6 Labiotomy incision: a common approach to the oral cavity when a transoral approach is inadequate.

lateral neck should be irradiated to 50 Gy followed by a boost to the involved nodal basin and primary tumor to 70 Gy.

Radiation of the buccal mucosa may be associated with significant complications. Trismus may occur if the muscles of mastication are irradiated to high doses. Care should be taken to limit radiation dose to the mandible. For oral commissure lesions, an intraoral stent may displace the tongue out of the field. A lead shield placed inside the mouth minimizes radiation dose to the contralateral parotid gland and mandible.

Tumors of the Palate

Surgical Treatment

Unlike other areas of the oral cavity where squamous cell carcinoma makes up the overwhelming majority of pathology, the palate is rich in minor salivary glands and therefore is the site of both benign and malignant salivary gland tumors. The principles of management of tumors of the palate are similar to those of the mandible; obtaining tumor-free margins is essential to achieving a good outcome. Preoperative imaging of this area is important to assess invasion of the sinus, palatal bone, and the nasal vault. The CT scan is ideal for assessing this because it offers a high-resolution image of the palatal and nasal bones. Lateral tumors may represent a risk to invasion and perineural spread via the palatine or trigeminal neurovascular bundle. Pain or anesthesia may suggest nerve invasion, and MRI with gadolinium may demonstrate enhancement or edema of the nerve suggesting nerve invasion. The depth of invasion will dictate the extent of the surgical resection. Superficial lesions of the palatal mucosa are best managed with a wide surgical resection including the underlying palatal periosteum. The periosteum serves as an early barrier to spread; however, as tumors become more invasive, tumors can vertically invade the nasal vault or sinus.

Tumors of the hard palate rarely metastasize to the neck, and therefore a neck dissection is rarely warranted in the absence of demonstrable regional disease. One exception is when there is tumor erosion through the posterior or posterior lateral sinus into the pterygopalatine fossa.

Radiation Therapy

Carcinomas of the hard palate are most commonly managed surgically; however, in select cases, radiation is an option for a superficial T1 lesion without bone invasion. When radiation therapy is applied, external beam radiation is directed at the primary tumor to 50 Gy followed by a 16- to 20-Gy boost to primary tumor. Local control after radiation is 65 to 70% for T1 to T2 cancers.[15,27] More advanced lesions[20] require external beam radiation to primary tumor to 50 Gy followed by a 20-Gy boost to primary tumor, with consideration of concomitant chemotherapy for those patients with T4 cancer. In this group, local control is 55 to 65% for radiation for T3 to T4 tumor.

Tumors of the Floor of the Mouth

Surgical Treatment

The floor of the mouth is rich in neural and vascular structures including the lingual and hypoglossal nerves, the submandibular duct, and the sublingual glands. The lack of any substantial fascial barrier means that early tumors of the floor of the mouth can quickly invade into the underlying structures and metastasize the first echelon lymph node basin. A careful preoperative clinical examination may reveal information such as submandibular sialoadenitis or lingual atrophy that may suggest submandibular duct or hypoglossal nerve invasion, respectively. The MRI is ideal for imaging the floor of the mouth because it is accurate in identifying soft tissue and perineural invasion.

Because of the density of neurovascular structures in the floor of the mouth, metastasis to the sublingual, submandibular, and level II lymph node basins are not uncommon. Sessions et al reviewed 280 cases and found a significant reduction in 5-year survival in the patients with involved margins, advanced clinical tumor stage, positive nodes, and tumor recurrence.[28] They suggested that in patients with no clinically positive nodes, patients can be observed safely for regional nodal disease because subsequent positive nodes can be treated with no adverse affect on survival. Others have found that a more aggressive approach to the N0 neck is warranted and that a selective neck dissection allows for early removal of occult metastases with acceptable morbidity.[29,30] Hicks et al found that as many as 21% of patients with T1 lesions or greater had occult metastatic dis-

ease. They suggested an elective neck dissection and adjunctive radiotherapy for increased regional control of disease for advanced tumors.[30] Given the high rate of occult metastasis, we advocate a selective neck dissection for all tumors of the floor of the mouth. Radiation therapy is reserved for advanced local disease or N2 or greater disease.

Radiation Therapy

T1 to T2 N0: Although surgery and radiation result in equivalent cure rates, most patients are treated by surgery because of concerns of late radiation complications. Primary radiation is most commonly recommended for medically inoperable patients. For T1 lesions less than 1.5 mm thick, interstitial implantation alone to a dose of 60 to 65 Gy with ^{192}Ir is adequate treatment. For deep T1 and T2 lesions, external beam radiation is administered at a dose of 45 Gy to the primary tumor + 2 cm + levels 1 to 2 followed by an ^{192}Ir interstitial implant for an additional 25 to 30 Gy. Local control is 85 to 95% for T1 lesions and 70 to 90% for T2 lesions. External beam radiation alone results in less promising local control.

T3 to T4 N0: Primary surgery is the preferred mode of treatment. For inoperable or unresectable T3 patients, external beam radiotherapy consists of primary tumor + 2 cm margin + levels 1 to 3 receiving 54 Gy (with spinal cord blocked after 45 Gy), and the primary tumor + 1 cm receives 72 Gy in 6 weeks. Local control is 55 to 75% for T3 lesions and ~25 to 40% for T4 lesions. To improve local control for T4 lesions, consideration should be given to concomitant chemotherapy with radiation.

Complications Doses in excess of 70 to 75 Gy to the mandible will result in unacceptable rates of osteonecrosis; however, with careful attention to technique, the University of Florida reported a 5% rate of severe complications with radiation alone compared with 17% for surgery alone and 15% for surgery followed by adjuvant radiation. For external beam radiation, an intraoral stent is constructed to displace the maxilla and upper lip and a rubber cork applied to a tongue blade is used to displace the lower lip and tongue (if not involved by tumor) out of the radiation field. For brachytherapy, care is taken to minimize dose to the mandible. The use of a dental prosthesis may provide protection to the mandible.

The Neck

Lymph node metastasis is one of the most important prognostic factors in squamous cell carcinoma of the head and neck. Management choices for the N0 neck include observation, elective neck dissection, or external beam radiation therapy. An evolution in the management of the N0 neck has occurred over the past 20 years. In the 1980s, observation was not uncommon; however, the data eventual demonstrated that nearly 30% of patients who were observed developed cervical metastasis.[1,31] Those patients that suffered from regional recurrence often required a modified or radical neck dissection and adjuvant therapy. The result was a higher degree of morbidity and a compromise in overall survival. As a result, the elective neck dissection was adopted in the 1990s for those patients at risk for occult disease; however, its role in the management of oral cavity cancer has been controversial.[32,33]

The elective neck dissection offers several important advantages over observation or radiation therapy. The elective neck dissection provides the only method of accurate staging and therefore the only accurate method to predict survival and disease-free interval.[34] This is largely because the elective neck dissection provides staging information that has the potential to identify those patients at high risk for systemic disease. In spite of high-resolution imaging, detecting occult disease is difficult. Several studies have demonstrated that pathologically positive lymph nodes can be found in 20 to 30% of patients, and extracapsular spread, a finding highly predictive of the development of distant metastasis, may occur in 8% of patients.[35-37] Whereas the majority of patients who undergo elective neck dissection will not have occult disease, those who are found to have regional disease and or extracapsular spread can be offered adjuvant therapy including radiation and chemotherapy. Currently, work is being done to evaluate the efficacy of sentinel lymph node biopsy; however, this technique remains experimental.

When there is no clinical evidence of lymph node metastasis and the risk of occult disease exceeds 15 to 20%, the ipsilateral neck should be addressed. Within the oral cavity, the oral tongue and floor of the mouth have been identified as sites with the highest risk for occult disease and therefore require management of the neck. The options include external beam radiotherapy or a selective neck dissection. Because it is optimal to treat patients with single-modality therapy and early carcinoma of the oral cavity is commonly treated surgically, surgical management of the neck is preferred. This approach reserves the use of external beam radiation in the event of a regional failure.

A selective neck dissection, in the setting of oral cancer requires that the lymph nodes in levels Ia, Ib, IIa, IIb, III, and IV be dissected and removed. There has been debate regarding the appropriateness of a supraomohyoid neck dissection in the management of the N0 neck. Proponents of the supraomohyoid neck dissection suggest a limited neck dissection can be used for staging with minimal risk of morbidity. Opponents of the supraomohyoid neck dissection express concern over the documented skip metastasis that has been documented in up to 15% of patients with carcinoma of the lateral tongue. Because the morbidity of a selective neck dissection, including level IV lymph nodes is not significantly greater than a supraomohyoid neck dissection, we advocate a selective neck dissection that addresses levels I to IV in such cases.

Reconstruction

The Oral Cavity

Reconstruction of the oral cavity has evolved over the past two decades. Prior to the introduction of microvascular free tissue transfer, skin grafts, local flaps, and pedicled regional flaps represented the reconstructive options available to head and neck surgeons. Although skin grafts, local and regional flaps are often acceptable for limited defects of the buccal and palatal region, larger defects and defects involving the tongue and floor of the mouth are more susceptible to tethering and contraction. Tethering of the tongue and floor of the mouth can compromise speech and swallowing. For this reason, the once popular tongue flap is seldom used for intraoral reconstruction.

The Tongue

The split-thickness skin graft has been used for many years for the management of superficial defects of the tongue; however, skin grafts have a tendency to contract. This may impair speech and swallowing especially if the graft is placed in the floor of the mouth and tongue. The radial forearm free flap has been used extensively in oral cavity reconstruction. The thin pliable tissue of the volar surface of the radial forearm is ideal for reconstruction of the oral cavity because it can be fashioned to reconstruct the complex three-dimensional anatomy. Additionally, the radial forearm flap can be reinnervated to provide sensation that may help rehabilitate swallowing. The radial forearm free flap is ideal for partial glossectomy and buccal and palatal defects; however, larger defects of the tongue require more bulk than the radial forearm can offer. This is particularly important for total glossectomy defects. Because the bulk and height of the oral tongue are essential for articulation and bolus transfer, it is imperative to preserve the oral volume during reconstruction. Additionally, if movement of the base of the tongue is preserved, functional rehabilitation of swallowing will be significantly improved. Movement of the base of the tongue will drive the food bolus posteriorly to initiate the swallow. It is therefore important to design the reconstruction in such a way that the neotongue is not tethered or impeded from moving with the base of the tongue.

The pectoralis myocutaneous flap has been advocated for reconstruction of oral defects; however, this technique has several shortcomings. Because the pectoralis flap is a pedicled flap, it has a tendency to draw down on the skin paddle. Coupled with the muscle atrophy, the pectoralis flap characteristically loses its bulk over time creating a gutter that can result in poor speech and aspiration. One of the advantages of free tissue transfer is the ability to reconstruct defects without the limitations associated with a vascular pedicle. There are several free flap donor sites available for reconstruction of an oral tongue defect. The optimal choice is predicated upon the size of the defect and the need for bulk and sensation. Donor sites like the anterolateral thigh and rectus abdominis offer excellent bulk for total glossectomy defects; however, the rectus abdominis flap lacks sensory innervation, but the anterolateral thigh has recently been reported to provide sensory restoration. The radial forearm and lateral arm free flap donor sites have the potential for sensory innervation that can be helpful for oral rehabilitation.

The Buccal Mucosa

Reconstruction of the buccal mucosa can be achieved with an adjacent tissue flap, a split-thickness skin graft, or a free flap reconstruction. Although an adjacent tissue flap is ideal, often defects are extensive and require more tissue than can be afforded by the adjacent mucosa. The split-thickness skin graft has been used successfully for buccal defects; however, contraction of the skin graft, especially in larger defects, can result in debilitating trismus. For this reason, the radial forearm free flap has provided an excellent source of donor tissue for buccal reconstruction. The radial forearm skin contracts very little, making it ideal for buccal reconstruction.

The Mandible

Reconstruction of the mandible can be achieved using a reconstruction plate without a bone graft, a nonvascularized bone graft, or the bone-containing free flaps. The use of a reconstruction plate without accompanying bone is discouraged because of the high rate of plate fracture, plate extrusion, and infection associated with his technique. A reconstruction plate can be used with a nonvascularized bone graft if the graft is not exposed to the intraoral milieu and if the patient has no history of prior radiation. Vascularized bone grafts have many advantages over plate or nonvascularized reconstruction. They are significantly more resistant to infection and resorption, and because they heal to the adjacent native mandible, they provide strength and stability to the mandibular complex (**Table 1–3**).

When considering the optimal donor site for mandible reconstruction, it is essential to consider the nature of the defect. Defects may range from a large bony defect with a small mucosal defect to a small bony defect with a large soft tissue defect. Most prioritize the soft tissue component of the flap because it is the soft tissue component that will most affect the functional outcome of the patient.[3] Whereas an isolated alveolar defect may require a bone graft and a small skin paddle for intraoral lining, a composite glossectomy-mandible defect will require donor tissue that provides an adequate bone graft and a skin paddle that will not tether the remaining native tongue. The ideal qualities of a flap for mandible reconstruction include a thin and pliable skin paddle, a skin paddle that is mobile relative to the bone segment, and a skin paddle that has the potential for sensory reinnervation.

The scapula donor site was first introduced as a vascularized bone containing free flap by Teot et al in 1981.[38] Based on the subscapular artery and vein, this donor site is unique in its ability to provide a large variety of soft tissue components including the scapular fasciocutaneous flap, latissimus dorsi myocutaneous flap, and serratus anterior flap. The scapula donor site has the potential to provide a large skin paddle with significant mobility relative to the bone segment. The versatility of this donor site and the mobility of the skin paddle relative to the bone segment make it ideal for complex three-dimensional reconstructions. We find this donor site an ideal choice for head and neck reconstruction in the elderly population because unlike the fibula and iliac bone-containing donor sites, the scapular vessels are very rarely affected by atherosclerosis. Additionally, using the upper extremity as a donor site ensures that the patients will ambulate more quickly in the postoperative period therefore decreasing the likelihood of a deep vein thrombosis.

The fibular donor site has been considered by many as the ideal donor site for oromandibular reconstruction. This flap provides the longest segment of bone that is available and is therefore the only donor site that can provide enough bone for a total mandible reconstruction. The peroneal vessels supply up to 25 cm of bone as well as a segment of skin along the lateral aspect of the lower leg. The skin paddle is often thin and pliable; however, the mobility relative to the bone segment can be limited. The straight segment of fibula bone can be contoured through numerous osteotomies to simulate the shape of the mandible. The iliac crest–internal oblique donor site provides vascularized bone of excellent quality; however, the skin paddle is not ideal for relining the oral cavity. The skin and associated subcutaneous tissue are often too thick for restoration of the oral cavity. Other shortcomings include the blood supply to the skin may be tenuous because it is derived from small musculocutaneous perforators making the skin paddle unreliable. In addition, the significant donor site morbidity related to gait disturbance and hernia have turned the attention of surgeons to other bony flaps.

The Palate

Rehabilitation of the palate can be achieved with a prosthetic obturator, a palatal flap, or free flap reconstruction. Prosthetic obturation has several advantages and disadvantages. Prosthetic reconstruction is immediate, it does not require further surgery, and it allows for direct visualization and surveillance of the operative bed. Many patients, however, complain about the inconvenience of daily hygiene, the persistent odor, and the social awkwardness associated with a prosthetic obturator. Elderly patients with arthritis or poor vision may find it difficult to manage an obturator and would prefer a permanent solution. Until recently, prosthetic obturation has been the traditional approach to management of palatal defects. More recently, local regional flaps and free flap reconstruction have been demonstrated to provide an improvement in quality of life by achieving permanent separation of the oronasal fistula and, in some cases, improving mastication and speech.[39]

Dissatisfaction with prosthetic restoration has led to the description of several local and regional soft tissue flaps for the closure of defects involving the non–tooth-bearing por-

Table 1–3 Characteristics of Bone-Containing Free Flaps

Donor Site	Bone Length (cm)	Skin Paddle Mobility Relative to Bone	Donor Site Morbidity	Bone Stock
Fibula	20–25	Marginal	Marginal	Good
Scapula	12–15	Excellent	Minimal	Marginal
Iliac crest	12–15	Poor	High	Excellent

tion of the hard palate. The mobility and accessibility of the oral tongue made the tongue flap a popular choice for reconstruction in the early 20th century. The obvious functional repercussions associated with the tongue flap have led to the use of several alternative donor sites including the temporalis flap, the buccal mucosal flap, and the palatal island flap. More recently, free tissue transfer has been applied effectively to the rehabilitation of these defects. In nonirradiated patients with small- to moderate-sized defects, the palatal island mucoperiosteal flap, first described by Millard[40] and later popularized by Gullane and Arena,[41] provides an excellent source of donor tissue. Based on a single greater palatine neurovascular pedicle, the donor palatal tissue can be rotated and safely transposed across the hard palate (**Fig. 1–7**). The mucoperiosteum associated with the flap serves as a barrier to effectively separate the oral and nasal cavities. The secondary defect, which results from harvesting a palatal island flap, remucosalizes over a 3- to 4-week period; however, patients can tolerate an oral diet between 2 and 4 days postoperatively. Harvesting the palatal island flap on a growing child can lead to disturbance in midface growth. As a result, this flap is contraindicated in the growing child. Similarly, exposure to prior palatal irradiation is a relative contraindication to using this flap.

In situations where a palatal island flap is contraindicated, either because the area has been previously exposed to irradiation or the palatal island flap does not offer sufficient tissue area for coverage, the submental island flap or a radial forearm free flap are appropriate options. The submental island flap, first described by Martin in 1993, is based on the

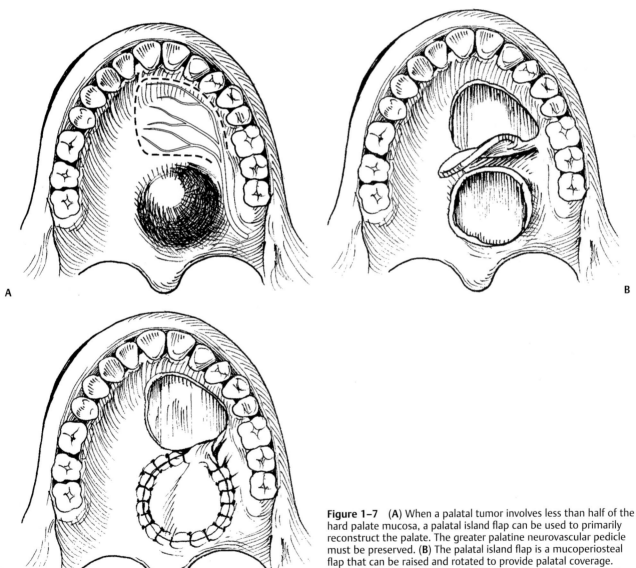

A

B

C

Figure 1–7 (**A**) When a palatal tumor involves less than half of the hard palate mucosa, a palatal island flap can be used to primarily reconstruct the palate. The greater palatine neurovascular pedicle must be preserved. (**B**) The palatal island flap is a mucoperiosteal flap that can be raised and rotated to provide palatal coverage. (**C**) The palatal flap can be sutured into position. The donor site is left to remucosalize secondarily.

submental artery, an anterior branch of the facial artery.[42] This donor site has been used to reconstruct a variety of defects including cutaneous, oral cavity, pharyngeal, and laryngeal defects, and it can offer an excellent source of tissue for reconstruction of buccal and palatal defects. This donor site is particularly useful in elderly or medically tenuous patients because the flap can be raised quite easily and, as a pedicled flap, it can be tunneled subcutaneously and used to cover a variety of hard palate, soft palate, and buccal defects with minimal donor site morbidity. When considering this donor site, it is imperative to consider the submental lymph node basin. Commonly, the submandibular triangle and the associated level I lymph nodes serve as the first echelon for drainage of oral cavity and palatomaxillary malignancies. We recommend a cautionary approach in primary reconstruction and a careful review of the preoperative imaging as well as intraoperative lymph node sampling before transferring the submental flap.

The fasciocutaneous radial forearm free flap offers an ideal source of donor tissue for the reconstruction of large palatal defects for a patient who seeks an alternative to prosthetic rehabilitation. The radial forearm free flap is designed such that the cutaneous paddle serves to reline the oral palatal surface, and a fascial component is raised adjacent to the cutaneous paddle so that it can be folded to provide nasal lining.[43] The pedicle can be passed through a subcutaneous tunnel to gain access to the facial vessels for the vascular anastomosis. In our experience, we find this method of reconstruction reliable and effective in achieving a permanent separation of the oral and nasal cavities, and it has become our primary choice for reconstructing these select defects of the palate in patients who have no medical contraindications.

Although nearly all palatal defects can be successfully managed with a prosthetic obturator, the inconvenience associated with maintaining oronasal hygiene and the necessity of relying on a prosthesis for communication and eating can compromise a patient's quality of life. Soft tissue reconstruction offers patients a single-staged procedure that obviates the need for a palatal obturator without interfering with the use of a tissue-borne denture.

The hemipalatectomy defect is the most common palatomaxillary defect and represents a controversial reconstructive dilemma. Until recently, prosthetic obturation has been considered the gold standard of therapy for such defects; however, several recent reports, including our own experience, demonstrate that single-stage reconstruction of these defects can be effectively accomplished with a bone-containing free flap.[3,44,45] Whereas some authors have advocated the prosthetic reconstruction of all hemipalatectomy defects,[46] others feel that defects involving any more than two thirds of the hard palate are functionally unstable.[47] The reconstruction of these defects with vascularized bone serves to stabilize these forces by providing a rigid infrastructure as well as by providing bone capable of retaining osseointegrated implants.

Similar to prosthetic restoration, soft tissue reconstruction using pedicled flaps or free tissue transfer can present adverse functional consequences in patients with palatomaxillary defects. Although soft tissue flaps are effective for relining the oral palate and separating the oral and nasal cavities, a soft tissue flap obliterates the retentive properties of the maxillectomy defect, which may prevent the retention of a tissue-borne palatal prosthesis for dental restoration. Furthermore, the absence of bone will prevent the placement of osseointegrated implants. As a result, patients are left without the opportunity for functional dental rehabilitation. Several attempts to combine a fasciocutaneous flap or a temporalis flap with free bone grafts have been used to address this problem. Choung advocated using a parietal osteofascial flap with vascularized cranial bone grafts for maxillary reconstruction.[48] Although cranial bone grafts can be stacked and wrapped in revascularized tissue to help preserve the bone stock and therefore accommodate osseointegrated implants, success with this technique is limited because of poor bone graft vascularization and resultant bone resorption. In addition, the reconstruction of extensive defects is limited by the amount of available donor bone. Whereas free nonvascularized bone grafts are an attractive alternative, our experience has been that this is an inadequate method to achieve long-term retention of osseointegrated implants particularly in extensive defects or in previously irradiated patients.

Reconstruction of the hemipalatectomy defect using vascularized bone-containing free flaps offers several unique advantages for orodental rehabilitation that cannot be realized with other forms of prosthetic or soft tissue reconstruction. Most importantly, free tissue transfer of a composite flap allows for the bony restoration of the absent maxillary alveolus (**Fig. 1–8**). The placement of osseointegrated implants and subsequent fitting of an implant-borne denture provides these patients with an optimal form of restoration without the inconvenience or instability associated with prosthetic appliances.

The role of the prosthodontist cannot be understated when considering the restoration of extensive composite defects of the palatomaxillary complex. Extensive resections involving the orbit, palate, skull base, and skin are best managed in a multidisciplinary fashion. Working with the prosthodontist and the oral maxillofacial surgeon, the combination of free tissue transfer, osseointegrated implants, and orbital prosthetics can yield an excellent functional and aesthetic result (**Fig. 1–9**). The coordination of care is essential because the fixation of bone, the placement of implants, and the development of an appropriate orbital cavity provides the foundation for maxillofacial restoration.

Dental Care

The dentist is an integral part of the multidisciplinary team caring for patients undergoing radiotherapy. Any indicated tooth extractions should be performed before radiation, and radiation should not begin for at least 10 to 14 days after extraction to allow for recovery of the gingiva. Muscle exercises are beneficial to decrease the likelihood of trismus. Brushing, floss, and daily fluoride gel applications with or without calcium application are useful to reduce the likelihood of dental caries in patients with xerostomia. If dental surgery is needed after radiation therapy, hyperbaric oxygen and antibiotics may be useful to prevent osteonecrosis.

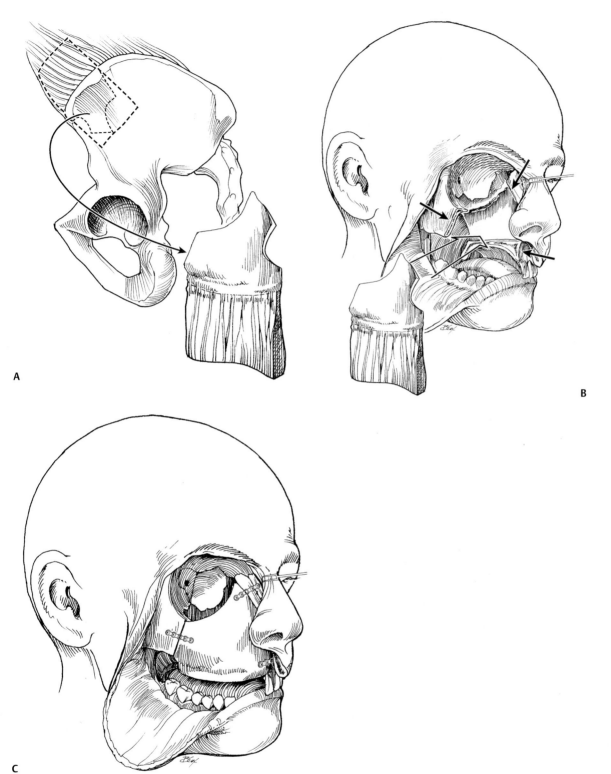

A

B

C

Figure 1–8 (**A**) The iliac crest bone and internal oblique muscle are harvested to reconstruct the maxilla. The bone is contoured to accommodate the nasal cavity, the orbital rim, and the zygoma. (**B**) The internal oblique muscle is used to reconstruct the palate. The vascular pedicle is placed into a subcutaneous tunnel to the neck where a vascular anastomosis can be performed with the facial artery and facial vein. (**C**) The iliac bone is secured into the maxilla with titanium miniplates.

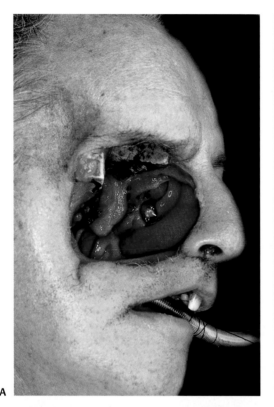

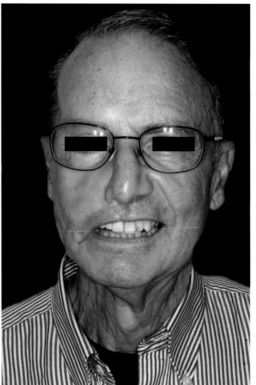

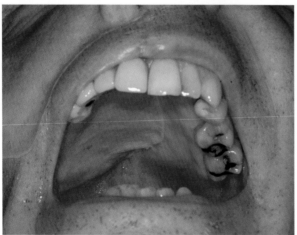

Figure 1–9 (**A**) Reconstruction of the extensive palatomaxillary defect requires intradisciplinary coordination. (**B**) The free tissue reconstruction serves as the foundation for the retention of an orbital prosthesis and (**C**) the placement of implants for dental restoration.

◆ Posttreatment Surveillance

The risk of recurrence or the development of a new primary warrants close follow-up for all patients treated for oral cavity carcinoma. We recommend follow-up examinations every 2 months for the first year, 3 months for the second year, 4 months for the third year, and 5 months for the fourth and fifth years.[3] Thereafter, patients are followed every 12 months. High-risk patients may be monitored more often, and low-risk patients may be monitored less frequently. We routinely see patients throughout the postoperative radiation course to provide support and surveillance.

All patients undergo CT imaging of the primary site and neck at 6 weeks after completion of therapy and undergo PET-CT 12 weeks after the completion of adjuvant therapy and every 6 months for 2 years.

◆ Clinical Cases

Case 1 T2 N0 M0 squamous cell carcinoma of the lateral border of the oral tongue.

Presentation A 72-year-old man with a 20 pack-year history of tobacco use presented with a 2-month history of a progressively enlarging tongue mass.

Physical Examination On examination, the patient had a 3.5-cm endophytic lesion on the lateral aspect of the oral tongue (**Fig. 1–10**). On palpation, the lesion was deeply invasive approaching, but not crossing, the midline. There was no evidence of mandibular fixation or palpable lymphadenopathy.

Diagnosis and Workup   A surgical biopsy was performed in the office with cupped forceps. A PET-CT scan was ordered to assess for depth of invasion and regional and distant metastasis. Given the patient's history of tobacco use, a pulmonary consultation was scheduled to evaluate the patient for chronic obstructive pulmonary disease.

Options for Treatment   The options for therapy for an early carcinoma of the oral tongue include surgery, radiation, or surgery and postoperative radiation. The appropriate choice of therapy is determined by stage of the tumor, the health and comorbid status of the patient, and the bias of the treating physician team. The addition of chemotherapy may also prove beneficial in select cases where there is high-risk disease or pathologic lymph nodes with extracapsular spread. Single-modality therapy is ideal when appropriate, particularly in the management of early disease of the oral cavity.

Treatment of the Primary Tumor   The patient underwent a partial glossectomy and radial forearm free flap reconstruction and ipsilateral selective neck dissection. This case represents a typical presentation of early oral tongue carcinoma. The tumor is easily accessible and can be optimally managed surgically. Although surgery and radiation result in equivalent cure rates, surgical therapy is often preferred due to concerns of severe late complications of external beam irradiation and the time and expense associated with brachytherapy. Exceptions would include inoperable patients and unresectable lesions.

Surgical access and reconstruction can be accomplished transorally, without the need for a labiotomy or mandibulotomy. It is essential to mark each of the peripheral and

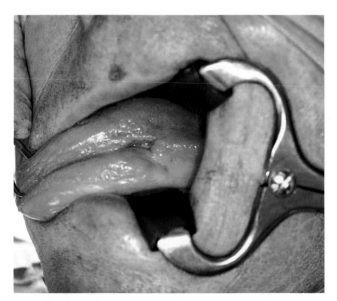

Figure 1–10   Oral tongue carcinoma.

deep margins carefully to facilitate pathologic analysis. Although there has been significant debate regarding the acceptable tumor-free clearance, most surgeons accept between 1 to 2 cm. Equally important, the deep margins must be carefully assessed.

Treatment of the Neck   In the case of a clinically negative neck, there are several options regarding management of the neck. The options include a selective neck dissection, radiation, or observation. High-risk histopathologic findings can reliably predict the presence of occult metastasis and therefore influence the decision-making process regarding management of the neck. The depth of tumor invasion represents the only variable that can be grossly assessed preoperatively. Factors such as tumor differentiation, pattern of infiltration, perineural invasion, angiolymphatic invasion, and lymphocyte response can only be determined histologically on final pathologic analysis. In contrast, depth of invasion can be grossly estimated on examination. In an effort to preoperatively counsel the patient, we often assess the depth of invasion during the initial office examination to determine if the patient would benefit from a neck dissection. Superficial lesions seldom lead to regional metastasis and tend to be highly responsive to either surgical or radiation therapy. In contrast, deeply invasive tumors are commonly associated with occult metastasis and mandate an elective neck dissection. In this case, a selective neck dissection was performed.

Reconstruction of the Oral Tongue   Reconstruction of the oral tongue may be accomplished through several methods. Superficial tumors that result in a mucosal defect with minimal deep resection can be closed primarily, left to heal by secondary intention, or resurfaced with a split-thickness skin graft. Larger defects have a tendency to contract using these methods. Wound contraction, particularly when it involves the floor of the mouth, may prove debilitating to speech and swallowing.

Free flap reconstruction of tongue defects may provide excellent results in speech and swallowing by resurfacing the defect, providing bulk, and allowing the remaining tongue to move without tethering. This is particularly true if the resection involves the floor of the mouth. The radial forearm free flap can be designed to match the defect and provide an excellent reconstructive alternative to a skin graft (**Fig. 1–11**). The thin pliable tissue of the radial forearm can be fashioned to reline the oral tongue and adjacent floor of the mouth. Additionally, innervation of the flap can provide sensation that may be beneficial to speech and swallowing; however, this remains speculative. Most importantly, free flap reconstruction provides "like tissue" that optimizes function.

Summary of Treatment   Early tumors of the oral tongue can be managed either surgically or with radiation therapy; however, early disease is best managed with surgery. Although radiation represents an option for select patients, tumors of the oral tongue are easily accessible and may be resected with minimal morbidity. Postoperative radiation is indicated in patient with high-risk histopathologic

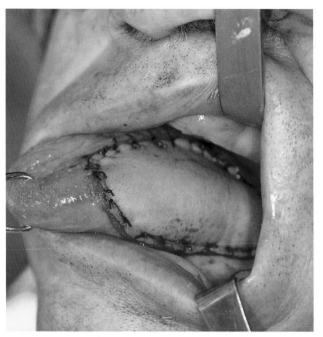

Figure 1–11 Oral cavity reconstruction. The radial forearm free flap is used to reconstruct the lateral tongue defect. The radial forearm provides a pliable source of skin that can be revascularized and reinnervated to provide sensory innervation.

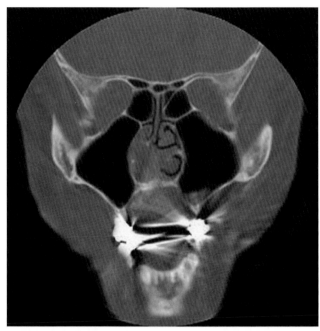

Figure 1–12 CT scan, coronal view. This scan demonstrates a lesion of the hard palate with extension into the nasal fossa.

features, N1 neck metastasis with ECS, or N2 or more advanced metastatic disease. Free flap reconstruction often provides patients with an optimal functional result.

Case 2 T4a N0 M0 adenoid cystic carcinoma of the hard palate.

Presentation A 32-year-old man with no significant risk factors for oral carcinoma presented with a history of a midline palatal ulcer that healed and reappeared spontaneously several times over the course of 4 months. The patient was seen by an oral surgeon who performed a biopsy in the office. The pathology revealed adenoid cystic carcinoma.

Physical Examination On examination, there was a subtle submucosal mass in the midline of the hard palate. The patient denied nasal obstruction, pain, or sensory loss. Nasal endoscopy revealed submucosal expansion of the inferior portion of the palatine-septal junction. There was no clinical evidence of a neck mass.

Diagnosis and Workup The diagnosis and workup was started with a review of the pathology slides to confirm the diagnosis. A CT scan was ordered and demonstrated erosion of the palate into the floor of the nose with expansion of the septum (**Fig. 1–12**). Given the predilection of adenoid cystic carcinoma for distant metastasis, an evaluation for pulmonary and bone metastasis was performed with a CT of the chest and a bone scan.

Treatment of the Primary Tumor Adenoid cystic carcinoma is a relatively rare tumor accounting for less than a quarter of salivary neoplasms. It most commonly occurs in the minor salivary glands of the palate. Adenoid cystic carcinoma is characterized by an indolent growth rate and rare

regional metastasis. Traditionally, surgical management is preferred for all minor salivary gland neoplasms including adenoid cystic. More recently, the addition of radiation and chemotherapy has been evaluated for local control. In this case, a resection of the palate and septum was necessary to gain tumor-free margins. The resection was performed through a combined transpalatal and facial degloving approach (**Fig. 1–13**). Because adenoid cystic carcinoma has a high affinity for perineural invasion, meticulous neural biopsies are essential to clear the disease. This is best obtained by performing a retrograde dissection until the frozen-section pathologic margins are free of disease.

Surgery alone is acceptable for a T1 lesion; however, improved control rates can be achieved for more advanced disease when surgery is followed by postoperative radiation.[49,50] Radiation therapy should be considered in advanced unresectable disease. In recurrent or unresectable disease, photon radiation has been demonstrated to improve locoregional control.[51]

Treatment of the Neck The neck was not addressed. The incidence of regional metastasis is extremely low; as a result, unless there is evidence of regional disease, management of the neck is not necessary.

Treatment of Distant Sites Distant disease is considerably more common than regional disease in adenoid cystic carcinoma; however, patients with distant metastasis can survive for many years even with extensive pulmonary disease. Currently, there is no evidence that systemic chemotherapy prevents distant metastasis or prolongs survival, and therefore chemotherapy is seldom administered.

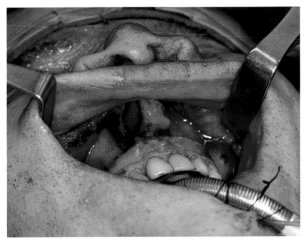

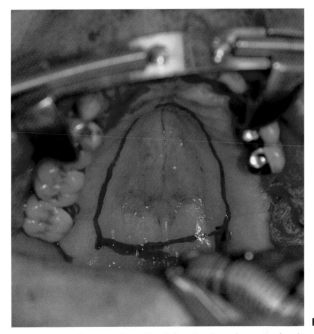

A   B

Figure 1–13 The resection is approached through (**A**) a facial degloving and (**B**) transoral approaches. The defect involves the entire hard palate, nasal septum, and floor of the nasal fossa.

Reconstruction of the Palate   A radial forearm free flap was used to reconstruct the palatal defect. Although dental obturation is always an option for rehabilitation of a palatal defect, flap reconstruction offers the advantages of a permanent closure of the oral nasal defect. Defects less than one half of the palatal surface area can be reconstructed with a palatal island flap. Defects greater than one half the palate such as the defect in case no. 2 require either obturation or a free flap reconstruction. The radial forearm free flap is used for rehabilitation of this defect because it allows for resurfacing the palate with "like" tissue. The skin paddle is designed to reline the palatal surface, and the fascia of the radial forearm is used to reline the floor of the nose (**Fig. 1–14**).

The radial forearm reconstruction provides excellent functional results. Additionally, during the course of radiation, mucositis and xerostomia may make wearing an obturator unpleasant. The radial forearm reconstruction obviates the need for an obturator and, therefore, improves a patient's quality of life.

Summary of Treatment   Adenoid cystic carcinoma is a rare nonepidermoid carcinoma that is locally aggressive and has an affinity for perineural invasion. Regional metastasis is rare; however, adenoid cystic carcinoma has a propensity for distant metastasis. Surgical resection is acceptable for early disease; however, advanced disease should be managed with surgery and postoperative radiation. Reconstruction may be accomplished through a variety of methods from prosthetic obturation to local or free flap reconstruction.

Case 3   T4 N2b MX squamous cell carcinoma of the mandibular alveolus.

Presentation   A 65-year-old man patient with a history of tobacco and ethanol use presented with an 8-week history

of progressive pain along the right side of the alveolus and decreased sensation along the right lip.

Physical Examination   On examination, there was a 3 × 2 cm ulcer along the right edentulous mandibular alveolus. The neck exam demonstrated a 2 × 2 cm jugulodigastric lymph node and several smaller firm lymph nodes in level III.

Diagnosis and Workup   A thorough head and neck exam was performed and contributed a great deal of information regarding the extent of the lesion and therefore the stage. Palpation of the mass and the neurologic deficit suggested that the tumor had eroded the mandible and invaded the inferior alveolar nerve. The palpable lymph nodes suggested that the tumor had regionally metastasized to level II. A biopsy of the oral cavity lesion was performed in the office with a small cupped forceps to confirm the diagnosis. A panoramic x-ray and CT scan (**Fig. 1–15**) with contrast demonstrated invasion of bone and the presence of regional disease. A PET-CT scan was done to assess for regional and distant disease.

Options for Treatment   The physical exam, panoramic x-ray, and CT scan suggested that this be staged as a T4 N2b MX tumor of the mandibular alveolus. The invasion of mandible mandates surgical therapy. Whereas radiation does not play a role in the primary management of this tumor, postoperative radiation therapy is indicated given the stage. Because the imaging does not demonstrate ECS, unless ECS is found on final pathologic analysis, systemic chemotherapy is not mandated.

Treatment of the Primary Tumor   A resection of the floor of the mouth and segmental resection of the mandible with ipsilateral selective neck dissection was performed through a transcervical approach (**Fig. 1–16**). Because there was invasion of tumor through the cortex and into

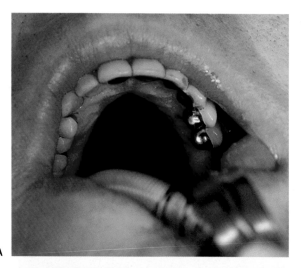

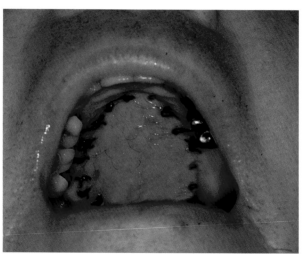

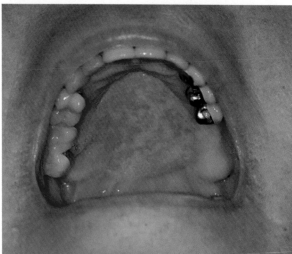

Figure 1–14 Reconstruction of oral cavity is achieved with a radial forearm free flap. (**A**) The surgical defect. (**B**) One week after surgery and (**C**) 1 week after completing radiation and chemotherapy.

the inferior alveolar nerve, a marginal resection was contraindicated. The resection was approached transcervically; however, if access were limited, a midline labiotomy and mandibulectomy could have been used. In addition to marking and analyzing mucosal margins, the marrow was sampled with a curette and sent for touch prep analysis to assess the bone margins.

Treatment of the Neck   An ipsilateral selective neck dissection was performed. Because there was no evidence of

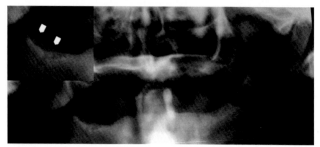

Figure 1–15 Panoramic radiograph demonstrating cortical erosion of the retromolar trigone (*arrows*).

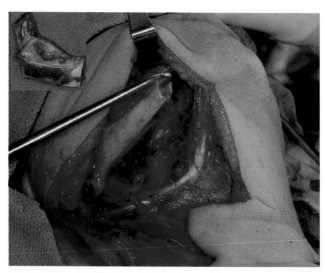

Figure 1–16 Segmental resection of mandible achieved through a transcervical approach.

ECS, a selective neck dissection is appropriate for managing the regional disease. The patient will require postoperative external beam radiotherapy. As a result, surgical management of the contralateral N0 neck is not required.

Reconstruction of the Mandible   Reconstruction of the mandible may be accomplished with either a reconstruction plate without vascularized bone or a bone-containing free tissue transfer. Although a reconstruction plate can be used, the rate of plate fracture and extrusion is relatively high, and when postoperative radiotherapy is administered, complications from plate fracture or exposure are extremely common. In most centers, a bone-containing free flap is the standard of care. In this case, a fibula, scapula, or iliac crest free flap will suffice.

Choosing the appropriate donor site is determined by patient factors and defect factors. Patient factors that may impact the choice of donor site include a history of injury to the lower extremity, shoulder, or pelvic girdle, a history of deep vein thrombosis, or a radical neck dissection. Patients that have suffered an injury or rely on an aid for ambulation can be disabled by a fibula or iliac crest free flap harvest. Similarly, patients that have sustained a shoulder deficit as a result of a radical neck dissection can be disabled by a scapular harvest. Patients that have a history of deep vein thrombosis may benefit from a scapular harvest so that the postoperative ambulation is not hindered by a healing donor site.

Summary of Treatment   The presence of mandibular erosion through the cortex requires a segmental resection and mandibular reconstruction. Advanced-stage disease and the presence of lymph node metastasis are indications for a neck dissection and postoperative radiation therapy.

Case 4   T4 N0 MX mucoepidermoid carcinoma of the maxillary alveolus.

Presentation   A 41-year-old man presented with a history of a slowly expanding hard palate mass located along the right maxillary alveolus. The mass was not associated with pain or numbness of the surrounding palate.

Physical Examination   The examination demonstrated a hard palate mass involving the right maxillary alveolus. The patient denied sensory deficit along the palate, face, or nasal vault. Nasal endoscopy did not demonstrate evidence of nasal mucosal ulceration or submucosal deformity.

Diagnosis and Workup   A cupped biopsy was performed demonstrating a low-grade mucoepidermoid carcinoma. A CT scan was obtained and demonstrated palatal bone erosion (**Fig. 1–17**). A PET-CT scan was ordered and demonstrated no evidence of regional or distant disease.

Options for Therapy   Grading a mucoepidermoid carcinoma is based on the cytologic atypia and the ratio of epidermoid to mucinous histologic elements. High-grade tumors exhibit a greater epidermoid component and extensive cellular atypia. A low-grade mucoepidermoid carcinoma is predominately mucinous with a small component of epidermoid features. Radiation therapy is a treatment option; however, surgical therapy is indicated based on

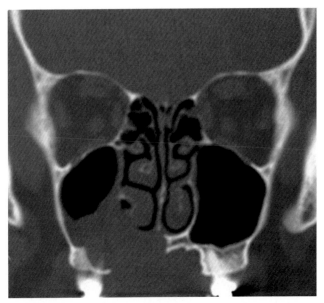

Figure 1–17   CT scan, coronal view. The CT scan demonstrates an erosive lesion of the palate and maxilla.

the grade of the tumor, the location, and the presence of bone invasion.

Treatment of the Primary Tumor   The surgical resection was accomplished transorally with a small lip split incision. The resection resulted in a hemipalatectomy defect with resection of the sinus and nasal infrastructure (**Fig. 1–18**).

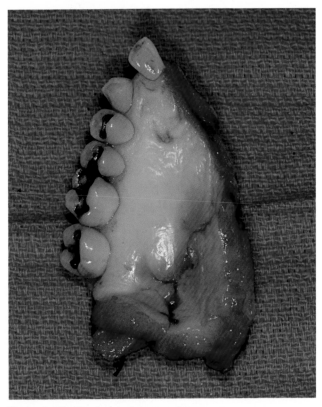

Figure 1–18   Hemipalatectomy specimen.

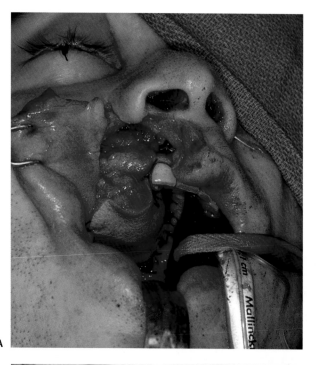

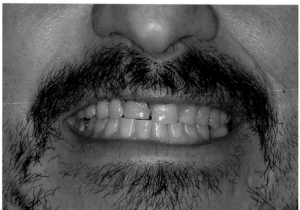

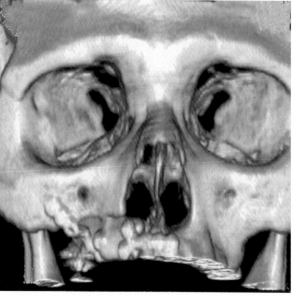

Figure 1–19 **(A)** Fibula free flap reconstruction. The fibula is used to reconstruct the alveolar arch. The skin paddle is used to reconstruct the palate mucosal defect. **(B)** Implant-borne dentures are placed and the oral reconstruction is complete. **(C)** Three-dimensional reconstruction of the mid-face demonstrates the reconstructed mid-face arch.

Treatment of the Neck The neck was not addressed. The low rate of regional metastasis associated with low-grade mucoepidermoid carcinoma does not warrant a neck dissection.

Rehabilitation of the Maxilla The maxilla can be rehabilitated with a prosthetic obturator or tissue reconstruction. It is important to counsel the patient regarding the options. If an obturator is chosen, a preoperative consultation with a prosthodontist enables the fabrication of a dental mold so that the obturator can be placed at the time of surgery.

Given the low-grade nature of the tumor and the patient's age, the patient was given the option of a bone-containing free flap reconstruction. Because the defect will entail an

infrastructure maxillectomy, a fibula free flap is an ideal donor site (**Fig. 1–19**). A fibula free flap was harvested with a skin paddle for palatal lining. Osseointegrated implants were placed secondarily for retention of an implant-borne denture (**Fig. 1–19A**). After osseointegration, the implant-borne dentures were placed (**Fig. 1–19B**). A three-dimensional CT scan demonstrates complete reconstitution of the alveolus (**Fig. 1–19C**).

Summary of Treatment Whereas high-grade mucoepidermoid carcinoma should be managed no differently than squamous cell carcinoma, low-grade mucoepidermoid carcinoma behaves less aggressively and seldom metastasizes regionally.

References

1. Whitehurst JO, Droulias CA. Surgical treatment of squamous cell carcinoma of the oral tongue: factors influencing survival. Arch Otolaryngol 1977;103(4):212–215
2. Brandwein-Gensler M, Teixeira MS, Lewis CM, et al. Oral squamous cell carcinoma: histologic risk assessment, but not margin status, is strongly predictive of local disease-free and overall survival. Am J Surg Pathol 2005;29(2):167–178
3. Brown JS, Rogers SN, McNally DN, et al. A modified classification for the maxillectomy defect. Head Neck 2000;22(1):17–26
4. Yuen AP, Lam KY, Wei WI, et al. A comparison of the prognostic significance of tumor diameter, length, width, thickness, area, volume, and clinicopathological features of oral tongue carcinoma. Am J Surg 2000;180(2):139–143
5. Asakage T, Yokose T, Mukai K, et al. Tumor thickness predicts cervical metastasis in patients with stage I/II carcinoma of the tongue. Cancer 1998;82(8):1443–1448
6. Fukano H, Matsuura H, Hasegawa Y, et al. Depth of invasion as a predictive factor for cervical lymph node metastasis in tongue carcinoma. Head Neck 1997;19(3):205–210
7. Alvi A, Johnson JT. Extracapsular spread in the clinically negative neck (N0): implications and outcome. Otolaryngol Head Neck Surg 1996;114(1):65–70
8. Greenberg JS, Fowler R, Gomez J, et al. Extent of extracapsular spread: a critical prognosticator in oral tongue cancer. Cancer 2003;97(6):1464–1470
9. Poate TW, Buchanan JA, Hodgson TA, et al. An audit of the efficacy of the oral brush biopsy technique in a specialist oral medicine unit. Oral Oncol 2004;40(8):829–834
10. Svirsky JA, Burns JC, Carpenter WM, et al. Comparison of computer-assisted brush biopsy results with follow up scalpel biopsy and histology. Gen Dent 2002;50(6):500–503
11. Lane AP, Buckmire RA, Mukherji SK, et al. Use of computed tomography in the assessment of mandibular invasion in carcinoma of the retromolar trigone. Otolaryngol Head Neck Surg 2000;122(5):673–677
12. Tsue TT, McCulloch TM, Girod DA, et al. Predictors of carcinomatous invasion of the mandible. Head Neck 1994;16(2):116–126
13. Shaha AR. Preoperative evaluation of the mandible in patients with carcinoma of the floor of mouth. Head Neck 1991;13(5):398–402
14. Johnson JT, Barnes EL, Myers EN, et al. The extracapsular spread of tumors in cervical node metastasis. Arch Otolaryngol 1981;107(12):725–729
15. Byers RM, Weber RS, Andrews T, et al. Frequency and therapeutic implications of "skip metastases" in the neck from squamous carcinoma of the oral tongue. Head Neck 1997;19(1):14–19
16. Ha PK, Hdeib A, Goldenberg D, et al. The role of positron emission tomography and computed tomography fusion in the management of early-stage and advanced-stage primary head and neck squamous cell carcinoma. Arch Otolaryngol Head Neck Surg 2006;132(1):12–16
17. Juweid ME, Cheson BD. Positron-emission tomography and assessment of cancer therapy. N Engl J Med 2006;354(5):496–507
18. Pellitteri PK, Ferlito A, Rinaldo A, et al. Planned neck dissection following chemoradiotherapy for advanced head and neck cancer: is it necessary for all? Head Neck 2006;28(2):166–175
19. Mendenhall WM, Van Cise WS, Bova FJ, et al. Analysis of time-dose factors in squamous cell carcinoma of the oral tongue and floor of mouth treated with radiation therapy alone. Int J Radiat Oncol Biol Phys 1981;7(8):1005–1011
20. Fein DA, Mendenhall WM, Parsons JT, et al. Carcinoma of the oral tongue: a comparison of results and complications of treatment with radiotherapy and/or surgery. Head Neck 1994;16(4):358–365
21. Decroix Y, Ghossein NA. Experience of the Curie Institute in treatment of cancer of the mobile tongue: I. Treatment policies and result. Cancer 1981;47(3):496–502
22. Wong RJ, Keel SB, Glynn RJ, et al. Histological pattern of mandibular invasion by oral squamous cell carcinoma. Laryngoscope 2000;110(1):65–72
23. Werning JW, Byers RM, Novas MA, et al. Preoperative assessment for and outcomes of mandibular conservation surgery. Head Neck 2001;23(12):1024–1030
24. Brown JS, Griffith JF, Phelps PD, et al. A comparison of different imaging modalities and direct inspection after periosteal stripping in predicting the invasion of the mandible by oral squamous cell carcinoma. Br J Oral Maxillofac Surg 1994;32(6):347–359
25. Holmstrup P, Thorn JJ, Rindum J, et al. Malignant development of lichen planus-affected oral mucosa. J Oral Pathol 1988;17(5):219–225
26. Vegers JW, Snow GB, van der Waall. Squamous cell carcinoma of the buccal mucosa. A review of 85 cases. Arch Otolaryngol 1979;105(4):192–195
27. Byers RM, White D, Yue A. Squamous carcinoma of the oral cavity: choice of therapy. Curr Probl Cancer 1981;6(5):1–27
28. Sessions DG, Spector GJ, Lenox J, et al. Analysis of treatment results for floor-of-mouth cancer. Laryngoscope 2000;110(10 Pt 1):1764–1772
29. McGuirt WF Jr, Johnson JT, Myers EN, et al. Floor of mouth carcinoma. The management of the clinically negative neck. Arch Otolaryngol Head Neck Surg 1995;121(3):278–282
30. Hicks WL Jr, Loree TR, Garcia RI, et al. Squamous cell carcinoma of the floor of mouth: a 20-year review. Head Neck 1997;19(5):400–405
31. Kowalski LP. Results of salvage treatment of the neck in patients with oral cancer. Arch Otolaryngol Head Neck Surg 2002;128(1):58–62
32. Wolfensberger M, Zbaeren P, Dulguerov P, et al. Surgical treatment of early oral carcinoma–results of a prospective controlled multicenter study. Head Neck 2001;23(7):525–530
33. Dias FL, Kligerman J, Matos de Sá G, et al. Elective neck dissection versus observation in stage I squamous cell carcinomas of the tongue and floor of the mouth. Otolaryngol Head Neck Surg 2001;125(1):23–29
34. Greenberg JS, El Naggar AK, Mo V, et al. Disparity in pathologic and clinical lymph node staging in oral tongue carcinoma. Implication for therapeutic decision making. Cancer 2003;98(3):508–515
35. Woolgar JA, Scott J, Vaughan ED, et al. Pathological findings in clinically false-negative and false-positive neck dissections for oral carcinoma. Ann R Coll Surg Engl 1994;76(4):237–244
36. van den Brekel MW, van der Waal I, Meijer CJ, et al. The incidence of micrometastases in neck dissection specimens obtained from elective neck dissections. Laryngoscope 1996;106(8):987–991
37. Duvvuri U, Simental AA, D'Angelo G, et al. Elective neck dissection and survival in patients with squamous cell carcinoma of the oral cavity and oropharynx. Laryngoscope 2004;114(12):2228–2234
38. Teot L, Bosse JP, Moufarrege R, et al. The scapular crest pedicled bone graft. Int J Microsurg 1981;3:257
39. Genden EM, Okay D, Stepp MT, et al. Comparison of functional and quality-of-life outcomes in patients with and without palatomaxillary reconstruction: a preliminary report. Arch Otolaryngol Head Neck Surg 2003;129(7):775–780
40. Millard DR Jr. Wide and/or short cleft palate. Plast Reconstr Surg 1962;29:40–57
41. Gullane PJ, Arena S. Palatal island flap for reconstruction of oral defects. Arch Otolaryngol 1977;103(10):598–599
42. Martin D, Pascal JF, Baudet J, et al. The submental island flap: a new donor site. Anatomy and clinical applications as a free or pedicled flap. Plast Reconstr Surg 1993;92(5):867–873
43. Genden EM, Wallace DI, Okay D, et al. Reconstruction of the hard palate using the radial forearm free flap: indications and outcomes. Head Neck 2004;26(9):808–814
44. Genden EM, Wallace D, Okay D, et al. Iliac crest internal oblique osteomusculocutaneous free flap reconstruction of the postablative palatomaxillary defect. Arch Otolaryngol Head Neck Surg 2001;127(7):854–861
45. Funk GF, Arcuri MR, Frodel JL. Functional dental rehabilitation of massive palatomaxillary defects: cases requiring free tissue transfer and osseointegrated implants. Head Neck 1998;20:38–51
46. Aramany MA. Basic principles of obturator design for partially edentulous patients. Part I: classification. J Prosthet Dent 1978;40(5):554–557
47. Funk GF, Arcuri MR, Frodel LR Jr. Functional dental rehabilitation of massive palatomaxillary defects: cases requiring free tissue transfer and osseointegrated implants. Head Neck 1998;20(1):38–51
48. Choung PH, Nam IW, Kim KS. Vascularized cranial bone grafts for mandibular and maxillary reconstruction. The parietal osteofascial flap. J Craniomaxillofac Surg 1991;19(6):235–242
49. Weber RS, Palmer JM, el-Naggar A, et al. Minor salivary gland tumors of the lip and buccal mucosa. Laryngoscope 1989;99(1):6–9
50. Prokopakis EP, Snyderman CH, Hanna EY, et al. Risk factors for local recurrence of adenoid cystic carcinoma: the role of postoperative radiation therapy. Am J Otolaryngol 1999;20(5):281–286
51. Laramore GE, Krall JM, Griffin TW, et al. Neutron versus photon irradiation for unresectable salivary gland tumors: final report of an RTOG-MRC randomized clinical trial. Radiation Therapy Oncology Group. Medical Research Council. Int J Radiat Oncol Biol Phys 1993;27(2):235–240

2

Carcinoma of the Oropharynx

Michael J. Odell, Bruce J. Walz, Hans-Joachim Reimers, and Mark A.Varvares

◆ Epidemiology

Incidence

The incidence of malignant tumors of the oropharynx was estimated by the American Cancer Society in 2004 at ~8300 new cases per year, with mortality estimated at 2000 deaths annually. According to National Cancer Institute (NCI) statistics, men are affected more often than women by a factor of approximately 3, with the majority of patients being diagnosed in their sixth decade.

Mortality

Survival statistics for patients with cancer of the oropharynx vary widely, depending on stage as well as site of the lesion. Early-stage disease generally carries a reasonable prognosis, whereas advanced disease continues to represent a significant treatment challenge. For the most part, early diagnosis of oropharyngeal carcinoma continues to be elusive; less than 10% of lesions are diagnosed in stage I, with greater than 70% presenting to cancer caregivers in stage III or IV.[1,2]

The association of prognosis with site of lesion is likely related not only to intrinsic anatomic factors such as increased lymphovascular supply and absence of barriers to tumor spread but also to the fact that tumors in some subsites (e.g., soft palate) are more likely to be diagnosed at an earlier stage.

Tumors of the base of tongue (BOT) are, in most series, the most frequently occurring oropharyngeal cancers, generally making up roughly 50% of all encountered cases. Five-year survival rates range from 70 to 75% for stage I disease, 60 to 70% for stage II, and 40 to 60% for stages III and IV. Unfortunately, most patients (>70%) present with advanced disease.

Tonsil cancer is the second most common malignant lesion of the oropharynx. Again, early-stage disease portends a favorable response to treatment with patients in stages I and II displaying 5-year survival rates of 80 to 90% and 70 to 80%, respectively. As is the case in cancer of the BOT, however, these patients represent the minority, with most patients again presenting in stage III or IV; 5-year survival rates average ~50% for stage III disease and 30% for stage IV.

Tumors of the soft palate make up around 20% of all cancers of the oropharynx but are often diagnosed at an earlier stage (>50% are diagnosed in stages I and II) than tumors in those subsites that are not directly visible. Unfortunately, compared with the BOT and the tonsil, palatal cancers are, stage for stage, less responsive to treatment. Early disease (stage I and II) cure rates at 5 years approach 60 to 70% in most series, with more advanced disease carrying a less favorable prognosis (reported 5-year survival rates range from less than 10% to 40%).

Tumors of the pharyngeal wall are the least prevalent in most Western series. As with tonsil and BOT cancers, these tend to present late, often with regional disease at presentation. Control and cure rates are similar to those of the soft palate and are generally poorer than those achieved in the tonsil and BOT.

◆ Etiology

Tobacco and Alcohol

Tobacco and alcohol use are both strongly associated with development of cancers of the oropharynx.[3] There appears to be a synergistic association between the two,[4,5] likely due to the ability of alcohol to increase the solubility and, hence, the penetration of the mutagenic substances found in tobacco products. The method of tobacco use also can influence the development of oropharyngeal cancer, as evidenced by the increased incidence of these tumors in populations where reverse smoking practices are prevalent.[6]

Human Papilloma Virus

There is an association between infection with human papilloma virus (types 2, 11, and 16) and development of oropharyngeal cancer[7]; however, the exact reason for this association has not been fully elucidated.

Genetic Factors

There is an increased incidence of patients with diseases characterized by defective DNA repair, such as xeroderma pigmentosum and ataxia telangiectasia.[8,9] Although many genetic alterations have been observed in patients with oropharyngeal malignancy, there is still relatively little clinical applicability for genetic analysis, although this is likely to change with increasing use of microarray analyses and the data produced by them.[10,11]

◆ Anatomy of the Oropharynx

The oropharynx extends craniocaudally from the level of the hard palate above to the hyoid below; in the anteroposterior dimension, the oropharynx is defined by the circumvallate

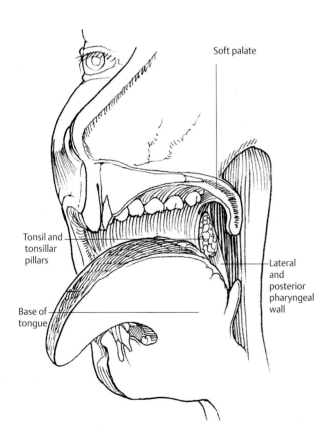

Figure 2–1   Anatomy of the opharnyx. Subsites include the tonsils and tonsillar fossae, the posterior and lateral pharyngeal walls, soft palate, and base of tongue.

line, the anterior tonsillar pillar, and the junction of the hard and soft palate anteriorly and the posterior pharyngeal wall posteriorly.

The oropharynx is subdivided into several subsites that include the tonsils and tonsillar fossae, the posterior and lateral pharyngeal walls, soft palate, and base of tongue (**Fig. 2–1**); these various sites can differ significantly in their clinical behavior and patterns of regional metastasis and influence the choice of therapy significantly.

Soft Palate

The soft palate extends from the junction of the hard and soft palate to the free edge of the soft palate and the uvula. Uvular tumors are included in the soft palate subsite. Only those tumors arising on the oral surface and not the nasal surface of the soft palate are considered to be oropharyngeal in origin.

Base of Tongue

The BOT extends from the circumvallate line to the vallecula and includes the glossoepiglottic fold and the paired lateral pharyngoepiglottic folds.

Tonsil and Tonsillar Pillars

The tonsil site includes not only the tonsil tissue proper and the anterior and tonsillar arches but also the glossotonsillar sulcus.

Lateral and Posterior Pharyngeal Wall

This subsite is defined anteriorly by the posterior tonsillar pillars and craniocaudally by the planes of the hard palate and the hyoid bone.

Lymphatic Drainage of the Oropharynx

Nodal groups of the neck have been divided into specific levels to facilitate the evaluation and treatment of regional metastasis of head and neck cancer.[12] Level I nodes are found in the submental and submandibular triangles, which are designated as levels Ia and Ib, respectively. Levels II through IV comprise the internal jugular chain from the posterior belly of the digastric muscle to the clavicle. The hyoid bone/carotid bifurcation and the cricoid cartilage/omohyoid muscle divide level II from III and level III from IV, respectively. Level II is divided by the accessory nerve into level IIa, which lies caudal to the nerve, and level IIb, which lies cranial to it. Level V is bound by the posterior edge of the sternocleidomastoid muscle anteriorly, the trapezius posteriorly, and the clavicle inferiorly. It is subdivided by the omohyoid muscle into Va, lying above the muscle, and Vb, lying below it.

Lymphatic drainage of the structures of the oropharynx is primarily to the nodal groups of the deep cervical chain (levels II to IV), although metastasis to the submandibular, submental (level I), posterior cervical (level V), and retropharyngeal nodes can be encountered (**Fig. 2–2**).

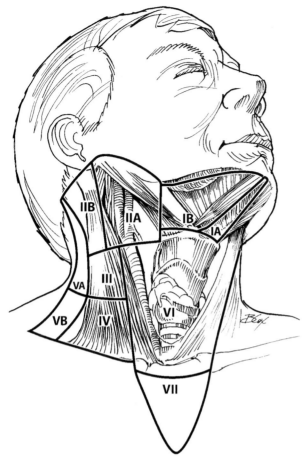

Figure 2–2 Lymphatics of the neck. (*IA*) Lymph nodes that lie within a triangle defined by anterior bellies of the digastric muscles and the hyoid bone (previously classified as submental nodes). (*IB*) Lymph nodes that lie within the triangle formed by the anterior belly of the digastric muscle, the stylohyoid muscle, and the body of the mandible (previously classified as submandibular nodes). (*II*) Level II lymph nodes are located adjacent to the upper third of the jugular vein and spinal accessory nerve. They exist in the area of the neck extending from the skull base and to the lower body of the hyoid bone. The anterior medial boundary is the stylohyoid muscle, and the posterior boundary is the sternocleidomastoid muscle. Radiographically, level II nodes lie anterior to a transverse line drawn on each axial image through the posterior edge of the sternocleidomastoid muscle and lie posterior to a transverse line drawn on each axial scan through the posterior edge of the submandibular gland. *IIA* refers to lymph nodes anterior to the spinal accessory nerve. *IIB* refers to lymph nodes posterior to the spinal accessory nerve. (*III*) Level III lymph nodes are adjacent to the middle third of the internal jugular vein extending from the hyoid bone to the lower margin of the cricoid cartilage. The medial border is the lateral border of the sternohyoid muscle, and the posterior border is the posterior border of the sternocleidomastoid muscle. (*IV*) Level IV lymph nodes are located around the lower third of the internal jugular vein extending from the inferior border of the cricoid cartilage to the clavicle. (*V*) Level V lymph nodes are located in the posterior triangle of the neck located along the spinal accessory nerve. The superior boundary is the convergence of the trapezius muscle and the sternocleidomastoid muscle. The inferior boundary is the clavicle. The anterior boundary is the posterior border of the sternocleidomastoid muscle. The posterior boundary is the anterior border of the trapezius. (*VI*) Level VI lymph nodes include pretracheal and paratracheal lymph nodes. The superior border is the hyoid bone, and the inferior border is the suprasternal notch. The lateral borders are the common carotid arteries.

The BOT, soft palate, and posterior pharyngeal wall are drained by lymph node groups on both sides of the neck; lesions of these subsites, as well as those that approach the midline due to tumor size, have the potential for contralateral or bilateral regional metastasis and must be investigated and treated accordingly.

◆ Classification

Malignant tumors of the oropharynx can be divided into those arising primarily in the oropharynx and those arising elsewhere but metastasizing to the oropharynx. The latter category is rare. Therefore, the majority of the focus will be on tumors arising in the tissues of the oropharynx.

Primary Tumors

Squamous Cell Carcinoma

The vast majority (>85%) of encountered tumors of the oropharynx are squamous cell carcinoma (SCC). Within this category are various histopathologic variants (**Table 2–1**) and varying degrees of cellular differentiation. Accurate histopathologic diagnosis is critical for appropriate staging, treatment, and prognostication. It is generally accepted that more-differentiated tumors behave in a less-aggressive fashion. Verrucous carcinomas, in particular, can follow a very indolent course, with regional and distant metastasis being extremely uncommon. Sarcomatous and dedifferentiated tumors can exhibit very aggressive behavior, both locally as well as in terms of metastatic potential. In addition, adenosquamous tumors must be accurately differentiated from minor salivary neoplasms, as their behaviors (especially in the case of adenoid cystic carcinoma) can be quite divergent. Pathologic review by a dedicated head and neck pathologist of referred biopsy material can add valuable information and can influence management decisions. This should arguably be done for all cases.

Lymphoid Tumors

The oropharynx contains a significant amount of lymphoid tissue (predominately within the structures of Waldeyer's ring) and can therefore give rise to tumors of lymphoid origin. These tumors are most commonly non–Hodgkin's lymphomas of B-cell origin, although T-cell lymphomas can also occur.[13] Mucosa-associated lymphoid tissue (MALT) cell lym-

Table 2–1 Variants of Squamous Cell Carcinoma in the Oropharynx

Keratinizing
Nonkeratinizing
Sarcomatous/spindle cell
Adenosquamous
Verrucous

phomas, plasmacytomas, histiocytosis X, as well as leukemic infiltration of oropharyngeal tissues are all described but are rare. In general, patients with lymphoid tumors of the oropharynx enjoy a more favorable prognosis than do those with epithelial tumors.

Salivary Gland Carcinoma

Malignant salivary tumors can arise from minor salivary glands found in the oropharynx. The most frequently encountered types are adenoid cystic carcinoma, mucoepidermoid carcinoma, polymorphous low-grade adenocarcinoma, and adenocarcinoma not otherwise specified (NOS). With ever-improving pathologic techniques, adenocarcinoma NOS is becoming increasingly rare. Acinic cell carcinoma is rarely encountered in the oropharynx.

Adenoid cystic carcinoma is classically a slow-growing but relentless tumor, characterized by failure both locally as well as distally. Local control can be difficult due to the propensity for perineural invasion. Survival can be prolonged, in spite of disease recurrence, both locally as well as distally. Distant metastasis is most commonly to the lungs.

The clinical behavior of mucoepidermoid carcinoma varies according to grade, which is, in turn, related to the proportion of tumor retaining salivary differentiation. Low-grade tumors, which exhibit a greater degree of salivary differentiation, generally have a more favorable prognosis than high-grade tumors, which resemble SCC more closely, both in terms of histopathologic appearance and clinical behavior.

Polymorphous low-grade adenocarcinoma (PLGA) is a relatively recently defined pathologic category, having been previously classified as adenocarcinoma NOS or adenoid cystic carcinoma, as well as by other names. PLGA is most commonly seen on the palate, and though it has a propensity for perineural involvement, it behaves like a low-grade neoplasm, with low rates of metastasis and generally good outcomes.

Mucosal Melanoma

Melanoma arising in the mucosa of the oropharynx is an uncommon, but very aggressive and often lethal, lesion. Both melanotic and amelanotic forms may be encountered. Immunohistochemical characterization is often necessary for accurate diagnosis. Outcomes of treatment for all but the earliest lesions are disappointing, with most patients eventually succumbing to relentless locoregional recurrence or distant metastasis.

Secondary Tumors

Although it is rare to encounter oropharyngeal lesions that have originated elsewhere, it is reported in the literature.[14] The most commonly encountered lesions include renal cell carcinoma, cutaneous melanoma, and papillary carcinoma of the thyroid. Pathologic suggestion of a lesion other than those listed above should prompt a search for another primary tumor.

◆ Presentation

Primary Sites

Clinical presentation varies somewhat according to location of the lesion. Painful nonhealing ulcers are common signs of cancers of the soft palate and palatine tonsils. These lesions are often noticed by the patient or the referring care provider (often the primary care physician or dentist). For those sites not visible to direct inspection, throat pain is often the presenting symptom. It is frequently associated with odynophagia and referred otalgia. The presence of otalgia suggests invasion of structures innervated by the glossopharyngeal nerve and has been shown to correlate with a higher radical radiotherapy failure rate.[15] Dysphagia and subsequent weight loss are also common findings in patients with tumors of the BOT, pharyngeal wall, and tonsil. Advanced tumors can also produce airway compromise due to bulk. Larger tumors of the soft palate can affect palatal function and therefore result in velopharyngeal insufficiency or frank oronasal fistulization. Invasion of the hypoglossal or lingual nerves can produce paresis or sensory disturbances of the oral tongue, respectively. Tumor extension into the nasopharynx can also interfere with eustachian tube function, resulting in middle ear effusion and hearing loss.

It is important when clinically evaluating tumors of the oropharynx to establish whether or not adjacent structures are invaded, as this can have significant impact on treatment decisions. Mandibular involvement is heralded by pain and tumor immobility; tooth loosening or loss also suggests growth into the mandible. Evaluation is often best accomplished under anesthesia, at the time of biopsy, where palpation and visualization are not compromised by attempts to minimize patient discomfort.

Neck

Neck metastasis is common in SCC of the oropharynx. Generally, the presence of metastasis correlates with tumor size (T stage) and thickness (or depth of invasion). Neck metastasis may occur with even early-stage tumors; in fact, many carcinomas of the oropharynx present initially with a neck mass and either very small primary lesion or an occult primary detected only with directed biopsy under anesthesia. As a group, patients with carcinoma of the oropharynx present with neck metastasis, either overt or occult, ~45 to 55% of the time.[1,2] This number can be even higher if only patients with cancer of the BOT or the tonsil are considered. Metastasis generally is discovered in the upper jugular chain nodal area (levels II and III), although metastasis to all levels is not uncommon.[16] Bilateral metastasis can occur with any subsite and can be present in up to 20 to 30% of patients, with tumors arising in the BOT, soft palate, and posterior pharyngeal wall.

Evaluation of the patient with neck metastasis must be comprehensive and bilateral and must include an evaluation of potential resectability. Large neck metastasis is not uncommon, and invasion of the carotid vessels, vertebral column, or the base of skull must be excluded if surgical resection is to be safely attempted.

Second Primary Tumors

Patients with oropharyngeal malignancies are at risk for second primary tumors, either synchronous or metachronous. This is secondary to the field cancerization effect of the inciting carcinogens alcohol and tobacco. The risk of second primary tumor is in the range 15 to 20%, with the annual risk being 2% per year. As an anatomic site, the oropharynx shows greatest risk for second primary tumor to occur elsewhere in head and neck mucosal locations.

Distant Metastasis

Fifteen percent to 20% of patients with oropharyngeal cancer will develop distant metastasis at some point during the course of their illness. The overwhelming majority of these will present in the lungs, although distant spread to bone, brain, and liver is not rare.

◆ Diagnosis and Workup

Diagnostic Imaging

Primary Site

Cross-sectional imaging modalities have largely replaced plain films in the evaluation of oropharyngeal lesions. Computed tomography (CT) and magnetic resonance imaging (MRI) both have features that make one or the other advantageous (**Fig. 2–3**). It is generally accepted that MRI provides superior soft tissue imaging and is therefore often the modality of choice for determining the soft tissue extent of the lesion. MRI is more sensitive in evaluating the possibility of intracranial extension, through the demonstration of dural enhancement, cerebral edema, or frank brain invasion. Conversely, determination of presence and/or extent of bony involvement by tumor is often best accomplished with CT, although presence of marrow enhancement on MRI can provide useful information. The addition of CT–panoramic x-ray (CT-panorex) algorithms has further enhanced the ability of CT to accurately delineate osseous involvement. Use of non-invasive angiographic imaging (either with CT [CTA] or magnetic resonance (MRA)] has largely supplanted traditional angiographic techniques for evaluation of carotid invasion.

There are other factors to consider when choosing an imaging modality for primary site evaluation. Metallic foreign bodies and pacemakers contraindicate MRI, as does significant claustrophobia. As CT technology evolves and acquisition times decrease, the applicability of this technique continues to expand. Improved software has resulted in improved three-dimensional imaging in CT, an area where MRI has traditionally had an advantage.

Other imaging modalities also serve various roles in evaluating and treating oropharyngeal malignancy. Panorex plain films continue to provide excellent cortical bony detail and can demonstrate subtle degrees of bony invasion that may be missed by CT. Although angiography is not generally used diagnostically, its role in providing preoperative embolization of certain tu-

mors has expanded as experience evolves and accumulates.

Imaging the Neck

Cross-sectional imaging continues to play the greatest role in evaluating the neck for regional metastasis. Although MRI and CT can provide valuable information, CT appears to be slightly superior when appropriate criteria are used.[17]

Distinguishing benign adenopathy from metastasis radiologically is based on several criteria. Size of the node and the presence of central necrosis are likely the most important, but demonstration of extranodal extension, invasion of arterial structures, and calcification also can add valuable information in deciding whether a node harbors metastasis.

Size criteria have been standardized and generally are considered to be as follows: for nodes in the jugulodigastric area as well as the submandibular triangle, nodes greater than 15 mm in longitudinal diameter are considered radiologically positive, whereas other nodes are considered positive if greater than 10 mm. The exception to this applies to the retropharyngeal nodes, where a node measuring >8 mm is considered abnormal. Axial diameters are also occasionally used, with 11 mm being the cutoff for jugulodigastric nodes and 10 mm being used for all others.

Nodal shape can be described using the ratio of the longitudinal and transverse diameters (the LT ratio). A ratio of less than 2 suggests metastasis (i.e., a round node vs. a kidney bean–shaped node).

Imaging for Distant Metastases

In the past, metastatic workup for SCC of the head and neck, oropharynx included, mandated a chest x-ray, an abdominal ultrasound to rule out liver metastasis, a bone scan, and blood work. Cost analyses have demonstrated that, given the frequency and likely sites of metastasis, only the chest need be imaged to effectively identify the majority of those who will present with asymptomatic metastasis. All patients presenting with symptoms or signs suggesting metastatic disease (e.g., jaundice, bone pain, headaches, seizures, etc.) should be comprehensively evaluated.

It has also been shown that CT scans of the chest are significantly more sensitive than standard radiography in their ability to discover chest metastasis. CT has generally replaced standard x-rays in both the initial workup as well as the investigation of pulmonary symptoms suggestive of new lung metastasis. Chest x-ray continues to play a role, however, in the routine posttreatment surveillance of asymptomatic patients and is generally performed at yearly intervals.

PET/PET-CT/PET-MRI

Positron emission tomography (PET) is a functional imaging modality used not only to localize a lesion but also to demonstrate its metabolic activity. Images obtained using PET can be fused with images from standard cross-sectional modalities (CT and MRI) to provide increased anatomic defi-

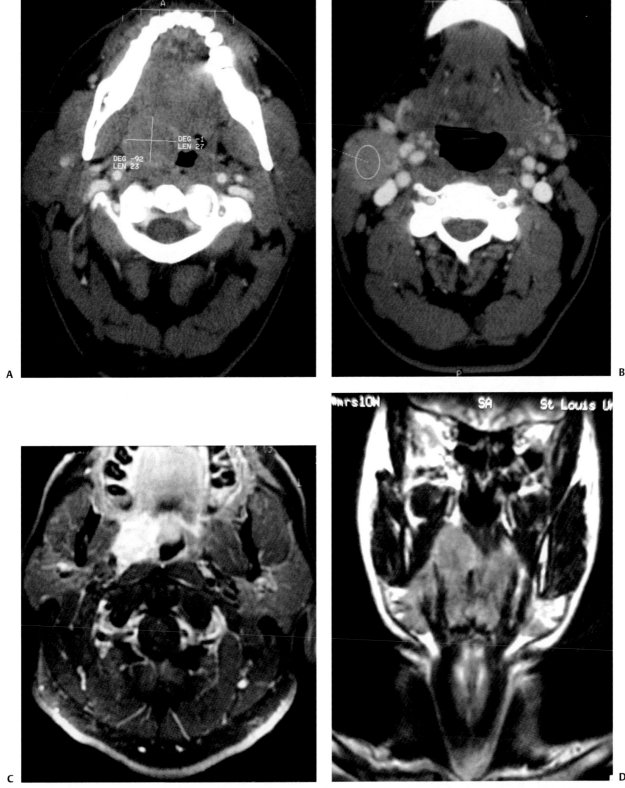

Figure 2–3 Radiologic appearance of oropharyngeal squamous cell carcinoma. (**A**) Axial contrast-enhanced computed tomography (CECT) demonstrating a tumor of the right tonsil extending into the tongue base. (**B**) Axial CECT demonstrating a metastatic level IIA lymph node; note the change in shape from kidney bean to a rounder profile. (**C**) Axial gadolinium-enhanced MRI scan demonstrating a tumor of the right palatine tonsil. (**D**) Coronal MRI of the tumor shown in (**C**).

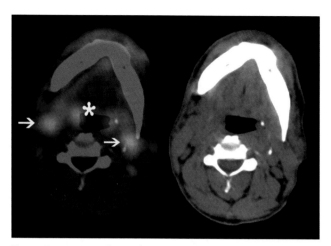

Figure 2–4 PET-CT fusion demonstrating increased [¹⁸F]fluoro-2-deoxy-d-glucose (FDG) uptake of a primary (*asterisk*) SCC of the right tonsil and bilateral cervical metastases (*arrows*).

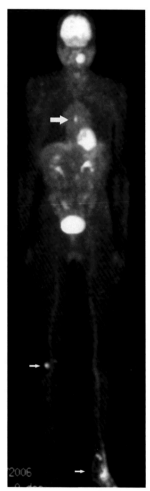

Figure 2–5 Whole-body PET-CT image demonstrating abnormal uptake in the thoracic esophagus (*large arrow*) as well as in the right knee and left ankle (*small arrows*). The esophageal lesion represented a synchronous primary SCC, whereas the other lesions were inflammatory.

nition. The use of PET has dramatically increased in recent years, and it is now being employed routinely by many centers for tumor staging as well as for posttreatment tumor surveillance (**Figs. 2–4** and **2–5**).

As data continue to emerge regarding the use of PET and fused PET, it is becoming clear that while PET can add important data during initial tumor staging that can potentially alter treatment approaches,[18,19] there remains a patient population in whom PET fails to accurately assess presence of the disease and/or its extent. When compared with conventional cross-sectional techniques, fused images appear to delineate tumors of the oropharynx more accurately.

There is also some evidence that PET can, as a stand-alone tool, provide some prognostic information, based on the degree of tracer uptake.[20] This ability has yet to be confirmed in large-scale studies with appropriate durations of follow-up.

There has also been significant investigation into the potential role of PET in monitoring tumor response posttreatment. This is especially typical in tumors of the tongue base and tonsil, where most patients present with cervical adenopathy and many are treated without surgery. In a significant number, complete responses are obtained at the primary site with clinical and/or radiologic persistence in the neck. This generally will prompt attempts at salvage neck dissection, where it is not uncommon to remove specimens with no viable tumor. Functional imaging has shown promise in reducing the number of false-positive studies.[21] It may allow the surgeon to follow some patients with small radiologic abnormalities that demonstrate no uptake on PET and avoid the potential problems associated with performing neck dissection in patients who have received a full therapeutic dose to the neck.

Sentinel Node Biopsy

Management of the N0 neck has long presented a challenge for head and neck surgeons. The determination of which patients require treatment of the neck and which do not can limit morbidity as well as the likelihood of regional recurrence. To this end, sentinel node biopsy (SNB) has been investigated as a method of providing an accurate pathologic stage in the neck.

SNB involves localization of first-echelon lymph nodes using radioactive tracers and/or colored dyes and subsequent histopathologic analysis. Identification of pathologically positive sentinel node(s) leads to more comprehensive neck dissection, whereas a negative result is generally used as evidence to support avoidance of further surgery of the neck.

A recent meta-analysis of studies evaluating SNB results in cancers of the oral cavity and oropharynx demonstrated that SNB was feasible in more than 97% of cases and that sensitivity was very high for SNB. A decision tree analysis was performed by the authors of the study comparing SNB with elective neck dissection (END); their results favored END in terms of cumulative survival by ~1%.[22] Randomized trials by the European Organization for Research and Treatment of Cancer (EORTC) and the NCI are currently under way and will provide more information to either validate or refute the use of SNB for SCCs of the oral cavity and oropharynx.

Head and Neck Cancer

◆ Treatment

In determining the most appropriate treatment for malignancies of the oropharynx, several considerations are at the forefront of the decision-making process. Across both early-stage and late-stage disease, both surgical and nonsurgical modalities have traditionally shown essentially equal overall survival rates. This includes nearly equivalent rates of local regional control and overall survival across both groups. As investigators delve more deeply into issues such as morbidity of treatment, functional results, and overall quality of life, it is hoped that this information will help clinicians to better advise patients as to the most appropriate approach to treat their tumors. As of yet, this information is not available.

As in all areas of head and neck oncologic disease management, the goal of the treating clinician is to offer the patient the greatest chance for cure with the lowest possible treatment-related morbidity. Oftentimes, an approach may be used in early-stage disease that utilizes a single modality, thereby limiting toxicity compared with multimodality treatment. In more advanced stage disease, a trimodality approach may be utilized that could conceivably result in a lower level of toxicity from each modality and improve overall quality of life and functionality of the patient. Further investigation into these possibilities and ongoing multicenter trials will soon shed more light onto these approaches.

Surgical Treatment

Early-Stage Disease

In general, early-stage presentation of an oropharyngeal carcinoma represents the minority of patients. However, when these patients do present to the head and neck team, it is possible that they may be treated with a single-modality therapy. The applicability of a surgical approach to these early-stage lesions is entirely dependent upon the subsite involved.

Primary Site Management Early-stage lesions may be managed by a transoral resection. This is particularly true of small lesions involving the tonsil, BOT, and posterior pharyngeal wall. For patients that present with an early tonsillar carcinoma, the primary site may be adequately treated surgically with a simple widefield tonsillectomy. In some cases, it may be necessary to take the constrictor muscles as a deep margin, thereby exposing the parapharyngeal fat. Even these defects, provided there is no vascular exposure, could be allowed to granulate and heal by secondary intention.

Similarly, lesions of the BOT may be resected transorally using advanced transoral endoscopic techniques either with laser surgery or using conventional Bovie cautery. Similarly, these lesions are left to granulate. Lesions of the posterior pharyngeal wall that present at an early stage are amenable to straightforward transoral resection with adequate margins. These lesions as well may be allowed to granulate or to be reconstructed with a split-thickness skin graft. Lesions of the soft palate, unless very small and requiring only a uvulectomy, are probably best treated with a nonsurgical approach because of the severe functional implications of soft palate resection.

For limited lesions involving the BOT, an appropriate and direct approach is a transhyoid or suprahyoid pharyngotomy. This has great utility for small lesions of the BOT that will not require flap reconstruction.

Management of the Neck In patients that present with an N0 neck after complete staging and with early-stage primary site disease, some type of treatment of the neck should be initiated in most cases. Most oropharyngeal primary sites, even at an early stage, will have a greater than 20% risk for metastasis. For this reason, in a patient who hopes to be treated with single-modality therapy, selective neck dissection of regions II, III, and IV at the very least should be employed. For unilateral lesions, such as tonsil, it would be appropriate to perform an ipsilateral selective neck dissection. However, for posterior pharyngeal wall lesions or lesions involving the BOT and soft palate, bilateral selective neck dissections would be appropriate.

Radiation Therapy Because the natural history of tumors of the oropharynx is different for the site, stage, and histology, treatment must be highly individualized. Some early-stage tumors may be managed by limited local therapy either by surgical excision or local irradiation.

Soft Palate Well-differentiated T1 and T2, N0 lesions may be managed by local irradiation (monotherapy), the analogy of transoral excision. Lateral opposed radiation fields designed by three-dimensional (3-D) technique or parotid-sparing intensity-modulated radiation therapy (IMRT) may be used. The goal is to deliver radiation doses of the order 6600 cGy in 33 fractions.[23,24]

If the tumor is very lateral, unilateral technique may be used. Either a mixed electron-photon beam may be used or IMRT, thus limiting the dose to the contralateral parotid and submandibular glands.

If the tumor is less than well differentiated, treatment of the level I and II lymph nodes should be included, even if the palpation of the neck and the PET scan are negative. These clinically and radiographically negative upper neck nodes should be treated to around 4600 to 5000 cGy in 23 to 25 fractions.

More advanced soft palate lesions may be treated with techniques similar to treatment strategies used for tonsillar carcinomas.[25,26]

Tonsil Early-stage T1 and T2, N0 tonsillar cancers may be irradiated similar to early soft palate cancers. The primary site should receive ~6600 cGy in 33 fractions. Usually, a diagnostic tonsillectomy will have been performed. Level I and II lymph nodal areas on the ipsilateral side are usually treated to ~5000 cGy if clinically and radiographically negative.[27]

It is worth mentioning that for early-stage lesions of the oropharynx, the disciplines of monotherapy by surgical resection or radiation therapy are generally competitive rather than complementary. The choice of whether or not to use radiation is based on patient age and comorbidities. In younger patients with a "good" life expectancy and early-stage disease, it may be desirable to withhold radiation therapy inasmuch as second primaries are common and radiation therapy may be required in the future.

Advanced-Stage Disease

Primary Site Management Traditional surgical approaches to the oropharynx or stage III and stage IV disease in the current era have largely become utilized for salvage procedures. In most centers treating a large volume of head and neck cancer, the approach to the primary oropharyngeal sites in advanced disease has almost uniformly become nonsurgical. The reason is the extreme functional implications of wide resection of the lateral pharyngeal wall, tonsil, and BOT.

For patients who elect for primary or salvage resection, it is first important to be certain that the lesion is locally and regionally resectable and that there is no evidence of distant disease. The appropriate radiographic evaluation that addresses these has been discussed previously.

In lesions involving the tonsil, lateral pharyngeal wall, soft palate, and BOT, there are several approaches that may be utilized. In a subset of cases, these lesions may still be approached transorally; however, there are limitations when there is deep BOT involvement and parapharyngeal space involvement from a tonsillar fossa cancer. Clearly, if there is mandibular involvement from a tonsillar fossa carcinoma, a transoral approach should be precluded because of the necessity of segmental mandibulectomy required to obtain clear margins.

Several open approaches may be used to address this area. If there is mandibular involvement, certain considerations need to be made to allow for segmental mandibulectomy in the area of involvement.

For patients with mandibular involvement, a lip-splitting incision with a cheek flap approach may be utilized. This provides a lateral mandibulotomy for exposure that includes mandibulectomy as part of the composite resection to encompass tonsillar fossa, lateral pharyngeal wall, and BOT (**Fig. 2–6**). With such an open approach, it is possible to place a reconstruction bar across the defect before resection. This allows maintenance of occlusion and serves as a template for bony reconstruction should that be elected. Primary site reconstruction requires soft tissue reconstruction either with a radial forearm free flap, which would allow 3-D reconstruction of the soft palate aimed at restoring velopharyngeal competence, or an anterolateral thigh flap. Soft tissue reconstruction may be accomplished using a pectoralis major myocutaneous flap, but the bulk and gravitational forces of this reconstruction lead to a less optimal result.

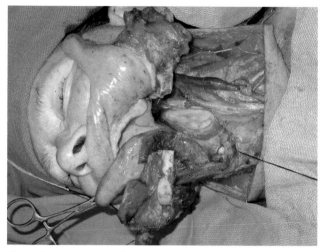

Figure 2–6 Resection of SCC involving the left palatine tonsil, with extension into the tongue base and invasion of the mandible. A segmental mandibulectomy was required and reconstruction performed with a free fibular osteocutaneous flap.

In selected cases, the reconstruction can be accomplished using an osseocutaneous flap, such as a free fibula, but often it is difficult to achieve the 3-D functional reconstruction necessary with the less than maneuverable fibula skin paddle. Many surgeons prefer to use a plate reconstruction for the mandibular defect and use a soft tissue free flap to repair the soft tissue defect.

For patients that do not require mandibular resection, midline mandibulotomy offers excellent closure to the BOT and lateral oropharynx. Soft tissue reconstructive options would be identical to those noted above.

An additional approach that allows resection and wide exposure of the BOT and oropharynx is the lingual release (**Fig. 2–7**). This utilizes an apron flap incision and obviates the need for a lip-splitting incision with mandibulotomy. In this approach, all the soft tissues on the lingual surface of the mandible are mobilized along the oropharynx to

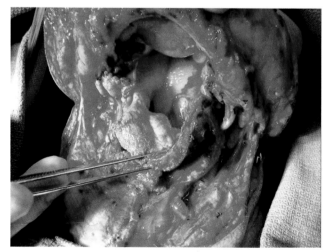

Figure 2–7 Lingual release approach to the oropharynx.

be dropped inferiorly into the neck for excellent exposure for the ablation and the reconstruction. Reconstructive options would be as noted above.

Neck Management In most patients undergoing a surgical approach for stage III and stage IV disease, at the very least the ipsilateral neck is addressed. In the N-positive neck, a comprehensive level 1 to 5 neck dissection would be most appropriate. In the N0 neck, it would be appropriate to perform a selective neck dissection involving regions II, III, and IV. In the majority of these patients who will be undergoing postoperative radiation therapy, it is not necessary to dissect the contralateral N0 neck.

Radiation Therapy Because T3 and T4 tonsillar cancers are often node-positive and surgical resection may result in significant functional deficits, treatment with definitive radiation, with induction (under investigation), and/or simultaneous chemotherapy is desirable.[27] Radiation fields must include the draining lymph nodes as well as the primary.[28,29] If fixed 3-D fields are used, care must be taken to limit the radiation dose to the spinal cord to less than 4600 cGy. A separate low-neck portal (radiation field) with a "notch" block to avoid an overlap between the upper and lower neck fields must be used lest there be a radiation "hot spot" on the spinal cord. If IMRT is used, the low neck may be irradiated with either an integral IMRT field or a separate fixed low-neck tangential portal. If a separate low-neck field is used, once again care must be taken to avoid a dose overlap over the spinal cord.

If the neck nodes are positive for metastases, they should be treated to 6600 to 7000 cGy using conventional fractionation or may be treated to 7200 cGy with concomitant chemotherapy and a hyperfractionated terminal boost. When treating with hyperfractionated chemoradiotherapy, the primary tumor and draining lymph nodes are included in a "large" IMRT field and given 180 cGy 30 times in 6 weeks, with a terminal boost to the radiographically and clinically positive primary site(s). The positive lymph nodes are included in the boost, which is given 150 cGy 12 times using twice-daily technique; that is, a total of 7200 cGy (180 cGy/fraction × 30 fractions [5400 cGy] + 150 cGy/fraction × 12 fractions [1800 cGy]) is given in 42 fractions in ~6 weeks elapsed time.[30]

In selected patients, induction chemotherapy, either one or two cycles, is given before the radiation, especially if tooth extractions are needed. (Because postradiation tooth extraction wound healing can be difficult after a full course of radiation therapy, it is highly desirable that any bad teeth be extracted before commencing radiotherapy and any marginal teeth be brought up to the level of good dental health. Induction therapy may be used to begin treatment of the disease while the dental issues are treated and resolved and before the onset of radiation therapy.) This has not been shown to have a survival advantage but is currently under investigation as part of a multicenter trial. Chemotherapy, when given concurrently with radiation, is administered on day 1 and day 22 of the radiation and is not given when the time comes for the twice-daily boost.

Severe mucositis and pharyngitis requiring nutritional support and often hospitalization are to be expected. A multidisciplinary team using hyperfractionated chemoradiation must be prepared to hospitalize and care for the patient. The acute mucosal reaction phase of chemoradiation for oropharyngeal cancer usually begins in the second or third week of radiation and may persist over 1 month after the end of the bimodality treatment, much longer than with radiation therapy alone.[31]

After chemoradiotherapy, elective neck dissection is usually reserved for either clinically or radiographically persistent neck nodal disease, as discussed elsewhere in this chapter.

An alternative to chemoradiation for tonsillar cancers is definitive radiation therapy alone without chemotherapy. The primary tumor is irradiated to 7000 cGy in 35 fractions in 7 weeks. Uninvolved neck areas at risk of recurrence are treated to ~5000 cGy and involved areas to 6600 to 7000 cGy at 200 cGy per day.

Base of Tongue BOT cancers may be treated with techniques similar to tonsillar cancer. Because of the high risk of cervical lymph nodes, including bilaterally positive occult nodes, both sides of the neck should be treated, usually to 5000 cGy to uninvolved areas with conventional techniques or if hyperfractionated with chemoradiotherapy in the 5400 cGy IMRT field. If positive, the nodes are included in the twice-daily boost, and the total dose will be 7200 cGy. Alternatively, if conventional radiation technique is used, the nodes are treated to 6600 to 7000 cGy in 33 to 35 sessions.

BOT cancers can usually be treated with fields that avoid full doses of the parotid glands, though if unusually high nodes are positive, the parotids may be too close to the nodes to be spared.

Lateral or Posterior Pharyngeal Wall The radiation therapy techniques used for pharyngeal wall tumors are very similar to tonsil and BOT cancers, but the incidence of ipsilateral nodes is high with lateralized lesions, as is the incidence of bilateral nodes for midline and near-midline lesions. Portals are individualized based on tumor location and clinical/radiographic evidence of nodal involvement.

Neck If there is evidence of residual nodal metastasis in the neck after either definitive radiation alone or combined chemoradiotherapy, therapeutic neck dissections should be considered. Controversy remains about whether or not neck dissection is beneficial if the PET scan has become negative after nonsurgical treatment.[21]

Postoperative Radiation Therapy With or Without Chemotherapy

Postoperative adjuvant radiation is considered for early-stage squamous cell oropharyngeal cancer (T1 to T2, N0 to N1) after excision of the primary and unilateral or bilateral neck dissection if there are positive nodes. If there is only one node without adverse features, adjuvant radiotherapy is optional (60 Gy [2 Gy/day] to the primary site; 50 Gy to low-risk nodal stations, 60 Gy to high-risk stations). Adverse features include close or positive margins; extracapsular spread; perineural, lymphatic, or vascular invasion; or multiple positive nodes. In the presence of any one of these features, adjuvant radiation treatment is indicated. In the presence of positive margins or extracapsular spread, adjuvant chemoradiation therapy (conventional fractionation >70 Gy [2 Gy/day], cisplatin 100 mg/m^2 days 1, 22, 43) has been shown to have a superior outcome compared with radiation treatment alone (category I recommendation) in patients with good performance status.[32]

More advanced disease (T3 N0 [stage III] or T4 N0 [stage IV]) in the absence of neck adenopathy can be approached in different ways. Although the preferred treatment would be concurrent chemoradiation therapy, surgery followed by adjuvant radiation therapy is an option.

Definitive Chemoradiotherapy

For locoregionally even more advanced lesions (any T, N2 to N3; T3 to T4, N+), concurrent chemoradiation therapy is also the preferred strategy (see above). However, if surgery is used as the initial modality, adjuvant radiotherapy (no adverse features, poor performance status) or adjuvant concurrent chemoradiation therapy are recommended (category I).

There is uniform consensus, based on high-level evidence, that concurrent chemoradiotherapy is the preferred treatment for locoregionally advanced stages III and IVA oropharyngeal cancer. Standard of care is the use of conventional fractionation concurrent with chemotherapy; however, altered fractionation techniques as well as IMRT technology are currently being studied in this setting with assessment of toxicity, quality of life parameters, and long-term outcome. Cisplatin (100 mg/m^2) on days 1, 22, 43 has been considered by some investigators the standard chemotherapeutic agent, but other chemotherapeutic drugs and schedules have been used successfully. Most recently, the epidermal growth factor receptor (EGFR) antibody cetuximab infused weekly with concurrent radiotherapy has shown promise.[33]

Concurrent chemoradiotherapy appears to prolong survival by improved locoregional control without impact on distant metastases. There is preliminary evidence that additional induction chemotherapy using cisplatin, 5-fluorouracil (5-FU), and a taxane results in significant improvement of survival due to diminished distant failure; sequential therapy and chemoradiotherapy are now being compared in phase III trials.[34]

Management of the Neck After Definitive Chemoradiotherapy

Management of the neck in patients that undergo definitive chemoradiotherapy for advanced oropharyngeal carcinoma continues to evolve.

In patients who have obvious residual nodal disease after definitive chemoradiation therapy, there is little debate as to the need to perform a salvage neck dissection. The pathologic findings in this scenario have important prognostic implications for the patient. In such a setting of residual disease after chemoradiotherapy, a comprehensive level 1 to 5 neck dissection is advised.

For the patient who presents with an N1 neck, undergoes chemoradiotherapy, and shows a complete response as assessed on physical exam and imaging studies including PET-CT, most investigators would agree that close follow-up is all that is warranted.

For the patients that present initially with a 3-cm or greater neck node, there is continued debate. There is an approach of performing a planned neck dissection in these patients regardless of their response. The rationale is that none of the means of assessing patients' pathologic disease status after chemoradiotherapy are perfect, and there will be both false-positives and false-negatives irrespective of the evaluative approaches used. The consequences of a false-negative assessment in these patients (lack of salvageability once the metastasis is clearly evident or progresses) are believed to justify the need for a planned neck dissection in all patients with this stage of neck disease. The low rate of salvage in patients who develop progressive neck disease in the setting of previous chemoradiotherapy has made this argument more compelling. The literature, however, is conflicted on this topic, and there has been no randomized prospective trial yet that truly shows the survival advantage to adding a planned neck dissection at the completion of therapy.[31] In addition, the predictive value of a truly negative PET-CT scan in determining the need to perform a neck dissection in this scenario is resulting in more centers observing the neck in this group of patients.

As to the type of dissection that should be done in this setting, opinions vary. For a truly N0 neck after chemoradiotherapy, selective neck dissection is believed in many centers to be adequate. Flexibility in the surgical approach is necessary so that if the surgeon finds obvious evidence of residual disease intraoperatively, this could be converted to a more comprehensive neck dissection. Others still advocate a comprehensive neck dissection in any patient after chemoradiotherapy as part of planned neck dissection.

Treatment of Recurrence

Chemoradiotherapy

The role of chemoradiotherapy in recurrent oropharyngeal cancer will usually be limited to locoregional recurrence in patients without prior radiotherapy if the tumor is unresectable.

Metastatic Disease

Single-agent chemotherapy and combination systemic chemotherapy regimens can be used. Response rates to single agents vary between 15 and 35%. Combination chemotherapy results in higher response rates of 30 to 40%. The most active regimens include cisplatin plus 5-FU or a taxane. The median survival with chemotherapy is ~6 months. One-year survival is ~20%. Achievement of a complete response is associated with longer survival. Patients with good performance status may be offered chemotherapy.

Treatment After Maximal Curative Treatment

Unfortunately, there are no good treatment modalities for patients that present with recurrent oropharyngeal carcinoma after maximal curative therapy, who have then failed in attempted surgical salvage. Protocols exist that are investigating the use of reirradiation of these patients with chemotherapy, but the toxicity is quite high and the long-term benefit low. Single-modality chemotherapy has been investigated but as of yet has shown no significant survival advantage or lengthening of the survival interval.

Complications

Myelopathy

Arguably, the most severe complication of radiotherapy in oropharyngeal (and other) cancers is spinal cord myelopathy resulting in weakness or paralysis.[35–37] The usually mild and transient minor complications of Lhermittes syndrome (the sensation of electric shocks with flexion of the neck) aside, weakness and/or paralysis, often a Brown-Sequard syndrome, is fortunately virtually unheard of with proper cord blocking techniques including "gaps" to avoid overlapping fields.[38]

Xerostomia and Dental Health

Xerostomia, pathologic salivary desiccation, with the concomitant loss of taste sensation (dysgeusia) and loss of the protective effects of antibodies and pH buffers, can result in loss of teeth. Postradiation extractions in an area that has been heavily irradiated may result in an unhealing "dry socket" and painful chronic abscesses.[39,40] Therefore, it is important to achieve good dental health before beginning radiotherapy and important to start an aggressive course of prophylactic posttreatment dental care. The dentist should be involved early in the patient's care as well as long-term. It is very important to educate the patient about the importance of dental hygiene and the patient's responsibilities regarding self-care under the guidance of the dentist.

Should extractions after radiation be required, preextraction hyperbaric oxygen treatment should be initiated and continued postextraction.[41] The usual recommendation is for 20 sessions ("dives") preextraction and 10 postextraction.

Artificial saliva and treatment with pilocarpine may be of some subjective value to the patient with severe posttreatment xerostomia.[42]

Dysphagia

Severe permanent posttreatment dysfunctional dysphagia may be avoided if the patient is coached and the services of the speech therapy team are employed early in the patient's course of radiation or chemoradiation. We try, when feasible, to avoid gastrostomy and encourage our patients to continue to swallow at least liquids or soft foods during the course of treatment. Even if a gastrostomy tube is placed, we encourage patients to continue to swallow liquids to help prevent severe long-term fibrosis or "frozen" laryngopharynx.

◆ Reconstruction

Reconstruction of ablative defects of the oropharynx has undergone significant change over the past 10 to 15 years. The introduction and increasing use of microvascular free tissue transfer has revolutionized the approach to oropharyngeal reconstruction. Reconstructive surgeons now have an unprecedented number of options available for minimizing postoperative morbidity and loss of function (**Table 2–2**). With so many tools, it is possible to tailor the reconstructive effort to the defect more than ever before.

The goal of oropharyngeal reconstruction is to provide tissue that most closely approximates that which was resected, in terms of structure and, if possible, function. Reconstruction-associated morbidity should be minimized and the techniques should be technically feasible for the average head and neck surgeon. The ideal technique can be completed at the time of initial surgery, obviating the need for a second anesthetic or procedure and should allow for simul-

Table 2–2 Reconstruction Options

Primary closure
Secondary-intention healing
Skin graft
   Split-thickness
   Full-thickness
Dermal
Local flaps
   Tongue
   Facial artery musculomucosal
Palatal island
Regional flaps
   Deltopectoral
   Forehead
   Latissimus dorsi
   Postauricular
   Pectoralis major
   Sternocleidomastoid
   Temporoparietal fascia
   Temporalis muscle
Trapezius
Free flaps
   Fasciocutaneous/myocutaneous
      Radial forearm
      Scapular/parascapular
      Latissimus dorsi
      Rectus abdominis
      Anterolateral thigh
   Osseous
      Fibula
      Iliac crest
      Radial forearm
      Scapular/parascapular
   Enteric
      Gastroomental
      Jejunum
   Fascial
Temporoparietal fascia

taneous harvest as ablation is being performed. Although it is rare for one technique to meet all these requirements, the challenge facing the reconstructive surgeon is to identify which of the available tools most closely approximates the ideal reconstruction.

Primary Closure

For relatively limited defects, primary closure should be attempted, provided the closure neither hinders postoperative function nor is under excessive amounts of tension. For bulky defects, serious consideration should be given to replacing the resected tissue volume, as failure to do so can result in unacceptable functional deficits.[43]

Secondary-Intention Healing

Secondary-intention healing has been used with increasing frequency with the more widespread use of endoscopic laser-assisted tumor ablation. Although endoscopic approaches do not provide the necessary access for many reconstructive techniques, there are reports demonstrating good postoperative function, even with bulkier tumors.[44,45]

Skin Grafts

For relatively shallow defects with an appropriate bed, skin grafts can provide excellent resurfacing and can help prevent cicatricial contraction and subsequent loss of function. Split- and full-thickness grafts as well as dermal grafts have all been used reliably for oropharyngeal defects.[46] Donor site morbidity is minimal, and the technique is highly reliable in any hands. As is the case with primary closure, careful evaluation of the need for tissue volume replacement is necessary to avoid compromising function. Measures should be taken to maximize the chances for graft survival, including the application of pressure on the graft to optimize take. In those tissue beds that have received radiation ± chemotherapy, the likelihood of graft take is significantly decreased and should likely prompt a search for a better vascularized reconstructive technique. Patients with bolsters should, in most instances, have a controlled airway to prevent the possibility of airway compromise should the bolster become dislodged.

Local Flaps

A variety of local flaps have been used to reconstruct oropharyngeal defects; with the increasing use of free tissue transfer, many of these techniques are used more sparingly than in past times. These techniques deserve strong consideration in those patients not considered suitable for more aggressive reconstruction for whatever reason(s).

Tongue rotation flaps provide a decent amount of well-vascularized tissue for reconstruction of small- to medium-sized defects. Whereas harvest is simple and relatively quick, the effects on the oral phase of swallowing and hence the overall swallow can be unpredictable.

The facial artery musculomucosal (FAMM) flap was described by Pribaz and has been used to reconstruct defects of the soft palate, tonsillar fossa, and BOT.[47] Although simultaneous harvest is not feasible, donor site morbidity is low. Experience with this flap is growing.

The palatal island flap[48,49] can provide reliable tissue that is easy to harvest. Donor site morbidity is not great, although healing can take several weeks. The principal limitation of this flap for oropharyngeal reconstruction is its limited arc of rotation and pliability. The tethering of the greater palatine vessels within the palatine canal can limit the distance that this flap can be rotated. This can, however, be somewhat overcome by using a drill to take down the canal and partially deliver the vessels from it.

Regional Flaps

A variety of regional flaps have been described for oropharyngeal reconstruction that offer different amounts of tissue as well as varying degrees of tissue pliability and mobility. As is the case with local flaps, many regional techniques have been supplanted where possible by free tissue transfer. It is important to be cognizant of these techniques, as they can be invaluable in those situations where microvascular reconstruction has failed or is not feasible.

Pectoralis Major Flap

Available as a muscle, a myocutaneous, or even a bone-containing (rib or sternum) flap, the pectoralis major still plays an important role in reconstruction of defects of the oropharynx. It can provide a large volume of tissue that can reach almost any oropharyngeal site with relative ease. It can also be designed with two skin paddles to allow for reconstruction of through-and-through defects. With appropriate positioning of the skin paddle, partial flap failure can be minimized. The muscle itself, however, is quite resilient, as evidenced by a very low failure rate. Its harvest is relatively fast and reliable, with acceptable donor site morbidity. Patient habitus can make use of this flap more challenging, although excessively thick flaps can be thinned by removing the skin, dermis, and subdermal fat and replacing them with a split-thickness skin graft applied directly to the muscle.

Free Tissue Transfer

A comprehensive discussion of the use of free tissue transfer for the reconstruction of defects of the oropharynx is outside the scope of this chapter. The goal here is to outline the free flaps commonly used in oropharyngeal reconstruction as well as to describe their advantages and disadvantages.

Fasciocutaneous

Fasciocutaneous flaps are widely used in reconstruction of oropharyngeal defects for many reasons. Large resections can be effectively resurfaced and, given the wide variety of donor site tissue types, many different thicknesses can be available to most accurately replace resected tissues.

Radial Forearm Free Flap

The radial forearm free flap (RFFF) is the most widely used free flap in head and neck reconstruction. Experience with this flap has repeatedly demonstrated its reliability and versatility. Successful reinnervation using the lateral antebrachial cutaneous nerve has been established. Flap elevation is straightforward and pedicle length and vessel caliber both facilitate the reconstructive effort. Simultaneous harvest is often possible, and donor site morbidity is generally very low.

Anterolateral Thigh Free Flap

The anterolateral thigh fasciocutaneous flap is becoming increasingly popular for the reconstruction of more extensive defects of the head and neck. Although flap elevation can be somewhat challenging because of the small size of the perforating vessels and the variable nature of the anatomy of the branches of the lateral circumflex femoral artery, donor site morbidity is negligible, and a two-team approach is easily possible. Reinnervation has been described as has the inclusion of vascularized vastus lateralis with the skin and fascia, making for a more versatile flap in terms of volume. As with the RFFF, pedicle length and vessel caliber are generally excellent (**Fig. 2–8**).

Scapular/Parascapular Free Flap

The subscapular arterial system provides a great number of flap options. The scapular/parascapular flaps have been used extensively for both straightforward and complex reconstruction. Minimal donor site morbidity and the ability to harvest multiple skin paddles, varying amounts of muscle and/or bone that can be rotated with respect to one another make the subscapular system of flaps extremely versatile. Although generally shorter than the RFFF, pedicle length is very good and vessel caliber is excellent. The absence of atherosclerosis in even the most vasculopathic patients can also be advantageous. This is offset by difficulties in patient positioning to allow for flap harvest and an inability to accommodate two surgical teams.

Lateral Arm Free Flap

The lateral arm flap based on the posterior radial collateral branch of the profunda brachii artery offers some of the advantages of both the radial forearm and the scapular flaps. It is of intermediate thickness and can often be closed without a skin graft. Pedicle length and caliber are acceptable although inferior to those of the RFFF in most cases. Care must be taken during harvest of the flap and care must be taken of the donor site to avoid postoperative radial nerve palsy, which has been reported.[50] Unfortunately, two-team harvest is often not possible.

Bone-Containing Flaps

Fibula Free Flap

After its introduction by Taylor in 1975, the free fibular flap has become the most commonly used bony flap in head and neck reconstruction in most centers. It offers excellent bone stock for lengths up to 25 cm, enough for total mandibular reconstruction. Pedicle length is excellent but shortens with longer bony harvests. Vessel caliber is good at both ends of the pedicle, allowing flow-through revascularization techniques where necessary. Reinnervation is possible, using the

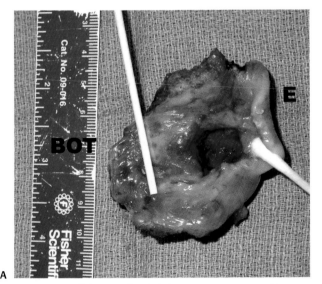
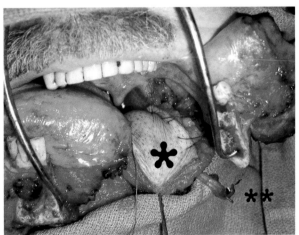

Figure 2–8 SCC of the BOT that failed primary treatment with concurrent chemoradiation. (**A**) The resection specimen. E, epiglottis; BOT, base of tongue. (**B**) Reconstruction of the ablative defect with a free anterolateral thigh flap. The skin paddle (*asterisk*) and the vascular pedicle (*double asterisk*) are shown.

lateral sural nerve as a recipient. Donor site morbidity is generally acceptable, although mild gait disturbances have been described, as have deficits in flexion of the great toe. The potential for ischemic injury to the foot mandates careful preoperative assessment of the vascular anatomy of the lower leg to avoid sacrificing the main arterial supply to the foot.

Radial Forearm Free Flap

Bone can be harvested along with RFFF (described above). In general, the amount of bone stock is limited compared with the other osseous flaps described. Donor site morbidity can also be significantly increased, especially if postoperative fracture of the radius occurs. For these reasons, osteocutaneous radial forearm flaps are not extensively used in oropharyngeal reconstruction.

Scapula Flap

The soft tissue aspects of the scapular system of flaps is described above. Ten centimeters to 15 cm of bone can be harvested along with the fasciocutaneous paddles. Although the bone stock is generally inferior to that of the fibula or the iliac crest, the increased mobility of the bony segment with respect to the cutaneous paddle(s), as well as the ability to harvest independently nourished bony segments with inclusion of the tip of scapula based on the angular branch of the thoracodorsal artery, makes this flap suitable for even the most complex of defects. Donor site morbidity is acceptable even when bone is harvested.

Iliac Crest Free Flap

The iliac crest was the first osseous flap to be used extensively in head and neck reconstruction. Although it has been replaced in most centers by the fibular flap, it continues to offer excellent and versatile bone stock as well as moderate amounts of muscle (the internal oblique) to provide soft tissue coverage over the neoalveolar ridge. Harvest is straightforward and can be performed simultaneously with the ablative procedure. The major disadvantage of the iliac crest flap relates to donor site morbidity, where pain, gait disturbances, and abdominal wall weakening and herniation can all occur.

Musculocutaneous Flaps

Latissimus Dorsi Flap

Based on the thoracodorsal branch of the subscapular artery, the latissimus dorsi myocutaneous flap offers the potential to transfer a large area of skin and large volumes of muscle. The thoracodorsal artery is generally resistant to atherosclerotic degeneration, regardless of patient age. Donor site morbidity is minimal, as most harvest sites can be closed primarily. Simultaneous harvest is generally not possible due to patient positioning. Muscle atrophy and subsequent volume loss must be taken into consideration when volume is important; reinnervation using the readily accessible thoracodorsal nerve has been described[51] and results in less atrophy than if a non-reinnervated flap is transferred. Excessive amounts of subcutaneous fat can be managed either by removing the skin and applying a skin graft to the underlying muscle or by allowing the muscle to mucosalize where appropriate. Mucosalization generally takes several weeks but results in excellent contouring over bony surfaces.

Rectus Abdominis Flap

The rectus abdominis flap, like the latissimus dorsi flap, can provide large volumes of muscle, subcutaneous tissue, and skin and is thus a versatile flap for a variety of soft tissue defects in the oropharynx. Positioning is straightforward, and simultaneous harvest is possible. Donor site morbidity is minimal if care is taken to reestablish the fascial layers of the abdominal wall to prevent postoperative herniation. Muscle reinnervation using the segmental neural supply is possible to minimize muscle volume loss.[52] Thinning of the flap can be accomplished much as described above for the latissimus dorsi.

Visceral Flaps

Gastroomental Flap

The initial transfer of the gastroomental flap was performed in 1979 by Beaudet[53]; subsequent reports have demonstrated the usefulness of this technique.[54] Gastric mucosa approximates that of the oropharynx well, and gastric secretions can somewhat alleviate postradiation xerostomia in those patients who have undergone radiation-based treatment regimens.

Perhaps the most useful aspect of this flap relates to the omental component. Composed of thin, pliable, and very well vascularized tissue, the omentum can supply nonradiated tissue to provide coverage of exposed vessels or accept a skin graft in cases of problematic neck wounds. Pedicle length and caliber are generally excellent.

The principal drawback of the gastroomental flap relates to the need for laparotomy for harvest. Multiple serious, potentially life-threatening, intraabdominal complications can arise and have led to a reduction in the use of this flap in preference for reasonable, less invasive alternatives. Previous laparotomy is a relative contraindication to this flap.

◆ Complications

Patients undergoing surgery for oropharyngeal cancer often require extensive surgical procedures and frequently present with one or more medical comorbidities. As a result, complications are not uncommonly encountered. **Tables 2–3** and **2–4** outline the various categories and specific complications most commonly facing patients after oropharyngeal surgery.

Myocardial Infarction/Cerebrovascular Accident

Many risk factors are common to both the development of vascular disease and upper aerodigestive malignancy; as a

Table 2–3 Major Complications of Oropharyngeal Surgery

Death
Cardiac
  Acute myocardial infarction
Cardiac arrhythmia
Thromboembolic
Deep venous thrombosis/pulmonary embolism
Pulmonary
Pneumonia
Renal
Acute renal failure
Vascular
Major vessel rupture
Free flap compromise/failure

result, many patients undergoing surgery are at significant risk for perioperative vascular complications. Careful preoperative evaluation, in conjunction with medical and anesthesia colleagues, can help identify those at greatest risk. For those with significant risk who are still fit to undergo surgery, it is important to formulate a surgical plan designed to minimize anesthetic duration where possible.

Deep Venous Thrombosis/Pulmonary Embolism

The true incidence of deep venous thrombosis/pulmonary embolism (DVT/PE) is difficult to assess, as many may be subclinical and, therefore, never detected. It is clear, however,

Table 2–4 Minor Complications of Oropharyngeal Surgery

Infectious
Urinary tract infection
Wound related
  Pharyngocutaneous fistula
  Orocutaneous fistula
  Osteonecrosis/osteomyelitis
  Plate exposure
  Malunion/nonunion
  Skin flap loss/major vessel exposure
Free flap donor site morbidity
Cranial nerve injury
  Trigeminal
  Facial
  Glossopharyngeal
  Vagal
  Accessory
Hypoglossal
Functional deficits
  Dysphagia
  Dysarthria
  Aspiration
Airway compromise
Postoperative hemorrhage

that when DVT/PE does become clinically apparent, morbidity, mortality, length of stay, and cost can be substantially increased. A review of DVT/PE by the group at the University of Iowa illustrated several important facts about DVT/PE in patients undergoing head and neck surgery.

Patients undergoing oncologic surgery of the head and neck are at significantly higher risk of DVT/PE when compared with other otolaryngologic subspecialties.[55] Two thirds of patients with proven DVT in this series went on to develop PE; mortality for those with proven PE was 10%. The authors identified age, obesity, and duration of surgery as important predisposing factors. The use of DVT prophylactic measures, either mechanical (pneumatic compression devices) or pharmacologic (low-dose heparin), was effective in reducing the incidence.

Wound Infection

Despite large numbers of potentially pathogenic bacteria and an inability to eradicate them, wound infection is uncommon in oropharyngeal surgery. Management of simple wound infection is generally uncomplicated, given timely drainage of suppurative collections and the appropriate culture-directed intravenous antibiotic(s) where necessary. Prophylactic antibiotics are indicated using a combination of a broad-spectrum cephalosporin with adequate gram-positive coverage and an anaerobic agent, such as metronidazole.

Mandibular Malunion/Nonunion

Failure of the mandible to heal at the site of mandibulotomy is a devastating complication. For this reason, the decision to perform mandibulotomy should be made only when no safe, oncologically sound alternative is available. It is unfortunately not rare in the setting of oropharyngeal cancer resection; it is increasingly problematic in the presence of significant radiotherapeutic doses to the mandibulotomy site. Prevention of failed bony union should include avoiding unnecessary devascularization of the bone at the osteotomy site and providing a stable fixation using accepted principles of open reduction and internal fixation.

Fistula

Fistulization is often a consequence of wound infection and underscores the need for expedient management of suspected infections. Treatment of established fistulas must be tailored to the site as well as to the patient. Orocutaneous fistulae will generally heal if the wound is appropriately managed, whereas oronasal and oroantral fistulae can be more persistent. Unfortunately, after significant doses of radiation, healing can be more problematic and can require secondary reconstruction. In this setting, introduction of nonradiated free tissue is advisable to aid in successful healing. In addition, orocutaneous fistula with a tract that passes over the great vessels in the previously irradiated patient significantly increases the risk for carotid hemorrhage and is a reason for interposition of vascularized tissue.

◆ Quality of Life Outcomes

Treatment of oropharyngeal lesions can have devastating consequences on many of the integral functions of the tongue, pharynx, and larynx. A not-insignificant proportion of patients undergoing treatment for advanced malignancies can be reliant on a tracheostomy tube for airway maintenance and/or a gastrostomy tube for nutritional support. Inabilities to phonate and/or swallow can place significant social restrictions on patients and hence severely affect their quality of life (QoL).

Although much attention has been focused on the topic of QoL in head and neck cancer therapy, interpretation of the literature can be a challenge, as no single device to measure QoL has gained universal acceptance. In addition, an inherent selection bias is encountered in many long-term QoL studies, given the increased likelihood of patients with early-stage disease experiencing prolonged control of their disease and therefore being available to complete QoL questionnaires.

Overall QoL for patients treated for oropharyngeal cancer is reasonable when general health indices are evaluated along with many oncologic symptoms.[56,57] In addition, patients with oropharyngeal lesions seem to maintain general domain QoL scores well during the course of therapy. Scores drop when domains relate to oropharyngeal structure and function (e.g., speech, taste, quantity of saliva, and swallowing).[58,59] This is especially true when patients requiring permanent gastrostomy tubes are included in the analysis. Although there is evidence to suggest that patients treated with surgery alone may enjoy a better QoL than those requiring multimodality therapy, this may relate more to initial disease stage than to any advantage of therapy.

Choice of reconstructive technique can also affect post-treatment QoL, in the case of patients treated surgically. There is evidence demonstrating improved function with microvascular free tissue techniques; many of these conclusions, however, are inferred from patients with oral cavity lesions.[43,60,61]

Pretreatment comorbidity status can have effects on the post-treatment QoL measures. A significant association between the American Society of Anesthesiologists (ASA) score and post-treatment QoL measures has been demonstrated in patients undergoing treatment for oropharyngeal malignancy.[57]

Overall, however, the majority of patients with oropharyngeal cancers who are successfully managed can expect an acceptable quality of life.

◆ Conclusions

Quality of life for patients successfully treated for cancers of the oropharynx is generally compromised compared with their pretreatment status, regardless of the method of treatment. Further studies are needed to determine which modalities leave the patient with the best chance for cure and most improved quality of life.

◆ Clinical Cases

Case 1   T2 N0 M0 squamous cell carcinoma of the tonsil.

Presentation   This patient was a 52-year-old African-American man who reported a 4-week history of right pharyngeal pain with otalgia, odynophagia, and jaw pain. Treatment with Amoxil (amoxicillin) by his primary care doctor did not relieve the symptoms. He had a history of smoking 1½ packs of cigarettes per day for 22 years, quitting 13 years prior to presentation. He had a previous history of alcohol use but none in 11 years.

Physical Examination   Examination of the head and neck was normal with the exception of the oropharynx and neck. There was a 3-cm³ mass of the right superior tonsillar fossa with extension into the soft palate. There was no trismus. The neck examination showed a 2.5-cm³ region II mass on the right.

Diagnosis and Workup   A CT scan of the neck showed a soft tissue mass of the right soft palate (**Fig. 2–3C,D**). There was no significant cervical lymphadenopathy. Biopsy of this lesion in the office showed it to be consistent with SCC, moderately differentiated.

Chest x-ray to rule out metastatic disease was negative.

Options for Treatment   The options for treatment of this lesion were discussed with the patient in detail. As this was a T2 primary lesion, the options were primary radiotherapy for cure or a surgical resection including neck dissection with immediate reconstruction. The patient opted for resection. This was approached through a midline mandibulotomy with resection of the lesion of the right soft palate and upper tonsillar fossa. A type I modified radical neck dissection was done as well. The lesion was reconstructed using a palatal island flap.

The patient's pathology showed clear primary resection margins and 1 of 29 nodes positive for metastatic SCC without extracapsular disease. The patient then underwent postoperative radiation therapy to a total of 6600 cGy in 33 fractions to the tumor bed and upper ipsilateral neck. The patient has remained disease-free 2½ years postoperatively.

Summary of Treatment   In this situation, the patient presented with a relatively early-stage lesion that ultimately required combined therapy because of the positive nodes in the neck noted on pathologic evaluation. This patient's primary site could have been treated with equal results with respect to disease control with radiation therapy alone. The patient, however, preferred an upfront surgical approach. This was offered to the patient, as the reconstructive options for a small lesion in this area were of acceptable morbidity and most likely to result in excellent function.

Case 2   T2 N1 M0 tonsil cancer.

Presentation   This patient was a 47-year-old White man who presented with a mass in the right neck and a persistent sore throat that was believed to be strep tonsillitis of 2 months duration. Ten days of antibiotic therapy did not relieve his symptoms. An outside CT scan was done, which showed a 3-cm mass in region II on the right side without obvious primary. A fine-needle aspirate biopsy was done of the neck mass at the referring office that showed the metastatic SCC.

The patient had no other symptoms except as noted above. He did have a 30-pack-year smoking history without any significant alcohol use.

Physical Examination Examination findings showed the right tonsil to be somewhat hyperemic, but there was no palpable mass in either tonsillar fossa. The hypopharynx was normal. The neck showed a 5-cm multilobulated region II mass on the right.

Diagnosis and Workup The patient had a PET-CT scan performed to rule out distant disease and to help localize the primary tumor. The PET-CT scan showed the lymph nodes in the right neck consistent with the patient's known right upper neck mass. There was some asymmetry in the oropharynx suggestive of a primary tonsil lesion.

Treatment The patient was taken to the operating room for a tonsillectomy and frozen section. The right tonsil showed invasive SCC, moderately to poorly differentiated. A right modified radical neck dissection (type I) was performed. The neck dissection specimen showed metastatic squamous cell carcinoma to 5 nodes in level II and one in level III, with extracapsular disease noted. He was treated with postoperative platinum-based (days 1 and 22) chemoradiotherapy to a total dose to the primary tumor site of 70 Gy with 50 Gy to the lower neck bilaterally and the contralateral upper neck. He has remained without evidence of recurrent disease. He did develop significant postoperative toxicity and remains marginally nourished but alimented completely by mouth.

Summary of Treatment This patient presented with an early tonsillar cancer whose primary site could have easily been managed with tonsillectomy and postoperative radiation therapy; however, because of the extent of nodal disease, his high-risk status mandated treatment with postoperative chemoradiotherapy to improve regional control and long-term survival. This did result in significant late toxicity manifest as severe dysphagia and cachexia.

Case 3 T3 N2c M0 squamous cell carcinoma of the palate

Presentation This patient was a 56-year-old African-American man referred for symptoms of throat pain of 8 months duration. This became more constant and the patient developed odynophagia and right-sided otalgia. He had a history of smoking one-half pack of cigarettes a day for 40 years and moderate alcohol use.

Physical Examination Examination showed an ulcerative lesion involving the right tonsil in its upper one-half extending up onto the soft palate to involve the entire soft palate to the junction with the hard palate. It also extended up to the superior pole of the left tonsil, and there was absence to the uvula because of autonecrosis. The neck was

remarkable for bilateral 2-cm region II lymph nodes and a 1-cm right region V lymph node.

Diagnosis Workup The patient underwent a CT scan of the neck with contrast, which showed bilateral cervical lymphadenopathy measuring up to 1.7 cm on the right and 1.4 cm on the left. No obvious primary site was seen. A PET-CT scan was done, which confirmed the primary oropharyngeal site and the bilateral neck disease (**Fig. 2–4**). Biopsy of the palate lesion showed squamous cell carcinoma.

Treatment After discussions regarding possible treatment, which included primary surgical resection with neck dissections and immediate reconstruction versus a chemoradiotherapeutic approach, the patient opted for chemoradiotherapy. Because of the need for dental extractions and the desire to begin therapy sooner rather than later, he was admitted for dental extractions and one cycle of induction therapy (platinum-based). This was followed with concurrent chemoradiotherapy to a total dose of 7,200 cGy, using terminal boost technique with twice-daily fractionation with concurrent platinum-based chemotherapy. The low neck received 5000 cGy. He has completed treatment and has remained disease-free.

Summary of Treatment This patient's primary site, if resected, would have resulted in significant morbidity as it would have required total soft palate resection. Reconstruction of his defect does not reliably restore oropharyngeal function. The patient was able to achieve disease control and maintain a very good oropharyngeal function with this nonsurgical approach. The toxicity was acceptable.

Case 4 T2 N2 M0 squamous cell carcinoma of the tonsil.

Presentation This patient was a 44-year-old White man who presented with a right-side neck mass of approximately 8 months duration. Initial treatment with an antibiotic resulted in a decrease in size of the mass. He had occasional otalgia. A CT scan was done prior to presentation, which showed a 2.5-cm mass in region II and a 3-cm enhancing mass in the right tonsil (**Fig. 2–3A, B**). He had no other complaints. He did have a history of smoking a pack of cigarettes a day for 10 years, having quit 16 years before, and moderate beer use.

Physical Examination Physical examination showed a 4-cm mass in the upper half of the right tonsillar fossa that did not involve the mucosa of the soft palate. There was no trismus. There was a 3-cm right region II lymph node.

Diagnosis and Workup An office biopsy was performed, which showed moderately differentiated invasive SCC involving the right tonsil. In addition to the initial CT scan done, CT scans of the chest and pelvis performed prior to his presentation were negative.

Treatment The patient was taken to the operating room for examination under anesthesia, which revealed that a resection of the primary lesion would have extensively involved the lateral oropharyngeal wall and soft palate. For this reason, it was elected not to resect the primary tumor but to proceed with immediate modified radical neck dissection and leave his primary lesion to be treated nonsurgically. His pathology showed 4 of 19 nodes positive in region II, the largest of which measured 4.5 cm with extracapsular spread. The remaining regions of the neck were negative. He then received concomitant platinum-based postoperative chemoradiotherapy (because the extracapsular disease placed him in a high-risk group) and definitive curative chemoradiation to the tonsillar primary. He received a total of 72 Gy in 42 fractions with the last 12 treatments being twice-daily. The last treatment of chemoradiotherapy was withheld during the twice-daily portion of his radiation therapy. He did develop significant toxicities—a neuropathy of the left upper extremity and narcotic addiction. Both of these eventually resolved completely, and the patient remains disease-free.

Summary of Treatment   This patient had a primary tumor whose resection would have resulted in significant morbidity related to swallowing. It was elected to treat his primary site with definitive chemoradiotherapy and the neck with postoperative chemoradiotherapy because of the high-risk nature of his neck pathology due to the extracapsular disease. This case also illustrates the severe toxicities involved when chemotherapy is added to aggressive accelerated postoperative radiation therapy.

References

1. Spiro RH, Alfonso AE, Farr HW, Strong EW. Cervical node metastasis from epidermoid carcinoma of the oral cavity and oropharynx. A critical assessment of current staging. Am J Surg 1974;128:562–567
2. Henk JM, A'Hern RP, Taylor K. Carcinoma of the oropharynx in the United Kingdom. In: Johnson JT, Didolkar MS, eds. Head and Neck Cancer. Vol. 3. Amsterdam: Exerpta Medica; 1992:779–784
3. Spitz MR, Fueger JJ, Goepfert H, Hong WK, Newell GR. Squamous cell carcinoma of the upper aerodigestive tract. A case comparison analysis. Cancer 1988;61:203–208
4. Graham S, Dayal H, Rohrer T, et al. Dentition, diet, tobacco, and alcohol in the epidemiology of oral cancer. J Natl Cancer Inst 1977;59:1611–1618
5. Szpirglas H. [Alcohol and oral cancer.] Actual Odontostomatol (Paris) 1976;115:448–454
6. Reddy CRRM. Hypothesis on the origin of the carcinoma of the hard palate. Oncology 1974;30:134–140
7. Puscas L. The role of human papilloma virus infection in the etiology of oropharyngeal carcinoma. Curr Opin Otolaryngol Head Neck Surg 2005;13:212–216
8. Shumrick KA, Coldiron B. Genetic syndromes associated with skin cancer. Otolaryngol Clin North Am 1993;26:117–137
9. Kraemer KH, Lee MM, Scotto J. Xeroderma pigmentosum. Cutaneous, ocular, and neurologic abnormalities in 830 published cases. Arch Dermatol 1987;123:241–250
10. Perez-Ordonez B, Beauchemin M, Jordan RC. Molecular biology of squamous cell carcinoma of the head and neck. J Clin Pathol 2006;59:445–453
11. Warner GC, Reis PP, Jurisica I, et al. Molecular classification of oral cancer by cDNA microarrays identifies overexpressed genes correlated with nodal metastasis. Int J Cancer 2004;110:857–868
12. Robbins KT, ed. Pocket Guide to Neck Dissection Classification and TNM Staging of Head and Neck Cancer. Alexandria, VA: American Academy of Otolaryngology Head and Neck Surgery Foundation; 2001
13. Chan JK, Ng CS, Lo ST. Immunohistological characterization of malignant lymphomas of the Waldeyer's ring other than the nasopharynx. Histopathology 1987;11:885–899
14. Shetty SC, Gupta S, Nagsubramanium S, Hasan S, Cherry G. Mandibular metastasis from renal cell carcinoma. A case report. Indian J Dent Res 2001;12:77–80
15. Beer KT, von Briel C, Lampret T, et al. [Predictive significance of reflex otalgia in local radical radiotherapy of oropharyngeal carcinomas.] Strahlenther Onkol 1998;174:306–310
16. Shah JP. Patterns of cervical lymph node metastasis from squamous carcinomas of the upper aerodigestive tract. Am J Surg 1990;160:405–409
17. Curtin HD, Ishwaran H, Mancuso AA, et al. Comparison of CT and MR imaging in staging of neck metastases. Radiology 1998;207:123–130
18. Zanation AM, Sutton DK, Couch ME, et al. Use, accuracy, and implications for patient management of [18F]-2-fluorodeoxyglucose-positron emission/computerized tomography for head and neck tumors. Laryngoscope 2005;115:1186–1190
19. Schöder H, Yeung HW, Gonen M, Kraus D, Larson SM. Head and neck cancer: clinical usefulness and accuracy of PET/CT image fusion. Radiology 2004;231:65–72
20. Allal AS, Slosman DO, Kebdani T, et al. Prediction of outcome in head-and-neck cancer patients using the standardized uptake value of 2-[18F]fluoro-2-deoxy-D-glucose. Int J Radiat Oncol Biol Phys 2004;59:1295–1300
21. Yao M, Graham MM, Hoffman HT, et al. The role of post-radiation therapy FDG PET in prediction of necessity for post-radiation therapy neck dissection in locally advanced head-and-neck squamous cell carcinoma. Int J Radiat Oncol Biol Phys 2004;59:1001–1010
22. Paleri V, Rees G, Arullendran P, Shoaib T, Krishman S. Sentinel node biopsy in squamous cell cancer of the oral cavity and oral pharynx: a diagnostic meta-analysis. Head Neck 2005;27:739–747
23. Wang MB, Kuber N, Kerner MM, et al. Tonsillar carcinoma: analysis of treatment results. J Otolaryngol 1998;27:263–269
24. Hicks WL Jr, Kuriakose MA, Loree TR, et al. Surgery versus radiation therapy as single-modality treatment of tonsillar fossa carcinoma: the Roswell Park Cancer Institute experience (1971–1991). Laryngoscope 1998;108:1014–1019
25. de Arruda FF, Puri DR, Zhung J, et al. Intensity-modulated radiation therapy for the treatment of oropharyngeal carcinoma: the Memorial Sloan-Kettering Cancer Center experience. Int J Radiat Oncol Biol Phys 2006;64:363–373
26. Layland MK, Sessions DG, Lenox J. The influence of lymph node metastasis in the treatment of squamous cell carcinoma of the oral cavity, oropharynx, larynx, and hypopharynx: N0 versus N+. Laryngoscope 2005;115:629–639
27. Fallai C, Bolner A, Signor M, et al. Long-term results of conventional radiotherapy versus accelerated hyperfractionated radiotherapy versus concomitant radiotherapy and chemotherapy in locoregionally advanced carcinoma of the oropharynx. Tumori 2006;92:41–54
28. Prins-Braam PM, Raaijmakers CP, Terhaard CH. Location of cervical lymph node metastases in oropharyngeal and hypopharyngeal carcinoma: implications for cranial border of elective nodal target volumes. Int J Radiat Oncol Biol Phys 2004;58:132–138
29. Bussels B, Hermans R, Reijnders A, et al. Retropharyngeal nodes in squamous cell carcinoma of oropharynx: incidence, localization, and implications for target volume. Int J Radiat Oncol Biol Phys 2006;65:733–738
30. Fu KK, Pajak TF, Trotti A, et al. A Radiation Therapy Oncology Group (RTOG) phase III randomized study to compare hyperfractionation and two variants of accelerated fractionation to standard fractionation radiotherapy for head and neck squamous cell carcinomas: first report of RTOG 9003. Int J Radiat Oncol Biol Phys 2000;48:7–16
31. Pellitteri PK, Ferlito A, Rinaldo A, et al. Planned neck dissection following chemoradiotherapy for advanced head and neck cancer: is it necessary for all? Head Neck 2006;28:166–175
32. Bernier J, Cooper JS, Pajak TF, et al. Defining risk levels in locally advanced head and neck cancers: a comparative analysis of concurrent postoperative radiation plus chemotherapy trials of the EORTC (#22931) and RTOG (# 9501). Head Neck 2005;27:843–850
33. Bonner JA, Harari PM, Giralt J, et al. Radiotherapy plus cetuximab for squamous-cell carcinoma of the head and neck. N Engl J Med 2006;354:567–578
34. Haddad R, Tishler R, Wirth L, et al. Rate of pathologic complete responses to docetaxel, cisplatin, and fluorouracil induction chemotherapy in patients with squamous cell carcinoma of the head and neck. Arch Otolaryngol Head Neck Surg 2006;132:678–681
35. Breen SL, Craig T, Bayley A, et al. Spinal cord planning risk volumes for intensity-modulated radiation therapy of head-and-neck cancer. Int J Radiat Oncol Biol Phys 2006;64:321–325
36. Jeremic B, Djuric L, Mijatovic L. Incidence of radiation myelitis of the cervical spinal cord at doses of 5500 cGy or greater. Cancer 1991;68:2138–2141
37. Marcus RB Jr, Million RR. The incidence of myelitis after irradiation of the cervical spinal cord. Int J Radiat Oncol Biol Phys 1990;19:3–8
38. Fein DA, Marcus RB Jr, Parsons JT, Mendenhall WM, Million RR. Lhermitte's sign: incidence and treatment variables influencing risk after

irradiation of the cervical spinal cord. Int J Radiat Oncol Biol Phys 1993;27:1029–1033

39. Kanatas AN, Rogers SN, Martin MV. A practical guide for patients undergoing exodontia following radiotherapy to the oral cavity. Dent Update 2002;29:498–503

40. Epstein JB, Stevenson-Moore P. Periodontal disease and periodontal management in patients with cancer. Oral Oncol 2001;37:613–619

41. Vissink A, Burlage FR, Spijkervet FK, Jansma J, Coppes RP. Prevention and treatment of the consequences of head and neck radiotherapy. Crit Rev Oral Biol Med 2003;14:213–225

42. Berk LB, Shivnani AT, Small W Jr. Pathophysiology and management of radiation-induced xerostomia. J Support Oncol 2005;3:191–200

43. Seikaly H, Rieger J, Wolfaardt J, et al. Functional outcomes after primary oropharyngeal cancer resection and reconstruction with the radial forearm free flap. Laryngoscope 2003;113:897–904

44. Christiansen H, Hermann RM, Martin A, et al. Long-term follow-up after transoral laser microsurgery and adjuvant radiotherapy for advanced recurrent squamous cell carcinoma of the head and neck. Int J Radiat Oncol Biol Phys 2006;65:1067–1074

45. Lippert BM, Teymoortash A, Folz BJ, Werner JA. Wound healing after laser treatment of oral and oropharyngeal cancer. Lasers Med Sci 2003;18:36–42

46. Schramm VL Jr, Myers EN. "How I do it"—head and neck. A targeted problem and its solution. Skin graft reconstruction following composite resection. Laryngoscope 1980;90:1737–1739

47. Pribaz J, Stephens W, Crespo L, Gifford G. A new intraoral flap: facial artery musculomucosal (FAMM) flap. Plast Reconstr Surg 1992;90:421–429

48. Millard DR, Batstone JH, Heycock MH, Bensen JF. Ten years with the palatal island flap. Plast Reconstr Surg 1970;46:540–547

49. Gullane PJ, Arena S. Palatal island flap for reconstruction of oral defects. Arch Otolaryngol 1977;103:598–599

50. Katsaros J, Tan E, Zoltie N, et al. Further experience with the lateral arm free flap. Plast Reconstr Surg 1991;87:902–910

51. Haughey BH. Tongue reconstruction: concepts and practice. Laryngoscope 1993;103:1132–1141

52. Urken ML, Turk JB, Weinberg H, Vickery C, Biller HF. The rectus abdominis free flap in head and neck reconstruction. Arch Otolaryngol Head Neck Surg 1991;117:857–866

53. Beaudet J. Reconstruction of the pharyngeal wall by free transfer of the greater omentum and stomach. Int J Microsurg 1979;1:53–59

54. Panje WR, Pitcock JK, Vargish T. Free omental flap reconstruction of complicated head and neck wounds. Otolaryngol Head Neck Surg 1989;100:588–593

55. Moreano EH, Hutchison JL, McCulloch TM, et al. Incidence of deep venous thrombosis and pulmonary embolism in otolaryngology-head and neck surgery. Otolaryngol Head Neck Surg 1998;118:777–784

56. Klug C, Neuburg J, Glaser C, et al. Quality of life 2–10 years after combined treatment for advanced oral and oropharyngeal cancer. Int J Oral Maxillofac Surg 2002;31:664–669

57. Rogers SN, Hannah L, Lowe D, Magennis P. Quality of life 5–10 years after primary surgery for oral and oro-pharyngeal cancer. J Craniomaxillofac Surg 1999;27:187–191

58. Borggreven PA, Verdonck-de Leeuw I, Langendijk JA, et al. Speech outcome after surgical treatment for oral and oropharyngeal cancer: a longitudinal assessment of patients reconstructed by a microvascular flap. Head Neck 2005;27:785–793

59. Lloyd S, Devesa-Martinez P, Howard DJ, Lund VJ. Quality of life of patients undergoing surgical treatment of head and neck malignancy. Clin Otolaryngol Allied Sci 2003;28:524–532

60. Urken ML, Buchbinder D, Weinberg H, et al. Functional evaluation following microvascular oromandibular reconstruction of the oral cancer patient: a comparative study of reconstructed and nonreconstructed patients. Laryngoscope 1991;101:935–950

61. Vaughan ED, Bainton R, Martin IC. Improvements in morbidity of mouth cancer using microvascular free flap reconstructions. J Craniomaxillofac Surg 1992;20:132–134

3

Carcinoma of the Hypopharynx

David P. Goldstein, Jonathan Clark, Patrick J. Gullane, Laura A. Dawson, Lillian L. Siu, and Jonathan C. Irish

Treatment options for early-stage hypopharyngeal cancer include radiation therapy and conservative or radical surgical procedures, whereas advanced hypopharyngeal cancer has preferentially been treated with a total laryngectomy with partial or total pharyngectomy, followed by radiation therapy. Over the past decade, there has been a growing trend toward organ preservation strategies with either altered fractionation radiotherapy or combined modality treatment with chemotherapy and radiation therapy. Technological advancements have occurred in radiation therapy, including intensity-modulated radiation therapy (IMRT) and image-guided radiotherapy (IGRT), which improve the dose delivered to the tumor while facilitating sparing of dose to normal tissues. Advances in conservation and reconstructive surgery have also occurred, enabling shorter hospital stay and better functional outcomes.

With multiple treatment options, there remains a lack of high-level evidence to guide optimal management.[1] The current literature on hypopharyngeal cancer is limited to retrospective reviews with relatively small numbers of patients. Comparisons between studies are difficult because of changes in the staging system over time,[1] inclusion of different subsites, and lack of uniform treatment approaches.[2] Treatment decisions for these complex tumors should incorporate a multidisciplinary team of surgical, radiation, and medical oncologists, radiologists, pathologists, and paramedical disciplines such as speech therapy, nutrition, nursing, and social work. This chapter will review the presentation, diagnosis, and multidisciplinary management of squamous cell carcinoma of the hypopharynx. Rather than provide an exhaustive summary of all studies on the different therapeutic approaches, our goal is to provide a general overview of the treatment options available and their indications.

◆ Epidemiology

Incidence

Carcinoma of the hypopharynx is uncommon in North America, accounting for ~4.3 to 7% of all head and neck cancers[3,4]

with a reported incidence of 1 case per 100,000 per year.[4] This varies worldwide with the highest rate in France at 9.4 per 100,000 per year.[5,6] Based on the Surveillance, Epidemiology, and End-Results (SEER) database, there has been a decrease in incidence over the past 3 decades.[7] Males account for 75 to 85% of all cases,[3,8–10] with the majority occurring in the sixth and seventh decades of life.[3,8,9] Squamous cell cancer accounts for more than 95% of all hypopharyngeal malignancies[3,4,11] and will be the focus of this chapter.

Mortality

The hypopharynx is divided into three subsites: the paired piriform sinuses, posterior pharyngeal wall, and postcricoid region.[12] In North America, 65 to 80% of hypopharyngeal cancers arise in the piriform sinus.[8,10,13,14] The posterior pharyngeal wall accounts for 25 to 35% of cases, whereas postcricoid cancers are less common, representing only 4 to 8% of cases.[8–10,13,14] The ratio of piriform sinus cancers to postcricoid cancers is 19:1, and in Europe this ratio decreases but still favors the piriform sinus.[15]

The prognosis of patients with hypopharyngeal cancer is poor, with survival rates lower than most other squamous cancers of the head and neck.[4,9,16–19] Explanations include late stage at presentation, early invasion of surrounding structures due to lack of supportive tissues and barriers, frequent nodal and distant metastases, and high rate of synchronous malignancies.[2,8,19–21] Management is complicated by the fact that patients are often older with multiple medical comorbidities and poor nutritional status.[22] Tumors tend to be locally advanced at presentation[10,13–15] with a tendency for submucosal spread,[13,23–26] and treatment can have a profound effect on quality of life.

◆ Anatomy of the Hypopharynx

The hypopharynx, which is situated posterior and lateral to the larynx, extends from the plane of the hyoid bone superiorly (or vallecula floor) to the lower border of the cricoid cartilage inferiorly, where it is contiguous with the cervical esophagus. **Figure 3–1** shows the subsites and anatomy of the hypopharynx.

The piriform sinuses conceptually are like inverted pyramids situated lateral to the larynx with their base superior and the lateral and anterior walls tapering to an inferior apex. The limit superiorly is the pharyngoepiglottic fold and the free margin of the aryepiglottic fold.[27] The medial wall is formed by the lateral surface of the aryepiglottic fold and arytenoids, posterior ventricle, and lateral aspect of the cricoid cartilage.[28] The lateral wall is bounded superiorly by the thyrohyoid membrane and inferiorly by the thyroid cartilage.

The posterior pharyngeal wall is bounded by the inferior constrictor muscle. It extends from the level of the hyoid bone to the inferior border of the cricoid and from the apex of one piriform sinus to the other.[12] Posteriorly, it is related to the bodies of the third through sixth cervical vertebra.[29] Potential spaces separate the posterior pharyngeal wall from the prevertebral fascia, vertebrae, and attached spinal musculature.[30] The postcricoid region is bounded anteriorly by the cricoid cartilage and arytenoids.[12] Inferiorly, it is contiguous with the cervical esophagus. Important relations include the cricoarytenoid joints, the intrinsic laryngeal muscles, and the recurrent laryngeal nerves.[28]

Neurovascular Supply

The sensory innervation of the hypopharynx is by the glossopharyngeal and vagus nerves via the pharyngeal plexus, superior laryngeal nerves (SLNs), and recurrent laryngeal nerves (RLNs).[28] The internal branch of the SLN synapses in the jugular ganglion along with vagal branches from the middle ear (Arnold's nerve), thus accounting for the referred otalgia seen in patients presenting with hypopharyngeal cancer.[27] Motor innervation is from the pharyngeal plexus and RLNs. The vascular supply is from the superior laryngeal, lingual, and ascending pharyngeal arteries.[21]

◆ Patterns of Tumor Spread

Local Patterns of Spread

Hypopharyngeal carcinomas have a tendency for multisite spread, particularly with large and undifferentiated tumors.[2] It is important for oncologists to have a fundamental knowledge of tumor growth patterns because it affects the type and extent of treatment.

Medial invasion of piriform sinus tumors tends to involve the aryepiglottic folds, supraglottis, arytenoids, intrinsic laryngeal muscles, and the paraglottic space[15,31,32] (**Fig. 3–2**). Lateral spread results in invasion of the thyroid cartilage[31] and with inferolateral extension the tumor may extend through the cricothyroid membrane to involve the cricoid cartilage and thyroid gland.[31] Thyroid gland involvement can also result from direct extension through the thyroid cartilage. In lateral piriform sinus tumors, thyroid gland and cartilage invasion occurs in up to 30% and 55% of surgical

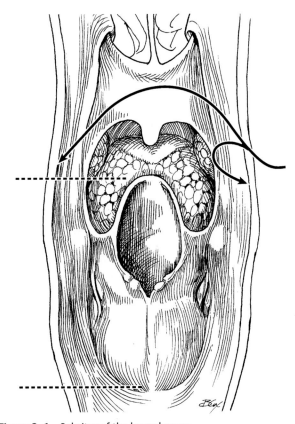

Figure 3–1 Subsites of the hypopharynx.

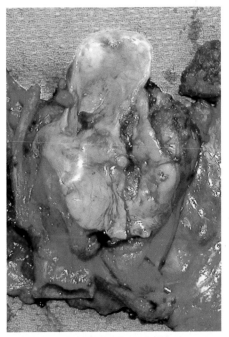

Figure 3–2 Gross pathologic specimen of a right piriform sinus cancer with gross invasion of the medial piriform and larynx.

specimens, respectively.[15,32,33] Kirchner noted that invasion of the thyroid and/or cricoid cartilage occurred most commonly with tumors involving the apex of the piriform sinus.[15] These observations of local spread have resulted in a recommendation of ipsilateral hemithyroidectomy for all patients requiring definitive surgery for hypopharynx cancer.[29] Large piriform sinus tumors may extend to the base of the tongue, soft tissues of the neck, posterior pharyngeal wall, or across the postcricoid region to the contralateral piriform. Invasion of the intrinsic laryngeal muscles, cricoarytenoid joint, and recurrent laryngeal nerves can all result in vocal cord immobility.[15,31,32,34]

Posterior pharyngeal wall tumors tend to remain on the posterior wall with superior and inferior spread, although extension into the cervical esophagus is uncommon.[21,27] Tumors may invade through the posterior wall to involve the prevertebral fascia and the vertebral bodies limiting resectability.

Postcricoid cancers frequently involve the arytenoids, intrinsic laryngeal muscles, RLNs, and the cricoid cartilage.[32,35] Inferiorly, the tumor may extend to the cervical esophagus or invade the trachea.[25] Hypopharyngeal cancers, particularly postcricoid cancers, exhibit skip lesion behavior and extensive submucosal spread,[23–25] which has been demonstrated in up to 60% of specimens.[13] The extent of submucosal spread is greatest in the inferior direction (up to 30 mm) followed by the lateral direction (between 10 and 20 mm) and least in the superior direction (between 5 and 10 mm).[13,24,25] Submucosal extension and skip lesions may not be evident macroscopically, particularly after radiotherapy.[13] These findings need to be taken into account when deciding on the extent of surgical margins or in planning radiation treatment fields.

Regional Patterns of Spread

The hypopharynx demonstrates a particularly rich network of lymphatic channels accounting for the high rate of regional disease. Lymphatics from the piriform sinuses drain through the thyrohyoid membrane following the superior laryngeal neurovascular pedicle to the jugulodigastric, midjugular (level II and III), and retropharyngeal nodes.[21,28,36] Lymphatics of the posterior pharyngeal wall pierce the inferior constrictor muscle and drain to the retropharyngeal and upper jugular nodes (level II), whereas lymphatics of the postcricoid region tend to follow the RLNs to the paratracheal, paraesophageal, and lower jugular nodes (level IV and VI), with on occasion extension to the posterior mediastinal nodes.[21,28,36,37] The posterior pharyngeal wall, postcricoid, and the medial piriform sinus have bilateral lymphatic drainage patterns.[19]

◆ Pathology

More than 95% of all hypopharyngeal malignancies are squamous cell carcinomas (SCCs),[3,4,11] which are often poorly differentiated.[2,9,21] Adenocarcinomas account for the majority of the remaining 5% of hypopharyngeal malignancies; however, other rare neoplasms such as malignant fibrous histiocytoma, liposarcoma, synovial sarcoma, and mucosal melanoma have been reported.[4,38–41]

◆ Etiology

Tobacco and Alcohol

Alcohol and tobacco are the major risk factors for the development of SCC of the hypopharynx,[5] with more than 90% of patients presenting with a history of tobacco use.[13,42] Alcohol consumption is more frequent in hypopharyngeal SCC than in laryngeal cancer.[13,43] Risk increases with both the quantity and duration of tobacco and alcohol use, and there is a synergistic effect when used together.[42] Smoking cessation is associated with a substantial risk reduction.[5]

Plummer-Vinson Syndrome

Plummer-Vinson syndrome, also termed Paterson-Brown-Kelly syndrome, is associated with the development of postcricoid cancers in women aged 30 to 50 without a history of tobacco or alcohol use.[44–46] The syndrome is characterized by dysphagia secondary to hypopharyngeal and esophageal webs, weight loss, and iron-deficiency anemia.[29] Additional findings include cheilosis, tooth loss, and glossitis.[29] Early diagnosis and treatment with supplemental iron and vitamin B, prior to cancer developing, can successfully reverse the process.[21] Today, the syndrome is rare due to improved nutrition, fortification of food with iron and vitamins, and better health service and maternal care.[47]

Human Papilloma Virus

The role of human papilloma virus (HPV) in the carcinogenesis of hypopharyngeal SCC is less well defined than with oropharyngeal and laryngeal carcinoma. Rates of detection of HPV in hypopharyngeal specimens range from 19 to 29%.[48–50] Epstein-Barr virus does not appear to be associated with hypopharyngeal cancer.[51,52]

Genetic and Molecular Markers

Abnormalities of the p53 oncoprotein are common in hypopharyngeal carcinoma, occurring in up to 70% of patients.[50,53] Mutations in the p21 gene have also been identified.[53] Amplification of the 11q13 region, which contains loci for oncogenes (cyclin D1, fibroblast growth factor [FGF]) and a cytoskeletal protein were identified in 78% of cases by Rodrigues et al.[50,54] Overexpression of oncogenes at the 11q13 locus appears to be more frequent in hypopharyngeal cancers compared with other head and neck cancer sites.[54–56]

◆ Staging

The TNM classification set forth by the American Joint Committee on Cancer (AJCC) is the main staging system used for hypopharyngeal SCC (**Table 3–1**).[57] The only change to the staging in the latest edition (6th edition, 2002)[57] was the subdivision of T4 lesions into T4a and T4b group. Any diag-

Table 3–1 American Joint Committee on Cancer Staging for Hypopharynx Cancer

T Staging

T1	Tumor limited to one subsite of the hypopharynx (piriform fossa or postcricoid region or posterior pharyngeal wall) and 2 cm or less in greatest dimension
T2	Tumor invades more than one subsite of hypopharynx or an adjacent site, or measures more than 2 cm but not more than 4 cm in greatest dimension, without fixation of the hemilarynx
T3	Tumor more than 4 cm in greatest dimension, or with fixation of the hemilarynx
T4a	Tumor invades any of the following: thyroid/cricoid cartilage, hyoid bone, thyroid gland, esophagus, central compartment soft tissue (includes prelaryngeal strap muscles and subcutaneous fat)
T4b	Tumor invades prevertebral fascia, encases carotid artery, or invades mediastinal structures

N Staging

NX	Regional lymph node status cannot be assessed
N0	No regional lymph node metastases
N1	Metastases in a single ipsilateral lymph node, 3 cm or less in greatest dimension
N2a	Metastases in a single ipsilateral node more than 3 cm but not more than 6 cm in greatest dimension
N2b	Metastases in multiple ipsilateral lymph nodes, none more than 6 cm in greatest dimension
N2c	Metastases in bilateral or contralateral lymph nodes, none more 6 cm in greatest dimension
N3	Metastases in a lymph node more than 6 cm in greatest dimension

Distant Metastases

MX	Distant metastases cannot be assessed
M0	No distant metastases
M1	Distant metastases

Source: Greene FPD, Fleming I, Page DL, et al. Cancer Staging Manual. 6th ed. New York, NY: Springer-Verlag; 2002:220. Adapted with permission.

nostic information that contributes to the overall accuracy of pretreatment assessment should be considered in the clinical staging.[58]

◆ Presentation

History

Hypopharyngeal cancers tend to remain asymptomatic for a long period of time with the majority of patients presenting with locally advanced disease. Between 70% and 84% of patients present with either T3 or T4 disease and more than 70% with stage III or IV disease.[4,10,13–15,59–63] Symptoms occur when the tumor reaches considerable size or invades surrounding structures and include progressive dysphagia, neck mass, odynophagia, and otalgia.[9,13,23, 64]

Less frequent symptoms include hoarseness, hemoptysis, cough, and weight loss. Patients with large retropharyngeal nodes may present with occipital or posterior neck pain radiating to the retroorbital region.[28] The average duration of symptoms before presentation to a physician is 2 to 4 months.[9,29,44] Other important elements of the history include nutritional status, comorbidities, and tobacco and alcohol consumption.

Physical Examination

The physical examination should focus on assessing the extent of the primary tumor, detecting regional disease, and excluding a synchronous malignancy. On flexible endoscopy, hypopharyngeal malignancies tend to appear as either an ulcerative or infiltrative lesion. Exophytic lesions are less common and tend to occur on the posterior pharyngeal wall. Pooling of secretions suggests piriform sinus apex or cervical esophageal involvement.[9,27] Examination of the larynx and assessment of vocal cord mobility are important for staging, prognosis, and treatment planning. Postcricoid tumors may be difficult to visualize if they have caused significant mucosal edema of the posterior larynx. As they enlarge, they displace the larynx forward producing a fullness in the anterior neck and loss of the palpable clicking that occurs when one rocks the larynx from side to side.[27] Careful examination of both sides of the neck is required to detect nodal metastases.

◆ Diagnosis and Workup

Panendoscopy and Biopsy

Biopsy of hypopharyngeal tumors is usually performed under general anesthesia in conjunction with a panendoscopy of the upper aerodigestive tract. If a neck mass is present, a fine-needle aspiration can be performed to confirm the suspicion of a metastatic node. Panendoscopy allows the physician to assess the full extent of the tumor and increases detection of synchronous tumors. Information obtained will influence treatment decisions and provide valuable information for the surgeon about the extent of resection and method of reconstruction. Deep fixation of posterior pharyngeal wall tumors may be assessed by moving the tumor on the cervical spine.[29] In postcricoid malignancies or those with cervical esophageal involvement, flexible esophagoscopy should be considered over rigid techniques because it allows for distal assessment of the tumor and decreases the risk of perforation.

Diagnostic Imaging

Computed tomography (CT) and/or magnetic resonance imaging (MRI) of the head and neck are vital for staging the primary tumor and neck, as well as for treatment planning. Imaging will up-stage a significant number of hypopharyngeal tumors[1] and ideally should be obtained prior to panendoscopy to evaluate areas of concern.[29] CT and/or MRI should also be used to assess laryngeal and pharyngeal spread, cartilage invasion, and nodal status. Tumors encasing the carotid artery or invading the cervical spine or skull base are generally incurable even with radical resection. CT and MRI have improved accuracy over physical examination in assessing the primary and detecting nodal metastases.[65]

CT is particularly valuable in assessing invasion of the laryngeal cartilages and is more specific than MRI.[1] MRI has the advantage of better soft tissue definition, multiplanar imaging, and no ionizing radiation.[66] Occult submucosal disease, tumor spread along the superior laryngeal neurovascular pedicle,[27] involvement of the intrinsic laryngeal musculature, and deep extension into the paraglottic and pre-epiglottic spaces may be detectable on MRI.[67] MRI and CT are complementary examinations providing detailed cross-sectional anatomy of the hypopharynx and tumor growth patterns that will aid in the detection and evaluation of the full extent of the tumor.

Positron emission tomography combined with CT (PET-CT) has an increasing role in the workup of patients with head and neck cancer and currently is a supplementary test to CT and MRI. PET-CT has been shown to be beneficial in the confirmation of the primary tumor, as well as in the assessment of cervical and distant metastases. The limitations to PET include false-positive results with active inflammation, cost, and availability.

Metastatic and Synchronous Tumor Workup

The rate of distant metastases at presentation is reported to be between 6% and 24%.[13,60, 62, 64,68–70] The lungs are the most common sites of metastases followed by the liver.[60] The incidence of second primary tumors at presentation is reported to be around 7%.[13,23,71] A limited metastatic workup is indicated including chest CT and PET scan where available.[1]

Nodal Metastases

Palpable nodal metastases are detectable in 50 to 75% of patients at presentation.[9,14,15,27,44,59, 64,72] Piriform sinus cancers have the highest rate of neck metastases, present in more than 75% of patients, compared with posterior pharyngeal wall and postcricoid cancers where the rate of nodal metastases is between 30% and 60% at presentation.[23,25,61, 64,73–76] A significant proportion of nodal metastases are advanced (N2 or N3) and/or bilateral.[1,14,27,60,63] Bilateral metastases are associated with large tumors, posterior pharyngeal wall involvement, and midline piriform sinus cancers.[77–79]

Levels II, III, and IV are the most common sites for nodal metastases in patients with clinically positive necks (N+).[25,80,81] Level I and level V metastases occur infrequently, with reported rates as high as 10% and 11%, respectively.[16,25,78,80–82] Greater than 75% of N1 necks will be upstaged pathologically to N2b.[25] The risk of contralateral nodal metastases in the node-positive neck is in excess of 30%.[1,78] In patients with clinically negative necks (N0), ipsilateral micrometastases occur in ~40% of patients.[8,9,25,76,78,82,83] Occult metastatic

disease most commonly involves levels II and III and is frequently bilateral (more than 30% incidence).[1,25,78] Metastases to the retropharyngeal nodes are common in posterior pharyngeal wall cancers, occurring in ~40% of patients, and increases with tumor stage.[37,84] Postcricoid tumors frequently metastasize to the paratracheal nodes with a 20% incidence of occult metastases in the N0 neck.[74,78,85,86] These nodes are also at risk in tumors involving the apex of the piriform sinus.[74,87]

Risk factors for nodal metastases include invasion of the thyroid cartilage, RLNs, and extrapharyngeal soft tissue, and large tumors (tumors <4 cm have a 50% chance of regional metastases while tumors >4 cm have an 85% chance of regional metastases).[82]

◆ Prognostic Factors

Hypopharyngeal SCC has the worst prognosis of all head and neck SCCs.[4,7,13] Overall survival at 5 years for all tumor stages ranges between 14% and 28% and rarely exceeds 35% regardless of treatment approach used.[4,7,13,88] The Swedish Cancer Registry from 1960 to 1989 reported an overall survival rate of 15%.[45] A National Cancer Database review reported a disease specific survival (DSS) of 31.4% between 1985 and 1989,[4] and Carvalho et al, using the SEER database, reported a 33.3% 5-year survival.[7] A survey on 1317 hypopharyngeal cancers treated in the United States by Hoffman et al found a 5-year DSS of 33.4%, with survival decreasing as stage increased (stage I, 63.1%; II, 57.5%; III, 41.8%; IV, 22%).[13]

Poor prognostic factors are presented in **Table 3–2**. The presence of nodal metastases is the strongest predictor of survival and is more important than the number of

Table 3–2 Poor Prognostic Factors for Hypopharyngeal Carcinoma

Clinical factors
  Advanced tumor stage
  Positive nodal status
  Older age (>50 years)
  Comorbidity
  Vocal cord paralysis
  Piriform apex and lateral wall
  Site: postcricoid cancers have a better prognosis than the other subsites, with posterior pharyngeal wall cancers having the lowest survival of all sites.
Pathologic factors
  Metastases to level IV
  Multiple nodes
  Nodes greater than 3 cm
  Extracapsular extension
  Close (i.e., <2 mm) or positive margins
  Lymphovascular and perineural invasion
  Basaloid and spindle cell SCC variants
  Thyroid cartilage invasion

nodes.[20,25,89] The poor prognosis in hypopharynx cancer is also due to the frequent development of distant metastases and second primaries.[90] The reported rates of the development of nonsynchronous (metachronous) primaries range from 7.4% up to 22%, the majority of which occur in the upper aerodigestive tract.[13,60,91–93] Distant metastases occur in 4 to 50% with most reports between 20% and 30%.[10,14,20,60,62,68,69,83,89,94] The incidence increases with locally advanced disease (T3/T4), uncontrolled tumor at the primary site, and nodal metastases.[10,14,62,69,83] The majority of distant metastases occur within 9 months of diagnosis with the lungs being the most common site followed by liver, mediastinum, bone, and skin.[13,60,69] The median survival of patients with distant metastases is under 1 year.[83]

◆ Treatment

After a patient has undergone a thorough workup, a decision needs to be made about the curability of the tumor. For patients deemed incurable, a palliative approach is taken with treatment of symptoms as they arise. For those patients with curable disease, optimal treatment depends upon tumor factors (extent of the primary and neck disease), patient factors (comorbidities, performance status, and a patient's wishes regarding treatment and quality of life), and physician/institution factors (infrastructure for radiation and chemotherapy and management of their toxicities and surgeons' experience with reconstructive and conservation surgery).

Treatment of early and advanced hypopharyngeal cancers remains controversial with experienced centers throughout the world adopting what would appear to be contradictory paradigms. For early cancers, some authors advocate conservation surgery with or without postoperative radiation, whereas other authors advocate radiation therapy alone. In advanced cancers, some authors prefer surgery with postoperative radiation, whereas others believe in organ preservation strategies with either altered fractionation radiation therapy or combined radiation and chemotherapy.

There are few randomized controlled trials comparing treatment modalities in hypopharyngeal cancer. Given this, we must rely on the available evidence while recognizing the inherent weaknesses of these studies when making treatment decisions. The general principles listed in **Table 3–3** represent the philosophical view of the authors regarding their approach to the management of this disease at the University of Toronto, Princess Margaret Hospital.

Table 3–3 Principles of Treatment for Hypopharyngeal Cancer

Single-modality treatment where possible
Multimodality treatment where there is either survival or functional benefit from the additional modality
Preservation of function rather than organ preservation
In most cases, management of the neck is mandatory.
Salvage surgery should focus not only on disease.

Surgical Treatment

Early-Stage Disease (T1/T2)

Although early stage tumors can be managed effectively by radiotherapy alone, surgery is an equally valid option.[33] Arguments against primary radiation for these lesions include resource allocation, length of treatment, and, in younger patients, the concern over second primary tumors and radiation-induced malignancy. T1/T2 tumors arising in the piriform sinus (medial and lateral walls) or posterior pharyngeal wall can be effectively managed with surgery using either transoral endoscopic or open approaches.[83,88,92,95–98] Postcricoid cancer, however, displays a particular propensity for invasion of surrounding structures such as the cricoid, posterior cricoarytenoid muscle, and RLNs, which limits its suitability for partial resections even in low-volume disease.[15,32] Where a surgical approach is chosen, in centers with appropriate expertise, transoral laser endoscopic resection (TOL) has several advantages over other surgical options. These include preservation of the SLNs and/or RLNs, reduced fistula and septic complications by eliminating communication with the neck, and avoidance of reconstruction, permitting early return to oral intake and discharge from hospital.[1,88,95,96] Proponents for open and endoscopic approaches will argue their relative merit; however, there are no studies to compare oncologic or functional outcomes. Treatment of epilarynx and hypopharynx tumors with partial surgery provides a 5-year local control ranging between 90% and 95% with a 5-year larynx function preservation ranging between 85% and 100% and total laryngectomy with a partial pharyngectomy demonstrating a 5-year local control rate of 85%.[99] **Table 3–4** lists some commonly referenced series on local control rates after conservation surgery for early lesions.

Table 3–4 Control Rates After Conservation Surgery for Early (T1 and T2) Hypopharyngeal Carcinoma

Author	Year	Study Number	T Stage	Treatment	Local Control Rate (%)
Laccourreye[98]	1993	34	T2	Supracricoid hemilaryngopharyngectomy	97
Steiner[88]	2001	33	Stage I & II (PS)	Transoral laser excision; 6 patients RT	89.9
Chevalier[97]	1997	48	T1/T2 (PS & aryepiglottic fold)	Supraglottic hemilaryngectomy + RT	T1: 78 T2: 38
Vandenbrouck[184]	1987	18	T1/T2 (PS)	Conservation surgery	89

Abbreviations: PS, piriform sinus; RT, radiotherapy.

Advanced-Stage Disease (T3/T4)

Organ preservation is difficult to achieve surgically in patients with advanced local disease. Select patients are suitable for surgery without total laryngectomy; however, this often requires partial laryngeal resection for adequate margins and is rarely possible as a single-modality treatment. Patients undergoing these complex resections require adequate pulmonary reserve to withstand early postoperative aspiration. Tumor-related constraints for laryngeal preservation are summarized in **Table 3–5**.[29] Locally advanced tumors in patients with intact swallowing, functioning larynges, and without extensive cartilage destruction are best managed with nonsurgical organ-preservation approaches. In contrast, when disease control with an adequate functional outcome is unlikely, the patient should be given the option of primary surgery and postoperative irradiation. Patients with marked functional impairment due to destruction of critical structures are very unlikely to improve after nonsurgical therapy regardless of tumor eradication. A patient free of disease with an intact larynx but dependent on a tracheostomy and feeding tube is functionally more impaired than one who has undergone laryngopharyngectomy who can tolerate a near-normal diet by mouth and communicate using tracheo-esophageal puncture speech. Disease control with radiation therapy or chemoradiation is also poor in patients with extensive cricoid or laryngeal cartilage erosion or extension into the soft tissue of the neck, and we believe that these patients should be offered combined surgery and radiation therapy. Kim et al examined patients with locally advanced disease and noted that overall survival at 5 years was 15.7% and 13.9% for radiotherapy alone, 46.8% for surgery and postoperative radiation therapy, and 30.7% for neoadjuvant chemotherapy and radiotherapy.[100] In the literature, the reported 5-year survival rates range from 25 to 60% in patients treated with surgery with or without postoperative radiation therapy.[101] **Table 3–6** summarizes the disease-related outcomes in several large surgical series of hypopharyngeal carcinoma.

Management of the Neck

There is little data on the incidence of nodal metastases in T1 hypopharynx tumors because of its rarity. Whether it is reasonable to manage the neck expectantly for these lesions is debatable. In all other stages, treatment of the neck is mandatory given the high rate of nodal metastases at presentation and the high risk of delayed metastases.[25,78,80] When the primary tumor is treated surgically, the ipsilateral lymph nodes are managed with a neck dissection. Bilateral neck dissections are performed for extensive disease or medial piriform sinus, postcricoid and posterior pharyngeal wall cancers.[19] In

the clinically N0 neck, a selective neck dissection incorporating the levels at risk (levels II, III, IV) should be performed. Level I and V metastases are infrequently involved, and dissection of these nodal groups is not justified due to the potential morbidity from accessory and marginal mandibular nerve injury.[16,19,78,102] Many patients will have multiple nodal metastases and will require adjuvant radiotherapy on this basis. Where there are no adverse features, however, the primary site can be excluded from the radiation fields and the neck treated to a microscopic dose, limiting the long-term morbidity of combination therapy.

In patients with clinical nodal metastases (N+), a comprehensive neck dissection is indicated with inclusion of levels I through V. Although the incidence of metastases to levels I and V remains low, the risk increases to a level to justify their dissection. Sacrifice of the internal jugular vein (IJV), sternocleidomastoid muscle, and accessory nerve are only performed if they are directly invaded with cancer. Every attempt to preserve the accessory nerve should be made, where oncologically sound, to avoid the shoulder morbidity that results from resection. If bilateral comprehensive neck dissections are performed, an attempt should be made at preservation of al least one IJV to avoid venous congestion and subsequent cerebral edema.

In the N0 and N1 neck, ipsilateral paratracheal nodes (level VI) should be dissected, especially in piriform sinus tumors and advanced disease.[25,74] Certainly, one of the advantages of radiotherapy is the inclusion of retropharyngeal nodes into the treatment fields that are at high risk in extensive posterior pharyngeal wall tumors and not normally included in standard lymph node dissections.[25,37,84]

Approaches for Primary Surgery

Table 3–7 lists common approaches used for surgical resection of hypopharyngeal cancers. The approach one chooses depends upon the location and extent of the disease, surgeon experience, patient anatomy, and comorbidity. The advancement of laser surgery and chemoradiation protocols have substantially limited the application of many of these procedures. Ultimately, survival in hypopharyngeal cancer is usually determined by distant disease and second primary tumors; hence, the surgical approach to the primary is unlikely to alter survival as long as it is oncologically sound.

Transoral Laser Endoscopic Resection Transoral laser endoscopic resection (TOL) using the carbon dioxide laser has been extensively applied with high success rates for laryngeal cancers. The published experience for hypopharyngeal malignancy is considerably less.[25,88,96,103–105] Local control and recurrence-free survival rates for T1/T2 hypopharyngeal malignancies are similar to those reported for radiotherapy alone[88,95,106] and partial open surgery.[1] Series using TOL for hypopharyngeal and laryngeal malignancies have incorporated routine adjuvant radiotherapy to both the primary site and the neck in the treatment algorithm.[1,88,95,96] The difficulty with this approach is that these patients could be treated with

---

Table 3–5 Requirements for Laryngeal Preservation Surgery

One mobile arytenoid/true cord
No piriform apex or cervical esophagus involvement
No extensive thyroid or cricoid cartilage involvement
No postcricoid or interarytenoid involvement

Table 3–6 Overall and Disease-Specific Survival for Surgery With or Without Radiation Therapy for Hypopharyngeal Carcinoma

Reference	N	Treatment	5-Year Overall Survival (%)	5-Year Disease-Specific Survival (%)	Comment
Bova[251]	180	Laryngopharyngectomy + postoperative RT	33	52	1979–2002:
		82 induction chemotherapy			68% T3/T4
Jones[131]	90	Laryngopharyngectomy	17	42	
		55 primary surgery			
		28 postoperative RT			
		35 salvage after RT			
Shah[8]	301	238 laryngopharyngectomy	26	—	Minimum 5-year follow-up (AJCC, 1975)
		35 preoperative RT	T1: 37		
		28 RT	T2: 25		
			T3: 16		
Wei[122]	317	Pharyngolaryngoesophagectomy	1979: 18	—	HP, L, CE
		145 hypopharynx primary	1995: 25		
Peracchia[252]	107	Pharyngolaryngoesophagectomy	32 (R0)	—	HP, L, CE
		26 induction chemotherapy			
		31 chemoradiation + surgical salvage			
Tribuoulet[253]	209	Pharyngolaryngoesophagectomy	29 (HP)	—	HP, CE
Clark[113]	138	66 laryngopharyngectomy + postoperative RT	38 (PS)	45 (PS)	1992–2002
			31 (S)	40 (S)	HP, L, CE
		72 salvage after RT	—	40 (HP)	
Steiner[88]	127	Transoral laser resection	Stage I–II: 71	—	1981–1996
			Stage III–IV: 47		Piriform sinus only
Hoffman[13]	691	All surgery with or without adjuvant therapy	—	Stage I: 63	Survey of USA
				Stage II: 58	1980–1985
				Stage III: 33	
				Stage IV: 22	
Eckel[70]	136	46 larynx preservation	40	56	1986–1997
		54 total laryngectomy	61 (larynx preservation)		
		36 laryngopharyngectomy			
Kraus[92]	132	93 total laryngectomy with pharyngectomy	30	41	1975–1985
		39 partial pharyngectomy			80% received postoperative radiation

Abbreviations: RT, radiotherapy; HP, hypopharynx; L, larynx; CE, cervical esophagus; PS, primary surgery; S, salvage surgery after radiotherapy.

Table 3–7 Common Surgical Approaches Used for Surgical Resection of Hypopharynx Cancers

Larynx preservation
   Transoral endoscopic (laser)
   Transhyoid pharyngotomy
   Mandibulotomy and median glossotomy
   Mandibulotomy and jaw swing
   Lateral pharyngotomy
   Partial laryngectomy and hypopharyngectomy
      Horizontal supraglottic laryngectomy
      Vertical hemilaryngectomy
      Supracricoid partial laryngectomy
Larynx extirpation
   Partial laryngopharyngectomy
   Total (circumferential) laryngopharyngectomy

radiotherapy alone for T1 to T2 disease. Unless a substantial disease-control advantage can be demonstrated, primary surgery should only be considered where adjuvant radiation therapy is not likely to be necessary.

Ideal lesions for TOL include T1 and T2 lesions of the lateral piriform sinus and posterior pharyngeal wall. Medial piriform lesions are more difficult to manage as they will frequently require resection of the paraglottic space and supraglottis.[95] Postcricoid cancers are less amenable to TOL due to the proximity of the cricoarytenoid joint, intrinsic laryngeal muscles, and RLNs.[32] In these patients, it is difficult to achieve adequate margins without inflicting substantial morbidity, except in very early stage disease.[104] There is very limited published experience in resection of postcricoid cancers using this technique.

After TOL, the defect is left to granulate and remucosalize. Initial studies of TOL report fewer complications and earlier return to normal swallowing than with open partial surgery.[1] Stricture is uncommon unless the resection is nearly circumferential and the risk of stricture is reduced with early swallowing and avoidance of prolonged tube feeding. TOL for hypopharyngeal tumors is more likely to induce aspiration than for laryngeal primaries and can be marked in patients with advanced local disease and where a partial laryngeal resection is necessary, but is usually temporary.[103]

The role of TOL in locally advanced hypopharyngeal cancers has not yet been established, and there are no studies to compare outcomes with other approaches. Selected advanced lesions may be amenable to TOL with postoperative radiotherapy (with or without chemotherapy) as an organ-preservation protocol. Considerable laser experience is required before tackling complex advanced hypopharyngeal resections.

Transhyoid Pharyngotomy and Median Labiomandibular Glossotomy The transhyoid approach is performed by dividing the suprahyoid musculature and either depressing the hyoid bone or excising its central portion followed by entry into the pharynx. Because of the limited exposure, only T1/T2 tumors of the upper posterior pharyngeal wall are suitable for this approach. The median labiomandibular glossotomy involves splitting the lip, followed by a midline mandibulotomy and dividing the tongue along the midline raphe. This approach provides wider exposure for posterior pharyngeal lesions than the transhyoid pharyngotomy and can be used where tumors extend to the oropharynx.

Lateral Pharyngotomy The lateral pharyngotomy is a more versatile approach that entails mobilizing the laryngopharyngeal complex unilaterally and making a longitudinal incision into the piriform sinus behind the thyroid ala. This allows access to all subsites of the hypopharynx and is most suitable for tumors of the lateral piriform sinus and posterior wall. An attempt should be made to identify and preserve the internal branch of the superior laryngeal nerve. We currently use this technique for localized recurrence after radiation or in the primary setting for early lesions where surgery is chosen and a TOL approach is not feasible due to inadequate visualization of the tumor. Postoperative aspiration is not usually problematic except where there is injury to the SLNs, vocal cord paralysis, extensive resection, or excessive flap bulk.

Pharyngectomy and Partial Laryngectomy Numerous combinations of open partial laryngectomy and pharyngectomy have been proposed and reported in small- to moderate-sized series.[97,107,108] Partial pharyngectomy can be combined with vertical hemilaryngectomy, supraglottic laryngectomy, supracricoid laryngectomy, and near-total laryngectomy.[98,109–112] Few patients are eligible for these complex techniques because of medical comorbidity and advanced local disease. Patients undergoing any form of open partial laryngeal surgery require adequate

pulmonary reserve to tolerate the inevitable early and sometimes extended postoperative aspiration. Aspiration is considerably worse when hypopharyngeal resection is combined with partial laryngectomy. Partial laryngeal surgery must be converted to a total laryngectomy if contraindications for partial surgery are identified intraoperatively, and patients must be counseled preoperatively about this possibility.

Total Laryngectomy and Partial Pharyngectomy Total laryngectomy and partial pharyngectomy is suitable for malignancies of the piriform sinus involving the larynx and most postcricoid malignancies. Traditionally, this operation has been the standard of care for any locally advanced hypopharyngeal cancers. This is a reliable and oncologically sound method of resection and is also a reasonable option for small lesions in patients who refuse nonsurgical management and are unable to tolerate partial laryngeal surgery. The extent of margins for hypopharyngeal malignancy is controversial.[2,25,32] Ho et al demonstrated the propensity for submucosal spread in a histologic study and recommended using 1.5 cm superior, 2.0 cm lateral, and 3.0 cm inferior margins.[13] No study has demonstrated a control or survival advantage over traditional margins using 1.0- to 1.5-cm margins most likely due to the use of adjuvant radiotherapy.[113] Submucosal spread and skip lesions should be considered in margin determination, particularly in the salvage setting, and intraoperative frozen sections taken along the margins of resection should be obtained.

Circumferential Laryngopharyngectomy With or Without Esophagectomy Circumferential laryngopharyngectomy is necessary when adequate margins cannot be achieved with partial pharyngeal resection. At our institution, it is most often performed for patients with extensive disease recurrence after radiotherapy and as primary treatment of advanced cancers where disease is unlikely to be controlled with good functional outcomes by chemoradiation. Total laryngopharyngectomy should be combined with esophagectomy for patients with tumor extension below the cervical esophagus.

Other considerations in these patients include a high incidence of hypothyroidism due to the combination of radiotherapy and partial thyroidectomy.[114] Routine thyroid hormone replacement is advisable because of the major adverse impact of hypothyroidism, particularly on wound healing, which is often already compromised in these patients. Hypocalcemia frequently occurs with circumferential resection and dissection of the paratracheal and mediastinal nodes and should be expected and treated early.[113] Where possible, the parathyroid glands should be preserved or reimplanted.

Reconstruction

The goals of reconstruction after surgical resection of hypopharyngeal cancers are to restore form (pharyngeal conduit), function (speech and swallow), and to prevent complications (pharyngocutaneous fistula and pharyngeal stricture). The choice of reconstructive technique depends upon several factors including the size of the defect, previous radiation or chemoradiation, comorbidities, and the surgeon's experience. There are no large series in the literature assessing the functional outcomes between different forms of reconstruction and with nonsurgical therapies. **Figures 3–3** and **3–4** describe the current approach to reconstruction of partial and circumferential pharyngeal defects after laryngopharyngectomy at the Princess Margaret Hospital. Despite advances in reconstruction, survival after laryngopharyngectomy remains disappointing, and this needs to be considered in the reconstructive algorithm.[115] Minimizing perioperative morbidity is important so that patients can enjoy quality time out of the hospital with early and reliable return to acceptable speech and swallowing.

Partial Pharyngectomy Defects (With or Without Laryngectomy) Small defects confined to the lateral piriform sinus with larynx preservation can be closed primarily, whereas larger defects require reconstruction with a regional or free flap. Preference should be given to thin pliable flaps such as the radial forearm free flap (RFFF) or anterolateral thigh (ALT) flap, depending on body habitus.[116–119] Free jejunum has also been used as a mucosal patch to reconstruct partial defects. Our practice has been to combine flap reconstruction with a Silastic salivary stent for 2 to 6 weeks when stricture is likely. Most patients require a tracheotomy until swelling subsides and the stent removed.

For total laryngectomy and partial pharyngectomy defects, primary closure of the pharynx is rarely possible. In patients who have undergone prior chemoradiation, consideration should also be given to a highly vascularized flap, such as a pectoralis major flap, to bolster the reconstruction. Either a regional or free flap can be used, with the choice of flap based on donor site preferences rather than recipient site outcomes. The pectoralis major flap continues to be a good option (**Fig. 3–5**), although some patients, particularly women, find the donor defect to be unacceptable. The rate of distal flap necrosis is around 10% and may result in a pharyngocutaneous fistula.[115,120] When a pectoralis flap is raised, the distal vascularity should be assessed in the position of the reconstruction and be abandoned if dubious. In centers with extensive microvascular expertise, a fasciocutaneous free flap (such as the RFFF or

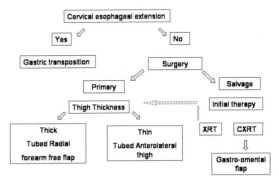

Figure 3–4 Reconstruction algorithm for total (circumferential) laryngopharyngeal defects.

ALT flap) avoids the donor site concerns in the chest and is associated with a lower rate of partial flap necrosis.[120] Functional outcomes after reconstruction of total laryngectomy with partial pharyngectomy defects in terms of swallowing are good, with lower stricture rates when compared with circumferential reconstructions.[120] Early and high-quality speech rehabilitation can be achieved using tracheoesophageal puncture (TEP), and long-term quality of life outcomes are acceptable when disease is controlled effectively.[121] Primary TEP may be performed in patients undergoing primary pharyngeal closure, whereas a secondary TEP is preferred when the pharynx is reconstructed with a regional or free flap.

Circumferential Laryngopharyngectomy Defects The introduction of free tissue transfer has increased the complexity but substantially reduced the morbidity and is preferred except in situations where there is significant cervical esophageal involvement.

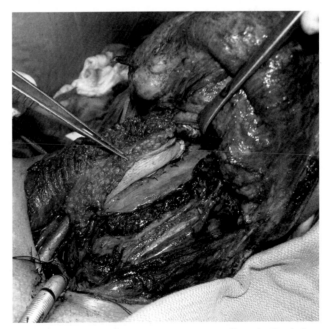

Figure 3–5 Picture of a myocutaneous pectoralis major flap being inset to reconstruct a total laryngectomy partial pharyngectomy defect.

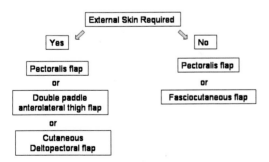

Figure 3–3 Reconstruction algorithm for partial laryngopharyngectomy defects.

Transposed Viscera Gastric pull-up is indicated for tumors extending to the cervical esophagus that require a laryngo-pharyngo-esophagectomy.[122] Gastric transposition has been extensively reported in the literature and is associated with a high morbidity and excessive mortality rate in some series.[23,44,123-125] Later series have reported lower but still significant mortality rates.[122,126-128] Wei et al reviewed 20 published series between 1966 and 1995 and found that the average major complication and mortality rates were 37% and 16%, respectively.[122] This was confirmed by reviews at our own institution in 1989 and 2005 as shown in **Table 3–8**.[129]

Pectoralis Major Flap The pectoralis major flap has mostly been abandoned for circumferential defects because of the difficulty with tubing the flap due to its bulk. Fabian described partial tubulation of the flap as an alternative combined with skin graft of the prevertebral fascia.[130] Several series exist in the literature and describe problems with partial flap necrosis, fistula in 13 to 63% of patients, poor swallowing, and long-term stricture.[115]

Enteric Free Flaps Free jejunal transfer is the most widely reported flap for circumferential pharyngeal reconstruction. Its popularity is related to the generally low stricture rates, large segments that can be taken for defects extending into the oropharynx or nasopharynx, and the lumen caliber match between jejunum and esophagus. **Table 3–9** presents a summary of a literature review by Shangold et al of free jejunal flaps,[116] as well as our own recent institutional experience.[120] It is difficult to accurately determine the morbidity associated with free jejunal transfer because the complication rates vary so widely in the literature even from institutions with extensive experience.[79,116,118,131-134] Institutional experience with these procedures has considerable bearing on morbidity-related outcomes. Donor site morbidity has been reduced by laparoscopic harvest techniques.[135,136]

The concerns with jejunum are that voice quality and swallowing are inferior to tubed fasciocutaneous flap reconstructions. The voice tends to have a "wet" quality, and patients often suffer intermittent dysphagia from uncoordinated peristalsis during deglutition.[137-139] There is

Table 3–8 Gastric Transposition at the University of Toronto

	Goldberg et al 1989[129]	Clark et al 2005[120]
N	41	21
Mortality	20%	0%
Major morbidity	46%	66%*
Fistula	22%	48%
Stricture	N/A	29%
Length of stay	Mean 31 days	Mean 34 days
	Median N/A	Median 22 days

*The increase in major morbidity (66%) in our most recent review corresponds with the increase in patients surviving the procedure (100%) and the use of chemotherapy and high-dose accelerated radiation.

Table 3–9 Summary of a Literature Review by Shangold et al of Free Jejunal Flaps and University of Toronto Experience with Free Jejunum

	Shangold et al 1991[116]	Clark et al 2005[120]
N	595	30
Mortality	4.4%	0%
Flap failure	8.9%	6.7%
Abdominal complications	5.8%	10%
Fistula	17.2% (67% spontaneously closed)	20% (67% spontaneously closed)
Stricture	10.9%	20%
Oral diet	82%	97%
TEP speech	14%	33%

little data to suggest that fistula rates are lower than with other reconstructive techniques.[121] Laparotomy may further compound preexisting comorbidities and malnourishment and can be associated with intraabdominal complications.

Where laparotomy is indicated, we favor the gastroomental free flap as the enteric reconstruction of choice. This flap has particular value in patients undergoing salvage surgery after high-dose accelerated radiotherapy or concurrent chemoradiation, where fistula rates exceed 50% in some series.[140] The unique feature of this flap is the abundant omentum that can be draped over the pharyngeal anastomoses and exposed vasculature, preventing major sequela such as high-volume fistulas, neck sepsis, and carotid rupture if a leak occurs. Early experience has demonstrated fistula rates between 0 and 16% in an extremely high risk group of patients.[113,140,141] Swallowing appears to be superior to the jejunal flap because there is no peristalsis and TEP speech does not have the typical wet character of jejunum. The flap is versatile in terms of length and width, easily harvested, and gastric donor complications are minimal as long as the prepyloric (antrum) region is avoided.

Fasciocutaneous Free Flaps The RFFF and ALT flap are the most commonly used fasciocutaneous free flaps for reconstruction of total laryngopharyngectomy defects. In thin patients, these flaps are pliable and easily tubed (**Figs. 3–6** and **3–7**). A less common reconstructive technique involves partial flap tubulation and securing it to the prevertebral fascia. In some centers, the ALT flap has replaced the RFFF as the workhorse for head and neck reconstruction because of its minimal donor site morbidity; however, it can be bulky in Western populations, particularly in women, making it difficult to tube.[142]

Large series of cutaneous flaps have emerged in the literature with varied fistula and late stricture rates. Most authors agree that fasciocutaneous flaps are superior to free jejunum with regard to TEP speech, lower failure rate, and avoidance of the morbidity of a laparotomy.[19,142-148] The fistula and stricture rates in some series are reported to be higher than

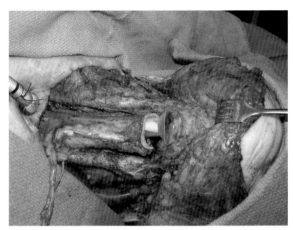

Figure 3–6 Picture of a tubed radial forearm flap being inset to reconstruct a total laryngopharyngectomy defect. A salivary bypass tube is used as a stent.

with jejunal flaps[1,117,118,143,145,149]; however, the routine use of a salivary bypass tube appears to reduce this problem.[120,150]

Salvage Surgery for Recurrent Disease Salvage surgery should be performed whenever recurrent disease is resectable and the patient is known to be free of distant metastatic disease and medically fit for surgery.[151-153] Only a limited number of patients (<40%), however, are suitable to undergo surgical salvage.[64,151-153] Long-term salvage is possible in select patients with reported survival in the head and neck literature ranging from 15 to 37%.[8,13,153-156] The 5-year survival rate after surgical salvage

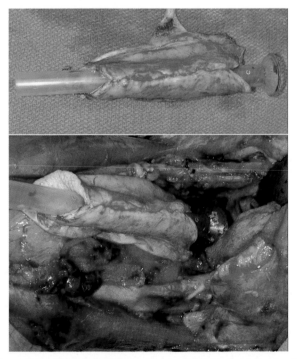

Figure 3–7 Picture of a tubed anterolateral thigh flap being inset to reconstruct a total laryngopharyngectomy defect. A salivary bypass tube is used as a stent.

for hypopharyngeal cancer ranges from 18 to 35%.[16,25,157,158] Tracheostomal recurrence tends to be associated with an even lower rate of successful salvage.[159]

Surgical salvage after radiation therapy or chemoradiation failure generally entails total laryngectomy with partial or total pharyngectomy and possible esophagectomy because it is the last opportunity to cure the patient of disease. Generous margins should be taken because of the risk of islands of microscopic residual tumor occurring beyond macroscopic disease. In the rare case of T1 and small T2 tumors developing very localized recurrences, conservation surgery or transoral laser surgery may be performed, thus preserving the larynx.[87,157] We advocate an aggressive approach and rarely perform partial resections for recurrent disease in the hypopharynx.

The morbidity of salvage laryngopharyngectomy continues to be problematic.[17,25,121,153,160-162] Achievement of a normal diet is not the typical outcome, and many patients may require long-term feeding tubes. A prolonged period of rehabilitation should be anticipated, and many patients will require weeks to months of swallowing therapy. Chemoradiation organ preservation protocols have increased pharyngocutaneous fistula rates after surgical salvage procedures. Novel approaches to minimize fistula rates include use of the gastroomental flap or bolstering pharyngeal anastomosis with musculocutaneous flaps even after simple laryngectomy.

Radiation Therapy

Radiation therapy has several established roles in the management of hypopharyngeal cancer. It can be used as single-modality treatment for early tumors, combined with surgery or chemotherapy in advanced disease, and in palliation of incurable locoregional or distant disease. Early series demonstrating superior locoregional control and survival for surgery over radiotherapy are difficult to interpret due to poor study design, selection bias, and variability in inclusion criteria of tumor subsites and stage. In addition, these early studies used suboptimal doses of radiation when compared with current standards, which accounts for the lower control rates seen in the past.[59]

To improve the therapeutic ratio of radiation therapy, doses have been increased above 60 Gy and altered fractionation schedules have been developed. Altered fractionation includes accelerated fractionation, hyperfractionation, or a combination of both. Altered fractionation regimens provide an increase in control rates over conventional fractionation in head and neck cancers, including hypopharynx cancer[1,163-167]. Most of the benefit from altered fractionation appears to be from improved control[168,169] at the primary site rather than the nodal site[168,169] although some trials have noted a survival advantage[165,167]

Early-Stage Lesions (T1/T2 with N0/N1)

Control and survival rates after radiation therapy for early hypopharyngeal cancers are similar to those reported for surgery[21,163,170]; however, there are no prospective trials comparing

Table 3–10 Local and Ultimate Control Rates in Early Hypopharynx Cancers Managed with Radiotherapy Alone

Author	Year	Study Number	T Stage	Treatment	Local Control Rate (%)	Ultimate Local Control After Salvage Surgery (%)
Bataini[172]	1982	90	T1/T2 (PS)	RT alone	68	
Dubois[254]	1986	60	T1/T2 (PS)	RT alone	73	
Amdur[170]	2001	101	T1/T2 (PS)	RT alone	T1: 90 T2: 80	
Garden[163]	1996	82	T1/T2 (all sites)	RT alone	T1: 89 T2: 77	
Mendenhall[173]	1987	29	T1/T2 (PS)	RT alone	T1: 89 T2: 75	T2: 90
Hull[255]	2003	60	T1/T2 (PW)	RT alone	T1: 93 T2: 82	T2: 87
Fein[164]	1993	41	T1/T2 (PW)	RT alone	T1: 100 T2: 92*	

Abbreviations: PS, piriform sinus; PW, posterior pharyngeal wall; RT, radiotherapy.

the two modalities.[1] Proponents for radiation therapy argue that functional outcomes are superior in terms of swallowing and speech when compared with surgery,[21] although evidence to support this is scant. A drawback to conservation surgery is that patients will often require postoperative radiation and therefore be subjected to toxicities from both therapies.[25]

Local control rates after radiation therapy for T1 hypopharyngeal cancers range from 68% to more than 90% for T1 lesions and more than 75% for T2 lesions.[106,163,164,171,172] Disease-specific survival for early tumors ranges from 50 to 100% at 5 years (**Table 3–10**). Treatment results for early-stage lesions are presented in **Table 3–10**. Control rates decrease with "high-risk" T2 tumors, which are defined as those larger than 2.5 cm, bulky tumors, or those that extend to the apex of the piriform sinus.[1,81,170,173] Exophytic, low-bulk, small (<2.5 cm) tumors with no vocal cord impairment are considered "low-risk" T2 tumors.[21,173] Conventional fractionated radiotherapy is indicated in patients with T1/T2 and N0/N1 disease. The dose per fraction is 1.8 Gy to 2 Gy per day delivered to a total dose of 66 Gy to 72 Gy over 6.5 to 7.5 weeks. Shorter fractionations, such as 50 Gy in 2.5 Gy per day over 4 weeks or 60 Gy in 2.5 Gy per day over 5 weeks, can be used in patients with substantial comorbidities and in those who cannot tolerate a longer treatment course. Patients with "high-risk" T2 lesions have improved local control with altered fractionation compared with conventional radiation.[21,163,170,174,175] Altered fractionation that can be used in this setting includes

76 to 81.6 Gy in 1.2 Gy per fraction twice daily over 6 to 7 weeks and 64 Gy in 1.6 Gy per fraction twice daily over 4 weeks. The latter radiation schedule (HARDWINS, or hyper-fractionated radiation delivered with integrated neck surgery) was investigated at Princess Margaret Hospital, as an altered fractionation with reduced overall treatment time. In a dose escalation study of 60 Gy, 62 Gy, and 64 Gy delivered with twice-daily radiation therapy over 4 weeks, 64 Gy was found to be associated with acceptable toxicity when used in combination with a planned neck dissection for N+ disease (irradiated to lower doses).[176]

Advanced Lesions (T3/T4, or Any T Stage with N2/N3)

Advanced-staged lesions are associated with local control rates between 38% and 80% (**Table 3–11**) and 5-year disease-specific survival from 0 to 12% treated with radiotherapy alone[19] (**Table 3–12**). Optimal treatment for advanced disease based on control and survival rates are concurrent chemoradiation or surgery with adjuvant radiation therapy. There is a limited role for radiotherapy only in the treatment of advanced hypopharyngeal cancer, due to the poor survival and high recurrence rates.[1,100,177,178] Single-modality treatment with radiation may be offered to patients who either refuse or cannot tolerate more aggressive therapy; however, disease-related outcomes are poor with this approach.[1,100,177,178] T3 N0/N1 lesions are amenable to altered fractionation techniques

Table 3–11 Local and Ultimate Control Rates in Advanced Hypopharyngeal Cancers Managed with Radiotherapy Alone

Author	Year	Study Number	T Stage	Treatment	Local Control Rate (%)	Ultimate Local Control After Salvage Surgery (%)
Bataini[172]	1982	344	T3 (PS)	RT alone	38	
Dubois[254]	1986	148	T3/T4 (PS)	RT alone	73	
Hull[255]	2003	88	T3/T4 (PW)	RT alone	T3: 59 T4: 50	T3: 61 T4: 50
Fein[164]	1993	58	T3/T4 (PW)	RT alone	T3: 80 T4: 50*	

Abbreviations: PS, piriform sinus; PW, posterior pharyngeal wall; RT, radiotherapy.

Table 3–12 Overall Survival and Disease-Specific Survival for Hypopharyngeal Cancers Managed With Radiotherapy With or Without Planned Neck Dissection

Author	Treatment	Overall Survival (%)	Disease-Specific Survival (%)
Bataini[172]	Radiation	T1: 21 T2: 28	T1: 49 T2: 48 T3: 39 Overall: 41
Hull[255]	Radiation with planned neck dissection	Stage I: 56 Stage II: 52 Stage III: 24 Stage IV: 22 Overall: 30	Stage I: 89 Stage II: 88 Stage III: 44 Stage IV: 34 Overall: 49
Tombolini[178]	Radiation	Stage III: 33 Stage IV: 5 Overall: 15.6	Stage III: 50 Stage IV: 16 Overall: 28.1
Amdur[170]	Radiation	Stage I: 57 Stage II: 61 Stage III: 41 Stage IVa: 29 Stage IVb: 25	Stage I/II: 96 Stage III: 62 Stage IVa: 49 Stage IVb: 33
Fein[164]	Radiation	Stage I: 50 Stage II: 36 Stage III: 26 Stage IVa: 28 Stage IVb: 5	Stage I: 100 Stage II: 72 Stage III: 56 Stage IVa: 75 Stage IVb: 29
Garden[163]	Radiation	T1/T2: 52	

alone; however, altered fractionation delivered with concurrent chemotherapy has been shown to improve locoregional control and progression-free survival in advanced head and neck cancers compared with altered fractionation alone.[168]

Postoperative radiotherapy is almost always indicated for locally advanced tumors and should be considered in patients with high-risk T2 cancers managed with surgery. Other indications for postoperative radiotherapy are listed in **Table 3–13**.[58,179–181] The addition of postoperative radiotherapy is associated with improved locoregional control, disease-free and overall survival in patients with advanced hypopharyngeal cancers.[74,106,179,182–184] It is recommended that postoperative radiation be initiated 4 to 6 weeks after surgery. Longer delays may allow tumor proliferation and diminish the benefits of adjuvant radiation. We recommend that the primary site and both sides of the neck be included in the radiation volumes with a dose of 50 to 60 Gy in 2 Gy per fraction. With

positive margins, the dose should be increased to 64 Gy to maximize control.[74] For very high risk disease, concomitant chemotherapy should be considered based on the results of recent randomized trials.

Complications

Radiation therapy is not only time intensive but can also be associated with substantial acute and late toxicity. Common acute and late toxicities are listed in **Table 3–14**. The majority of acute toxicities are transient, improving within 6 weeks after completion of radiation therapy; however, xerostomia is often permanent and associated with an increased risk of dental caries and altered speech and swallowing. Feeding tubes are sometimes permanently required because of dysphagia or aspiration risk. This risk is increased with concurrent chemotherapy.

Advances in Radiation Therapy

Therapeutic advances in the field of radiation oncology over the past 2 decades include the development of CT-based high-precision radiation planning and delivery (e.g., conformal radiotherapy and IMRT) and image-guided radiotherapy (IGRT). Conformal radiation and IMRT allow high doses to cover irregularly shaped target volumes with steep dose gradients near critical structures in close proximity to the target volumes and reduced dose to adjacent normal tissues (including the spinal cord and salivary glands). Such technological advancements allow better coverage of the tumor while reducing morbidity from treatment. These techniques facilitate dose escalation to the primary tumor, as the volume of normal tissue irradiated to high doses is reduced

Table 3–13 Indications for Postoperative Radiotherapy

Advanced-stage disease (T3/T4)
Microscopically involved margins of resection
Pathologically N2 or N3 disease
Extracapsular nodal extension
Perineural invasion
Microvascular tumor emboli

Table 3–14 Common Acute and Late Toxicities of Radiation

Acute toxicities
Fatigue
Reduced blood counts
Oral mucositis/esophagitis, dysphagia
Aspiration
Xerostomia
Altered taste
Skin erythema
Dry and moist desquamation
Alopecia (in the irradiated volume)
Hoarseness
Late toxicities
Xerostomia
Altered speech
Dysphagia
Esophageal stricture
Neck fibrosis
Skin pigmentation
Chondronecrosis
Osteoradionecrosis
Hypothyroidism

compared with conventional radiation techniques. One example of how these advancements contribute to improve quality of life is in the ability to minimize the dose to the parotid glands. With a reduced dose to one parotid gland, saliva flow can be preserved, substantially reducing the adverse impact of xerostomia on quality of life.[185] There is little data yet demonstrating that local control is improved in hypopharyngeal cancer due to the introduction of high-precision radiation therapy; however, recurrences after these techniques occur most often within the high dose volumes, providing rationale for dose escalation.[186] It is expected that these technological advances will result in improved locoregional control and survival of patients with both early and advanced hypopharynx cancer treated with radiation, with or without chemotherapy.

Chemotherapy

Locally Advanced Disease

The addition of chemotherapy to radiation therapy in the management of locally advanced cancers of the head and neck has demonstrated locoregional control and survival rates better than treatment with radiation alone and comparable with combined surgery and radiation therapy.[174,187,188] However, combining chemotherapy and radiation therapy has the advantage of organ preservation when compared with surgery for hypopharyngeal cancer. The primary goals of organ preservation are maintenance of oral alimentation, protection of a laryngeal airway, and intelligible laryngeal speech.[174,178] The main chemotherapeutic agent used for head and neck cancers is cisplatin with or without 5-fluorouracil (5-FU). Common side-effects of these agents are listed in **Table 3–15**.

Two major treatment strategies have been pursued in organ-preservation protocols: induction chemotherapy and concomitant chemotherapy. Induction chemotherapy consists of administration of two to three cycles followed by radiation therapy in partial or complete responders, whereas nonresponders usually go on to surgery. A meta-analysis of three larynx preservation randomized trials comparing induction chemotherapy with cisplatin and 5-FU followed by radiotherapy in responders (or surgery in nonresponders) with surgery and postoperative radiation was conducted by

Table 3–15 Side Effects of Chemotherapy

Cisplatin
Nausea and vomiting
Myelosuppression
Ototoxicity
Nephrotoxicity
Peripheral neurotoxicity
5-FU
Myelosuppression
Mucositis
Diarrhea
Cardiac toxicity

Pignon et al.[187] Two of the trials included only advanced laryngeal cancers[189,190] and the third included only hypopharyngeal cancers.[191] The results of the meta-analysis failed to show a significant control or survival benefit of induction chemotherapy; however, 23% of patients retained their larynx at 5 years in the induction chemotherapy group. The European Organization for Research and Treatment of Cancer (EORTC) phase III trial included in the above meta-analysis, which accrued only piriform sinus cancer patients (T2 to T4, N0 to N3), found no significant difference in survival rates (30% vs. 35%) or local (19% vs. 12%) and regional (23% vs. 17%) recurrence rates between the induction chemotherapy arm and the immediate surgery arm. A lower incidence of distant metastases in the induction chemotherapy arm (25% vs. 36%) was identified; however, this did not translate into an overall survival benefit. The 5-year estimate of retaining a functioning larynx was 35%. Results showing similar control rates with laryngeal preservation have been found in other studies evaluating induction chemotherapy in head and neck cancers, including hypopharyngeal cancers.[35,87,192,193] Thus, although there is no survival benefit, some patients may be able to retain their larynx with neoadjuvant therapy, although laryngeal preservation rates appear to be lower than those reported for laryngeal cancer. Practice guidelines set forth by the Cancer Care Ontario (CCO) Program in Evidence Based Medicine (www.cancercare.on.ca) recommend that neoadjuvant chemotherapy alone followed by radiation therapy not be used in the management of patients with locally advanced squamous carcinoma of the head and neck if the main objective is improved survival.[194] However, there are current ongoing phase II and III trials evaluating the safety, feasibility, and efficacy of induction chemotherapy followed by concurrent chemoradiation in patients with locally advanced disease, in the hope of combining the benefits of induction and concurrent chemotherapy strategies in a tolerable manner.

Concurrent chemoradiation therapy involves administering chemotherapy during the course of radiation therapy. The standard schedule used in North America is cisplatin given at 100 mg/m^2 for 3 cycles on days 1, 22, and 43 with standard fractionation radiotherapy. Other schedules of combining cisplatin and radiotherapy have been examined, and daily concurrent administration at 6 mg/m^2 with standard radiation fractionation has also been used by some centers.[195] There is no consensus on the optimal radiation fractionation regimen when combined with chemotherapy, and therefore standard fractionation is recommended until further trials determine the role for altered fractionation. Contraindications to concomitant chemoradiation include poor performance status and significant baseline organ dysfunction.

Concurrent chemoradiation therapy has shown a benefit in advanced head and neck cancers in terms of survival, local and regional control, and larynx preservation over radiation-alone and induction chemotherapy regimens.[187–189,196,197] A meta-analysis on concomitant chemoradiation trials by Pignon et al reported an absolute survival benefit at 2 and 5 years of 8% for patients undergoing concomitant chemotherapy[187]; however, given the heterogeneity between the studies, the authors commented that the size of the benefit remains uncertain. Similarly, other meta-analyses and systematic reviews have found that survival of patients with locally advanced stage III or IV head and neck SCC is improved with concomitant chemotherapy compared with conventional fractionation radiotherapy alone.[187,198,199] The CCO Program in Evidence Based Medicine recommends concomitant chemotherapy with conventional fractionation radiotherapy as the treatment of choice for patients with advanced head and neck SCC.[199] Having adopted these guidelines, Princess Margaret Hospital offers concurrent chemoradiation to patients with locally advanced (T3 or T4) hypopharyngeal cancer, regardless of neck nodal status, and concomitant chemotherapy is considered in patients with early local (T1/T2) but advanced neck disease (N2 to N3).

It must be recognized that organ preservation strategies are not for all advanced cancers, and patients must be carefully selected.[174] Patients with significant baseline organ dysfunction and poor performance status are unlikely to do well. Adequate baseline organ function is a prerequisite for functional organ preservation, as patients who cannot swallow well before treatment will rarely swallow better after therapy.[174,200] Laryngeal and pharyngeal dysfunction has been reported by several authors after concomitant therapy.[19,201–204] Even though the larynx may be preserved, it may not remain functional after combined modality treatment.[19] Pretreatment vocal cord fixation has been found to be a predictor of poor functional outcome.[205]

Concurrent chemoradiation therapy has also been assessed in the postoperative setting for tumors considered to be at high risk of recurrence (**Table 3–13**).[189,206,207] A meta-analysis of four trials comparing postoperative radiation therapy alone with concurrent chemoradiation for stage III or IV cancers or early-stage cancers with high-risk pathologic features showed significant improvements in locoregional control and survival benefit in favor of chemoradiotherapy.[181] Based on these results, postoperative concurrent chemoradiation should be considered for patients who have pathologic features suggestive of a high risk of recurrence (**Table 3–10**) and who are able to tolerate the addition of chemotherapy.

The trade-off with concomitant chemoradiation is the increase in acute and long-term toxicity, including long-term dysphagia and G-tube dependence, irreversible side effects of chemotherapy such as nephropathy and neurotoxicity, and increased risk of postoperative complications after salvage surgery. Acute toxicity, such as severe mucositis or dysphagia, skin reaction, nausea and vomiting, weight loss, and hematologic toxicity can lead to interruptions and/or failure of completion of the full course of treatment. The toxicity carried with the treatment is not insignificant, and patients should be cared for at a center experienced with managing these toxicities. Patients must be involved in their treatment decision and informed of the benefits and drawbacks of organ-preservation treatment.

Management of the Neck After Radiation or Chemoradiation

Complete response rates of cervical nodes to radiation therapy is reported to be between 59% and 83% and is dependant on lymph node size, with nodes greater than 3 cm having poorer response rates.[208–212] A planned neck dissection is usually not indicated in N0 or N1 disease because there is a high likelihood of control with radiation therapy.

Management of advanced neck disease (N2 or N3) with surgery after radiation therapy or chemoradiation depends upon response to treatment and in some centers the pretreatment nodal size. Patients with clinically or radiographically detectable incomplete responses should undergo a neck dissection for regional control. Planned neck dissection for N2 to N3 disease that completely responds to therapy is controversial; options include observation and surgical salvage for recurrence or a planned neck dissection 4 to 6 weeks after treatment.[213,214] Proponents of a planned neck dissection claim that a complete response (CR) does not predict pathologic status,[211] with more than 30% of patients with N2 or N3 disease harboring residual microscopic disease after radiotherapy,[19] and when recurrences do occur, they often are not salvageable.[215–217] Furthermore, planned neck dissection appears to result in improved regional control and possibly causes specific survival.[82,171,218–220] If a neck dissection is planned, the radiation dose can be reduced from 70 Gy to 50 Gy in 2 Gy per fraction. For low-lying nodal disease, this may reduce the risk of brachial plexus injury from high-dose radiation. Despite achieving regional control, survival is influenced by the high rate of distant metastases.[83,214] Therefore, only a minority of patients subjected to the morbidity of a planned neck dissection will have a survival benefit.

The role of PET is helping to define patients most appropriate for neck dissection after radiation therapy or chemoradiation. Current results of PET-CT studies suggest that neck dissection can be safely withheld for patients who have a CR or small residual lymphadenopathy and a negative PET scan 12 weeks posttreatment. For patients with large residual lymphadenopathy (i.e., greater than 2.0 to 3.0 cm in size) and a negative posttreatment PET-CT, a neck dissection is warranted at present until further studies with longer follow-up are performed to determine the appropriateness of withholding a neck dissection.[214,221–223]

Treatment of Recurrence

Most local recurrences present more advanced than the original tumor, often making salvage surgery impossible.[157] If surgery cannot be offered, treatment options are usually palliative. Unresectable recurrent or metastatic disease has traditionally been managed with chemotherapy, with the intent of either palliation of symptoms and/or achieving measurable reduction in tumor size.[151,188,224] For patients with adequate performance status and organ function, participating in a clinical trial is an appropriate option. Cisplatin and 5-FU based therapy remains standard treatment in an off-trial setting but has achieved a median survival of only 6 months, and long-term survival beyond 2 years is rare.[13,42,224–226]

Reirradiation with or without chemotherapy is a further option to be considered for recurrent disease. Although long-term survivors have been reported with this approach for selected recurrent nasopharyngeal or laryngeal cancer, the efficacy of reirradiation for hypopharyngeal cancer is limited with most of the data coming from series of highly heterogeneous patients. For all patients treated with reirradiation, 5-year survival rates range from 13% in unselected to 93% in highly selected series, and local control rates range from 12.5 to 42%. Severe or fatal complication rates occurred in 9 to 32% of patients.[224] With the addition of chemotherapy to reirradiation, the median survival of patients has only marginally improved survival but may substantially increase toxicity.[152] Oncologists therefore must balance the risk of severe complications from reirradiation and their detriment to quality of life with only a small possibility for long-term survival.

Given the limited treatment options for recurrent and/ or metastatic head and neck cancers, the development of novel targeted agents in this population is of high priority. These agents exert their anticancer effects against specific proteins or pathways that are overexpressed or abnormally activated in malignant cells such that normal tissues might be spared. Targeted agents against the epidermal growth factor receptor (EGFR) have been the most developed in head and neck cancers, including monoclonal antibodies (e.g., cetuximab) and small molecular tyrosine kinase inhibitors (e.g., erlotinib, gefitinib). In head and neck cancers, EGFR is overexpressed in 80 to 90% of cases, and its overexpression by immunohistochemistry has been associated with worse prognosis.[227,228] Binding of ligands to the extracellular domain of EGFR results in the autophosphorylation of its tyrosine kinase domain and triggers downstream cascades of events leading to cellular proliferation, survival, angiogenesis, and metastasis.[229] Several phase II trials of EGFR inhibitors such as cetuximab, erlotinib, and gefitinib in patients with recurrent and/or metastatic head and neck cancers, including those with platinum-resistant disease, have demonstrated objective response rates in the range of 4 to 13% and disease control rates in the range of 40 to 50%, whether given as single agents or in combination with platinum.[230–233] The development of EGFR inhibitors in head and neck cancers has also been evaluated in combination with radiotherapy in patients with nonmetastatic, locally advanced cancers. In a potential landmark study, Bonner et al reported the results of a phase III randomized trial comparing definitive radiotherapy with or without cetuximab, where a 3-year relapse-free survival and overall survival were superior in the combined therapy arm.[234] Toxicities observed were comparable between the two arms with the exception of skin rash, which is a class effect of EGFR inhibitors. The implications from the findings of this important study are significant as current interests include how to optimally incorporate molecularly targeted agents into concurrent chemoradiation regimens, in the primary therapy and in the postoperative settings. Various molecularly targeted agents besides EGFR inhibitors, such as antiangiogenic agents, multitargeted kinase inhibitors, among others, are undergoing active investigations for their antitumor activity in head and neck cancers.

◆ Posttreatment Surveillance

Regular posttreatment follow-up is required to evaluate treatment response, detect early recurrence, and identify second primary tumors. Most local recurrences occur within 2 years of treatment, and early diagnosis is essential to initiate curative treatment.[15,26,235] History, physical examination, endoscopic exam, and imaging techniques are important aspects of surveillance. Symptoms suggestive of recurrence include otalgia, odynophagia, dysphagia, and worsening neck pain. Suspicious findings on endoscopic exam include persistent edema in the region of the arytenoids, hypopharyngeal ulceration, and development of a fixed vocal cord.[27] It is often difficult to differentiate persistent disease and recurrence from postoperative changes and inflammation associated with radiation therapy/chemoradiation, chondronecrosis of the laryngeal cartilages, or continued nicotine exposure in the postradiation setting.[236–240] The risk of edema after radiation therapy is associated with total dose and field size and can persist for up to 18 months.[235,241,242] Examination for regional recurrence can be similarly difficult due to changes in the neck such as fibrosis.

Diagnostic imaging should be obtained for routine assessment of response to treatment and in any patient with a suspicion of recurrence. The posttreatment diagnosis of local residual disease or recurrence may also be difficult to establish on a single CT or MRI scan; however, serial examinations are more reliable. PET-CT has proved to be particularly beneficial in this setting and has improved accuracy over CT and MRI.[235,236,243,244] **Table 3–16** lists the diagnostic accuracy of PET in detecting persistent or recurrent disease.

As part of routine surveillance, CT or MRI and/or PET-CT scans should be obtained at 3 months after treatment.[245] A PET-CT scan performed at least 3 months after treatment is more specific, reducing false-positive scans that can result from active inflammation after treatment.[1] A negative PET-CT scan reliably excludes residual or recurrent disease, whereas a positive scan necessitates a diligent search including endoscopy and biopsy. Regardless of PET or other imaging results, if there is strong clinical suspicion of persistent disease, biopsy is mandatory. Multiple endoscopies and biopsies may be needed to differentiate recurrence from posttreatment changes or chondronecrosis. PET-CT scanning, with its improved diagnostic accuracy, has the potential to substantially reduce the number of endoscopies and biopsies. Metastatic surveillance is of unproven benefit; however, an annual chest x-ray is reasonable.

◆ Conclusions

In summary, patients with T1 and favorable T2, N0 to N1 disease achieve excellent local control with either radiation

Table 3–16 Diagnostic Accuracy of Positron Emission Tomography in Detecting Recurrent or Persistent Head and Neck Cancer

PET Scan	Ranges Reported in Literature (%)
Sensitivity	85–100
Specificity	63–93
Positive predictive value	46–92
Negative predicative value	87–100

therapy as a single-modality treatment or conservation surgery. Patients with unfavorable T2 or exophytic T3 tumors with N0 to N1 disease are better served with altered fractionation radiation therapy based on the consistent finding that locoregional control is improved. Patients with advanced nodal disease can achieve excellent regional outcomes with radiation therapy and a planned neck dissection.[91-94] Concurrent chemoradiation improves locoregional control and reduces the risk of distant metastases. Patients with unfavorable T3 cancers with nodal status N2+ are ideal candidates for concurrent chemoradiation. Patients with T4 lesions may best be served with radical surgery with postoperative radiation therapy.

◆ Clinical Cases

Case 1 T2 N2b M0 squamous cell carcinoma right piriform sinus.

Presentation This patient is a 63-year-old man with a 6-month history of right-side neck mass and some odynophagia. He has no history of otalgia, dysphagia, or weight loss. He has a significant smoking and alcohol history. There was no history of significant medical comorbidity. Flexible endoscopic examination performed revealed a nodular lesion of the right piriform sinus, mobile cords bilaterally, and no pooling of secretions.

He was referred by his family physician to an otolaryngologist who performed a fine-needle aspiration of the right neck mass, which was positive for a poorly differentiated carcinoma. He was subsequently taken to the operating room for a panendoscopy. A complete direct endoscopic assessment was performed under general anesthetic, including flexible esophagoscopy, bronchoscopy, and laryngoscopy. Direct endoscopy revealed a nodular lesion of the right piriform sinus with extension to the lateral surface of the right aryepiglottic fold. There was no extension to the piriform apex or cervical esophagus. There was no evidence of a second primary lesion. Biopsy was obtained and confirmed to be a poorly differentiated SCC on final pathology. He was subsequently referred to a tertiary care oncology center.

Diagnosis, Workup, and Staging CT scan of the head and neck with fine cuts through the larynx were performed (**Fig. 3–8**). Findings included thickening of the right piriform sinus and aryepiglottic fold. There was no cartilaginous or boney erosion, no invasion of the paraglottic space, or cervical esophageal extension. A right level III necrotic node was present measuring 2.1 cm and a 1.0 node in level II. Chest CT was also performed, which was negative. The tumor was staged as a T2 N2b M0 SCC of the right piriform sinus.

Options for Treatment The options for early carcinoma of the hypopharynx (T1 to T2, N0 M0) include primary radiotherapy or surgery. Radiotherapy using conventional or altered fractionation can be used as a single-modality therapy with similar control and survival rates to surgery. The addition of chemotherapy may provide a marginal survival advantage and could be considered in this patient due to

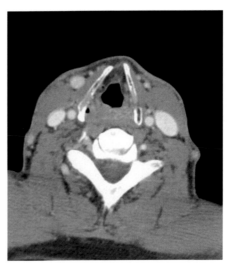

Figure 3–8 Case 1: Axial CT scan of a T2 N2b M0 piriform sinus cancer.

the advanced stage based on nodal disease; however, the additional morbidity must be anticipated.

Surgical options include transoral laser excision or standard partial pharyngectomy using a lateral pharyngotomy approach. Total laryngectomy is not indicated for early-stage lesions, except in selected cases not suitable for organ-preservation (surgical and nonsurgical) protocols. In centers with experience in laser surgery, this would be the optimal surgical approach for lesions limited to the lateral piriform sinus. Surgical excision would be made more difficult in this patient because of aryepiglottic fold involvement. For patients where the primary is managed surgically, the neck also needs to be treated using either neck dissection or postoperative radiotherapy. In patients with adverse pathologic features, postoperative radiotherapy would also be indicated.

Treatment of the Primary Tumor and Neck The patient was discussed in a multidisciplinary tumor board conference, and both primary surgical and radiotherapy options were offered to the patient. Our recommendation was to offer primary radiotherapy to both the primary site, both necks, and the paratracheal nodes. IGRT was performed to a dose of 70 Gy in 35 fractions. Radiation was chosen for this patient because of equivalent disease-related outcomes and minimal functional sequelae and also because of the probability of requiring adjuvant radiotherapy due to the likelihood of multiple nodal metastases. In this case, with the use of image-guided techniques, the tumor coverage is better than it would be with conventional radiation, and the dose is reduced to one of the parotid glands, allowing preservation of saliva flow that would not be possible after conventional radiation therapy.

Case 2 T4a N2a M0 squamous cell carcinoma of the piriform sinus.

Presentation This patient is a 60-year-old man with a 4-month history of progressive dysphagia associated with a 20-lb weight loss. His dysphagia was with both solids and liquids. Associated symptoms included odynophagia and right otalgia. He also noted a right-sided neck mass ~1 month prior to presentation that had slowly increased in size. He had a 40-pack/year smoking history and consumed two to three beers per day. There was no significant comorbidity history. On examination, he had mild stridor but did not appear to be in respiratory distress. He was thin and cachetic. Examinations of his oral cavity and oropharynx were normal. Otoscopic examination did not show any evidence of middle ear disease. Palpation of his right neck revealed a 3.5-cm level II/III node that was firm but not fixed. There were no palpable left neck masses. Flexible endoscopic examination found a large right-sided piriform sinus mass extending to involve the posterior pharyngeal wall. The right aryepiglottic fold appeared to be involved with reduction in the right vocal cord mobility.

Diagnosis, Workup, and Staging CT scan (**Fig. 3–9**) showed a large exophytic mass filling the right piriform fossa with involvement of the right aryepiglottic fold, posterior pharyngeal wall, and left lateral piriform fossa. There was no extension to the cervical esophagus. Posteriorly, the mass abutted the prevertebral space with no evidence of invasion of the paraspinal muscles or cervical spine vertebrae. There was abnormal soft tissue around the lateral thyroid cartilage suggesting erosion. A 3.1-cm necrotic lymph node was noted in right level III and a left retropharyngeal node measuring 1.5 cm. Chest CT did not show any evidence of pulmonary metastases.

The patient was then taken to the operating room for panendoscopy and tracheotomy. Direct endoscopy confirmed CT scan and flexible laryngoscopy findings. The cervical esophagus appeared grossly normal on flexible esophagoscopy. There was no evidence of a synchronous primary tumor. A biopsy was performed, which confirmed a poorly differentiated SCC. The tumor was staged as T4a N2a M0. A G-tube was also placed percutaneously at the time of his admission.

Treatment Options This patient requires combined-modality therapy with either the traditional approach of

surgery and postoperative radiotherapy or an organ-preservation protocol with concurrent chemoradiation. Surgery would require a total laryngopharyngectomy with bilateral neck dissections and reconstruction with a free flap (jejunum or tubed fasciocutaneous flap). This patient requires discussion at a multidisciplinary tumor board conference, and both options need to be discussed with the patient. There is no comparative data to indicate which approach has superior disease-related or functional outcomes for this extent of disease. Both primary surgery or chemoradiation are reasonable approaches for extensive disease. Surgery would be recommended for T4 tumors with soft tissue extension because of the lower complication rate associated with primary surgery over salvage after chemoradiation. If surgery is performed, the patient is likely to require a flap (regional or free) reconstruction and adjuvant radiotherapy or chemoradiotherapy. Although chemoradiation may offer cure and larynx preservation for this patient, long-term functional outcomes are unpredictable given the pretreatment functional status. Vocal cord fixation, marked dysphagia, and cartilage erosion are predictors of adverse outcome after chemoradiation. This patient is at high risk of distant metastases, which may be reduced by the addition of chemotherapy; however, there is no conclusive data to demonstrate an overall survival benefit.

Treatment of the Primary Tumor and Neck The patient was assessed at a multidisciplinary tumor board and a recommendation of surgical therapy was made; however, this patient elected to undergo an organ-preservation approach with concurrent chemoradiation. Patients need extensive performance status workup prior to chemotherapy including assessment of hematologic, liver, and renal function. The concurrent chemoradiation regimen given was 100 mg/m^2 cisplatin for 3 cycles on days 1, 22, and 43 with standard fractionation radiotherapy (70 Gy in 2 Gy per fraction over 7 weeks).

The nodal disease was managed with bilateral irradiation. Clinically, this patient had a complete response; however, on a follow-up PET-CT scan at 3 months, there was persistent uptake in the ipsilateral neck consistent with persistent nodal disease. There was no uptake at the primary site. A fine-needle aspiration was suspicious for persistent nodal disease. A salvage neck dissection was recommended. A direct endoscopy was performed prior to the neck dissection to assess the response at the primary site. Examination showed a complete response and frozen-section analysis of biopsies from the primary site were negative, and therefore we proceeded with a modified radical neck dissection performed with preservation of the accessory nerve. Final pathology found metastatic SCC in 4 of 52 lymph nodes. Although his tracheotomy was able to be decannulated, his vocal function was impaired and he was able to maintain a soft diet only.

Case 3 Recurrent T4 N0 M0 postcricoid carcinoma after concurrent chemoradiation.

Presentation This third patient is a 62-year-old man who was treated in 2003 for a T3 N2b M0 postcricoid SCC with

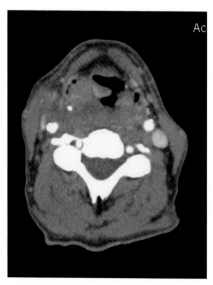

Figure 3–9 Case 2: Axial CT scan of right piriform sinus cancer.

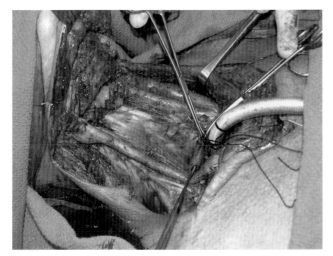

Figure 3–10 Case 3: Total (circumferential) laryngopharyngectomy defect.

concurrent chemoradiation. He required a G-tube and tracheotomy during treatment and was unable to be decannulated or have the G-tube removed after the completion of treatment. Approximately 6 months after treatment, he developed progressive odynophagia. On flexible endoscopy, persistent edema and ulceration of the postcricoid region was noted. Vocal cord mobility was severely limited bilaterally. Neck examination was difficult because of fibrosis.

Diagnosis and Workup A PET-CT scan was obtained, which revealed uptake at the primary site and neck. CT scan of the neck showed soft tissue thickening in the postcricoid region extending to the inferior aspect of the cricoid. Direct endoscopy was performed under general anesthesia confirming the findings seen on flexible examination. There was no extension of the lesion to the cervical esophagus. Biopsy of the ulcer was obtained, and frozen-

section confirmed recurrent squamous cell cancer. Based on the imaging and endoscopy, the recurrent disease was deemed to be resectable.

Treatment Options Surgical salvage, where possible, is the preferred modality for managing recurrent hypopharyngeal cancer. Reirradiation with or without chemotherapy is associated with significant morbidity and was not recommended for this patient. The main clinical decision for this patient is the best method of reconstruction, which will depend upon the extent of resection and previous therapy (radiation with or without chemotherapy). Options for reconstruction of a circumferential laryngopharyngeal defect without esophagectomy include regional and free tissue flaps. The most widely used regional flap is the pectoralis major flap; however, we would not recommend this reconstruction due to the difficulty tubing this flap and the poor functional outcome. Free flap options include either fasciocutaneous or enteric flaps. The anterolateral thigh is our preferred fasciocutaneous flap reconstruction because of the low donor site morbidity and fistula rate. The most widely used enteric flap is free jejunum; however, our preference for these high-risk reconstructions is the gastroomental free flap. Patients who have undergone prior chemoradiation are at high risk of fistula, wound complications, and potential major vessel rupture. The gastroomental flap has the advantage of highly vascular omentum to wrap around the pharyngeal anastomoses and major vessels, and we believe that the speech and swallowing outcomes are superior to jejunum.

Treatment of the Primary Tumor and Neck Referral was made to a speech therapist to discuss voice rehabilitation, and the patient was in agreement with the management plan. A total laryngopharyngectomy was performed along with bilateral level II to IV neck dissections for potential occult disease and vessel preparation (**Fig. 3–10**). A gastroomental flap (**Figs. 3–11, 3–12,** and **3–13**) was chosen

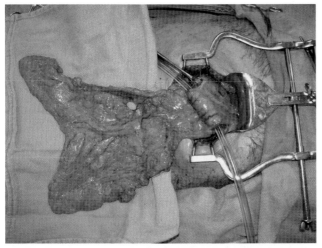

Figure 3–11 Case 3: Gastroomental flap being harvested. The greater curvature and omentum are taken. A chest tube is placed through the stomach, and a gastrointestinal anastomosis (GIA) stapler is then used to divide the stomach above the chest tube.

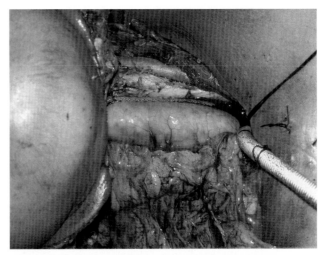

Figure 3–12 Inset of the gastroomental flap into the total laryngopharyngectomy defect.

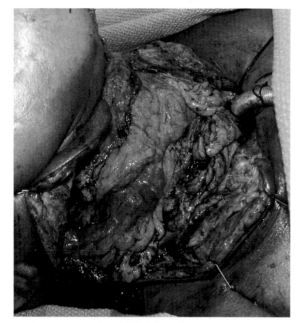

Figure 3–13 Gastroomental free flap inset with omentum draped over the flap and the necks providing coverage of the carotid arteries and left internal jugular vein.

for reconstruction because of the poor wound-healing abilities of chemoirradiated tissue. The patient recovered without any complications, and a secondary TEP was performed at a later date.

References

1. Roboson A. Evidence-based management of hypopharyngeal cancer. Clin Otolaryngol 2002;27:413–420
2. Helliwell TR. ACP Best Practice No 169. Evidence based pathology: squamous carcinoma of the hypopharynx. J Clin Pathol 2003;56:81–85
3. Muir C, Weiland L. Upper aerodigestive tract cancers. Cancer 1995;75:147–153
4. Hoffman HT, Karnell LH, Funk GF, Robinson RA, Menck HR. The National Cancer Data Base report on cancer of the head and neck. Arch Otolaryngol Head Neck Surg 1998;124:951–962
5. Menvielle G, Luce D, Goldberg P, Bugel I, Leclerc A. Smoking, alcohol drinking and cancer risk for various sites of the larynx and hypopharynx. A case-control study in France. Eur J Cancer Prev 2004;13:165–172
6. Parkin DMWS, Ferlay J, Raymond L, Young J. Cancer Incidence in Five Continents. Lyon, France: International Agency for Research on Cancer; 1997
7. Carvalho AL, Nishimoto IN, Califano JA, Kowalski LP. Trends in incidence and prognosis for head and neck cancer in the United States: a site-specific analysis of the SEER database. Int J Cancer 2005;114:806–816
8. Shah JP, Shaha AR, Spiro RH, Strong EW. Carcinoma of the hypopharynx. Am J Surg 1976;132:439–443
9. Carpenter RJ, DeSanto LW. Cancer of the hypopharynx. Surg Clin North Am 1977;57:723–735
10. Pingree TF, Davis RK, Reichman O, Derrick L. Treatment of hypopharyngeal carcinoma: a 10-year review of 1,362 cases. Laryngoscope 1987;97:901–904
11. Wenig B. Atlas of Head and Neck Pathology. Philadelphia, PA: W.B. Saunders; 1993
12. Sobin LHWC. TNM Classification of Malignant Tumors. New York, NY: Wiley-Liss; 2002
13. Hoffman HT, Karnell LH, Shah JP, et al. Hypopharyngeal cancer patient care evaluation. Laryngoscope 1997;107:1005–1017
14. El Badawi SA, Goepfert H, Fletcher GH, Herson J, Oswald MJ. Squamous cell carcinoma of the pyriform sinus. Laryngoscope 1982;92:357–364
15. Kirchner JA. Pyriform sinus cancer: a clinical and laboratory study. Ann Otol Rhinol Laryngol 1975;84:793–803
16. Davidson J, Briant D, Gullane P, Keane T, Rawlinson E. The role of surgery following radiotherapy failure for advanced laryngopharyngeal cancer. A prospective study. Arch Otolaryngol Head Neck Surg 1994;120:269–276
17. Van den Bogaert W, Ostyn F, Lemkens P, van der Schueren E. Are postoperative complications more frequent and more serious after irradiation for laryngeal and hypopharyngeal cancer? Radiother Oncol 1984;2:31–36
18. Arriagada R, Eschwege F, Cachin Y, Richard JM. The value of combining radiotherapy with surgery in the treatment of hypopharyngeal and laryngeal cancers. Cancer 1983;51:1819–1825
19. Gourin CG, Terris DJ. Carcinoma of the hypopharynx. Surg Oncol Clin N Am 2004;13:81–98
20. Son YH, Habermalz HJ. Prognostic factors in pyriform sinus carcinoma. Acta Radiol Oncol Radiat Phys Biol 1979;18:561–571
21. Pfister DGHK, Lefebvre JL. Cancer of the hypopharynx and cervical esophagus. In: Harrison LB SR, Hong WK, eds. Head and Neck Cancer: A Multidisciplinary Approach. Philadelphia, PA: Lippincott Williams & Wilkins; 2004:404–454
22. Schechter GL, Kalafsky JT. Cancer of the hypopharynx and cervical esophagus: management concepts. Oncology 1988;2:17–34
23. Stell PM. Cancer of the hypopharynx. J R Coll Surg Edinb 1973;18:20–30
24. Davidge-Pitts KJ, Manne IA. Pharyngolaryngectomy with extrathoracic esophagectomy. Head Neck Surg 1983;6:571–574
25. Kraus DH, Pfister DG, Harrison LB, et al. Salvage laryngectomy for unsuccessful larynx preservation therapy. Ann Otol Rhinol Laryngol 1995;104:936–941
26. Ho CM, Lam KH, Wei WI, Yuen PW, Lam LK. Squamous cell carcinoma of the hypopharynx–analysis of treatment results. Head Neck 1993;15:405–412
27. Million RRCN, Mancuso AA. Hypopharynx: pharyngeal walls, pyriform sinus, postcricoid pharynx. In: Million RRCN, ed. Management of Head and Neck Cancer. Philadelphia, PA: J.B. Lippincott; 1994:505–532
28. Montgomery PQ, Henk JM. Tumors of the hypopharynx. In: Rhys Evans PHMP, Gullane PJ, eds. Principles and Practice of Head and Neck Oncology. London, UK: Martin Duntz; 2003:253–277
29. Adams GL. Malignant tumors of the larynx and hypopharynx. In: Cummings CWFJ, Harker LA, Krause CJ, Richardson MA, Schuller DE, eds. Otolaryngology Head and Neck Surgery. St. Louis, MO: Mosby; 1998:2130–2175
30. Sinnatamby C. Last's Anatomy: Regional and Applied. Philadelphia, PA: Churchill Livingstone; 1999
31. Deleyiannis FW, Piccirillo JF, Kirchner JA. Relative prognostic importance of histologic invasion of the laryngeal framework by hypopharyngeal cancer. Ann Otol Rhinol Laryngol 1996;105:101–108
32. Olofsson J, van Nostrand AW. Growth and spread of laryngeal and hypopharyngeal carcinoma with reflections on the effect of preoperative irradiation. 139 cases studied by whole organ serial sectioning. Acta Otolaryngol Suppl 1973;308:1–84
33. Wei WI. The dilemma of treating hypopharyngeal carcinoma: more or less: Hayes Martin Lecture. Arch Otolaryngol Head Neck Surg 2002;128:229–232
34. Tani M, Amatsu M. Discrepancies between clinical and histopathologic diagnoses in T3 pyriform sinus cancer. Laryngoscope 1987;97:93–96
35. Kraus DH, Pfister DG, Harrison LB, et al. Larynx preservation with combined chemotherapy and radiation therapy in advanced hypopharynx cancer. Otolaryngol Head Neck Surg 1994;111:31–37
36. Sessions RBPC. Malignant cervical adenopathy. In: Cummings CWFJ, Harker LA, Krause CJ, Richardson MA, Schuller DE, eds. Otolaryngology Head and Neck Surgery. St. Louis, MO: Mosby; 1998:1737–1755
37. Ballantyne AJ. Significance of retropharyngeal nodes in cancer of the head and neck. Am J Surg 1964;108:500–504
38. PunT GD, Perez-Ordonez B, Rafferty M, Irish J. Mucosal melanoma of the hypopharynx. Univ Toronto Med J 2005;82:183–189
39. Nakamizo M, Yokoshima K, Sugisaki Y. Malignant fibrous histiocytoma of the hypopharynx: a case report in a young adult. J Nippon Med Sch 2004;71:301–305
40. Mouret P. Liposarcoma of the hypopharynx. A case report and review of the literature. Rev Laryngol Otol Rhinol (Bord) 1999;120:39–42
41. Artico R, Bison E, Brotto M. Monophasic synovial sarcoma of hypopharynx: case report and review of the literature. Acta Otorhinolaryngol Ital 2004;24:33–36

42. Forastiere A, Koch W, Trotti A, Sidransky D. Head and neck cancer. N Engl J Med 2001;345:1890–1900

43. Maier H, Sennewald E, Heller GF, Weidauer H. Chronic alcohol consumption–the key risk factor for pharyngeal cancer. Otolaryngol Head Neck Surg 1994;110:168–173

44. Jones PH, Farrington WT, Weighill JS. Surgical salvage in postcricoid cancer. J Laryngol Otol 1986;100:85–95

45. Wahlberg PC, Andersson KE, Biorklund AT, Moller TR. Carcinoma of the hypopharynx: analysis of incidence and survival in Sweden over a 30-year period. Head Neck 1998;20:714–719

46. Wynder EL, Hultberg S, Jacobsson F, Bross IJ. Environmental factors in cancer of the upper alimentary tract; a Swedish study with special reference to Plummer-Vinson (Paterson-Kelly) syndrome. Cancer 1957;10:470–487

47. Larsson LG, Sandstrom A, Westling P. Relationship of Plummer-Vinson disease to cancer of the upper alimentary tract in Sweden. Cancer Res 1975;35:3308–3316

48. Mineta H, Ogino T, Amano HM, et al. Human papilloma virus (HPV) type 16 and 18 detected in head and neck squamous cell carcinoma. Anticancer Res 1998;18:4765–4768

49. Rodrigo JP, Alvarez I, Martinez JA, Lazo PS, Ramos S, Suarez C. Relationship of human papillomavirus to ploidy in squamous cell carcinomas of the head and neck. Otolaryngol Head Neck Surg 1999;121:318–322

50. Rodrigo JP, Gonzalez MV, Lazo PS, et al. Genetic alterations in squamous cell carcinomas of the hypopharynx with correlations to clinicopathological features. Oral Oncol 2002;38:357–363

51. Shimakage M, Sasagawa T, Yoshino K, et al. Expression of Epstein-Barr virus in mesopharyngeal and hypopharyngeal carcinomas. Hum Pathol 1999;30:1071–1076

52. Zhou L, Miyagi Y, Hiroshi E, Tanaka Y, Aoki I, Tsukuda M. Evaluation of Epstein-Barr Virus infection in hypopharyngeal carcinomas from 37 Japanese patients. Mod Pathol 1998;11:509–512

53. Chien CY, Huang CC, Cheng JT, Chen CM, Hwang CF, Su CY. The clinicopathological significance of p53 and p21 expression in squamous cell carcinoma of hypopharyngeal cancer. Cancer Lett 2003;201:217–223

54. Rodrigo JP, Suarez C, Gonzalez MV, et al. Variability of genetic alterations in different sites of head and neck cancer. Laryngoscope 2001;111:1297–1301

55. Nimeus E, Baldetorp B, Bendahl PO, et al. Amplification of the cyclin D1 gene is associated with tumour subsite, DNA non-diploidy and high S-phase fraction in squamous cell carcinoma of the head and neck. Oral Oncol 2004;40:624–629

56. Meredith SD, Levine PA, Burns JA, et al. Chromosome 11q13 amplification in head and neck squamous cell carcinoma. Association with poor prognosis. Arch Otolaryngol Head Neck Surg 1995;121:790–794

57. Greene FPD, Fleming I, Page DL, et al. Cancer Staging Manual. 6th ed. New York, NY: Springer-Verlag; 2002:220

58. Irish J, Siu L, Lee A. Head and neck cancer. In: Pollock RE, Nakao A, O'Sullivan BO, eds. UICC Manual of Clinical Oncology. Hoboken, NJ: John Wiley & Sons; 2004:335–358

59. Spector JG, Sessions DG, Emami B, et al. Squamous cell carcinoma of the pyriform sinus: a nonrandomized comparison of therapeutic modalities and long-term results. Laryngoscope 1995;105:397–406

60. Stefani S, Eells RW. Carcinoma of the hypopharynx–a study of distant metastases, treatment failures, and multiple primary cancers in 215 male patients. Laryngoscope 1971;81:1491–1498

61. Jones AS, Stell PM. Squamous carcinoma of the posterior pharyngeal wall. Clin Otolaryngol Allied Sci 1991;16:462–465

62. Spector JG, Sessions DG, Haughey BH, et al. Delayed regional metastases, distant metastases, and second primary malignancies in squamous cell carcinomas of the larynx and hypopharynx. Laryngoscope 2001;111:1079–1087

63. Pene F, Avedian V, Eschwege F, et al. A retrospective study of 131 cases of carcinoma of the posterior pharyngeal wall. Cancer 1978;42:2490–2493

64. Godballe C, Jorgensen K, Hansen O, Bastholt L. Hypopharyngeal cancer: results of treatment based on radiation therapy and salvage surgery. Laryngoscope 2002;112:834–838

65. Katsantonis GP, Archer CR, Rosenblum BN, Yeager VL, Friedman WH. The degree to which accuracy of preoperative staging of laryngeal carcinoma has been enhanced by computed tomography. Otolaryngol Head Neck Surg 1986;95:52–62

66. Teresi LM, Lufkin RB, Hanafee WN. Magnetic resonance imaging of the larynx. Radiol Clin North Am 1989;27:393–406

67. Wenig BL, Ziffra KL, Mafee MF, Schild JA. MR imaging of squamous cell carcinoma of the larynx and hypopharynx. Otolaryngol Clin North Am 1995;28:609–619

68. Spector GJ. Distant metastases from laryngeal and hypopharyngeal cancer. ORL J Otorhinolaryngol Relat Spec 2001;63:224–228

69. Kotwall C, Sako K, Razack MS, Rao U, Bakamjian V, Shedd DP. Metastatic patterns in squamous cell cancer of the head and neck. Am J Surg 1987;154:439–442

70. Eckel HE, Staar S, Volling P, Sittel C, Damm M, Jungehuelsing M. Surgical treatment for hypopharynx carcinoma: feasibility, mortality, and results. Otolaryngol Head Neck Surg 2001;124:561–569

71. Dalley VM. Cancer of the laryngopharynx. J Laryngol Otol 1968;82:407–419

72. Barkley HT Jr, Fletcher GH, Jesse RH, Lindberg RD. Management of cervical lymph node metastases in squamous cell carcinoma of the tonsillar fossa, base of tongue, supraglottic larynx, and hypopharynx. Am J Surg 1972;124:462–467

73. Lefebvre JL, Castelain B, De la Torre JC, Delobelle-Deroide A, Vankemmel B. Lymph node invasion in hypopharynx and lateral epilarynx carcinoma: a prognostic factor. Head Neck Surg 1987;10:14–18

74. Peters LJ, Goepfert H, Ang KK, et al. Evaluation of the dose for postoperative radiation therapy of head and neck cancer: first report of a prospective randomized trial. Int J Radiat Oncol Biol Phys 1993;26:3–11

75. Hahn SS, Spaulding CA, Kim JA, Constable WC. The prognostic significance of lymph node involvement in pyriform sinus and supraglottic cancers. Int J Radiat Oncol Biol Phys 1987;13:1143–1147

76. Ogura JH, Biller HF, Wette R. Elective neck dissection for pharyngeal and laryngeal cancers. An evaluation. Ann Otol Rhinol Laryngol 1971;80:646–650

77. Marks JE, Devineni VR, Harvey J, Sessions DG. The risk of contralateral lymphatic metastases for cancers of the larynx and pharynx. Am J Otolaryngol 1992;13:34–39

78. Buckley JG, MacLennan K. Cervical node metastases in laryngeal and hypopharyngeal cancer: a prospective analysis of prevalence and distribution. Head Neck 2000;22:380–385

79. Schusterman MA, Shestak K, de Vries EJ, et al. Reconstruction of the cervical esophagus: free jejunal transfer versus gastric pull-up. Plast Reconstr Surg 1990;85:16–21

80. Candela FC, Kothari K, Shah JP. Patterns of cervical node metastases from squamous carcinoma of the oropharynx and hypopharynx. Head Neck 1990;12:197–203

81. Pameijer FA, Mancuso AA, Mendenhall WM, et al. Evaluation of pretreatment computed tomography as a predictor of local control in T1/T2 pyriform sinus carcinoma treated with definitive radiotherapy. Head Neck 1998;20:159–168

82. Newkirk KA, Cullen KJ, Harter KW, Picken CA, Sessions RB, Davidson BJ. Planned neck dissection for advanced primary head and neck malignancy treated with organ preservation therapy: disease control and survival outcomes. Head Neck 2001;23:73–79

83. Yao M, Graham MM, Hoffman HT, et al. The role of post-radiation therapy FDG PET in prediction of necessity for post-radiation therapy neck dissection in locally advanced head-and-neck squamous cell carcinoma. Int J Radiat Oncol Biol Phys 2004;59:1001–1010

84. Hasegawa Y, Matsuura H. Retropharyngeal node dissection in cancer of the oropharynx and hypopharynx. Head Neck 1994;16:173–180

85. Timon CV, Toner M, Conlon BJ. Paratracheal lymph node involvement in advanced cancer of the larynx, hypopharynx, and cervical esophagus. Laryngoscope 2003;113:1595–1599

86. Martins AS. Neck and mediastinal node dissection in pharyngolaryngoesophageal tumors. Head Neck 2001;23:772–779

87. Clayman GL, Weber RS, Guillamondegui O, et al. Laryngeal preservation for advanced laryngeal and hypopharyngeal cancers. Arch Otolaryngol Head Neck Surg 1995;121:219–223

88. Steiner W, Ambrosch P, Hess CF, Kron M. Organ preservation by transoral laser microsurgery in piriform sinus carcinoma. Otolaryngol Head Neck Surg 2001;124:58–67

89. Mamelle G, Pampurik J, Luboinski B, Lancar R, Lusinchi A, Bosq J. Lymph node prognostic factors in head and neck squamous cell carcinomas. Am J Surg 1994;168:494–498

90. Futrell JW, Bennett SH, Hoye RC, Roth JA, Ketcham AS. Predicting survival in cancer of the larynx or hypopharynx. Am J Surg 1971;122:451–457

91. Marks JE, Freeman RB, Lee F, Ogura JH. Pharyngeal wall cancer: an analysis of treatment results complications and patterns of failure. Int J Radiat Oncol Biol Phys 1978;4:587–593

92. Kraus DH, Zelefsky MJ, Brock HA, Huo J, Harrison LB, Shah JP. Combined surgery and radiation therapy for squamous cell carcinoma of the hypopharynx. Otolaryngol Head Neck Surg 1997;116:637–641

93. Haughey BH, Gates GA, Arfken CL, Harvey J. Meta-analysis of second malignant tumors in head and neck cancer: the case for an endoscopic screening protocol. Ann Otol Rhinol Laryngol 1992;101:105–112

94. Alvi A, Johnson JT. Development of distant metastasis after treatment of advanced-stage head and neck cancer. Head Neck 1997;19:500–505

95. Rudert HH, Hoft S. Transoral carbon-dioxide laser resection of hypopharyngeal carcinoma. Eur Arch Otorhinolaryngol 2003;260:198–206

96. Vilaseca I, Blanch JL, Bernal-Sprekelsen M, Moragas M. CO2 laser surgery: a larynx preservation alternative for selected hypopharyngeal carcinomas. Head Neck 2004;26:953–959

97. Chevalier D, Watelet JB, Darras JA, Piquet JJ. Supraglottic hemilaryngopharyngectomy plus radiation for the treatment of early lateral margin and pyriform sinus carcinoma. Head Neck 1997;19:1–5

98. Laccourreye O, Merite-Drancy A, Brasnu D, et al. Supracricoid hemilaryngopharyngectomy in selected pyriform sinus carcinoma staged as T2. Laryngoscope 1993;103:1373–1379

99. Lefebvre JL. What is the role of primary surgery in the treatment of laryngeal and hypopharyngeal cancer? Hayes Martin Lecture. Arch Otolaryngol Head Neck Surg 2000;126:285–288

100. Kim S, Wu HG, Heo DS, Kim KH, Sung MW, Park CI. Advanced hypopharyngeal carcinoma treatment results according to treatment modalities. Head Neck 2001;23:713–717

101. Chu PY, Wang LW, Chang SY. Surgical treatment of squamous cell carcinoma of the hypopharynx: analysis of treatment results, failure patterns, and prognostic factors. J Laryngol Otol 2004;118:443–449

102. Wenig BL, Applebaum EL. The submandibular triangle in squamous cell carcinoma of the larynx and hypopharynx. Laryngoscope 1991;101:516–518

103. Bernal-Sprekelsen M, Vilaseca-Gonzalez I, Blanch-Alejandro JL. Predictive values for aspiration after endoscopic laser resections of malignant tumors of the hypopharynx and larynx. Head Neck 2004;26:103–110

104. Glanz H [Pathomorphological aspects of transoral resection of hypopharyngeal carcinoma with preservation of the larynx. Patient selection, treatment results.] Laryngorhinootologie 1999;78:654–662

105. Zeitels SM, Koufman JA, Davis RK, Vaughan CW. Endoscopic treatment of supraglottic and hypopharynx cancer. Laryngoscope 1994;104:71–78

106. Amdur RJ, Parsons JT, Mendenhall WM, Million RR, Stringer SP, Cassisi NJ. Postoperative irradiation for squamous cell carcinoma of the head and neck: an analysis of treatment results and complications. Int J Radiat Oncol Biol Phys 1989;16:25–36

107. Florant A, Berreby S, Gilain L, et al. [Functional surgery of cancer of the hypopharynx. Hemilaryngopharyngectomy, posterior pharyngectomy by bilateral cervical approach.] Ann Otolaryngol Chir Cervicofac 1986;103:443–453

108. Lecanu JB, Monceaux G, Perie S, Angelard B, St Guily JL. Conservative surgery in T3-T4 pharyngolaryngeal squamous cell carcinoma: an alternative to radiation therapy and to total laryngectomy for good responders to induction chemotherapy. Laryngoscope 2000;110:412–416

109. Ogura JH, Jurema AA, Watson RK. Partial laryngopharyngectomy and neck dissection for pyriform sinus cancer. Conservation surgery with immediate reconstruction. Laryngoscope 1960;70:1399–1417

110. Ogura JH, Mallen RW. Partial laryngopharyngectomy for supraglottic and pharyngeal carcinoma. Trans Am Acad Ophthalmol Otolaryngol 1965;69:832–845

111. Pearson BW. Subtotal laryngectomy. Laryngoscope 1981;91:1904–1912

112. Dumich PS, Pearson BW, Weiland LH. Suitability of near-total laryngopharyngectomy in piriform carcinoma. Arch Otolaryngol 1984;110:664–669

113. Clark J dA J, Gilbert R, Irish J, Brown D, Neligan P, Gullane P. Primary and salvage hypo(pharyngectomy): analysis and outcome. Head Neck 2006;28:671–677

114. Thorp MA, Levitt NS, Mortimore S, Isaacs S. Parathyroid and thyroid function five years after treatment of laryngeal and hypopharyngeal carcinoma. Clin Otolaryngol Allied Sci 1999;24:104–108

115. Spriano G, Pellini R, Roselli R. Pectoralis major myocutaneous flap for hypopharyngeal reconstruction. Plast Reconstr Surg 2002;110:1408–1413; discussion 1414–1406

116. Shangold LM, Urken ML, Lawson W. Jejunal transplantation for pharyngoesophageal reconstruction. Otolaryngol Clin North Am 1991;24:1321–1342

117. Takato T, Harii K, Ebihara S, Ono I, Yoshizumi T, Nakatsuka T. Oral and pharyngeal reconstruction using the free forearm flap. Arch Otolaryngol Head Neck Surg 1987;113:873–879

118. Nakatsuka T, Harii K, Asato H, Ebihara S, Yoshizumi T, Saikawa M. Comparative evaluation in pharyngo-oesophageal reconstruction: radial forearm flap compared with jejunal flap. A 10-year experience. Scand J Plast Reconstr Surg Hand Surg 1998;32:307–310

119. Makitie AA, Beasley NJ, Neligan PC, Lipa J, Gullane PJ, Gilbert RW. Head and neck reconstruction with anterolateral thigh flap. Otolaryngol Head Neck Surg 2003;129:547–555

120. Clark J, Gilbert R, Irish J, Brown D, Neligan P, Gullane PJ. Morbidity following flap reconstruction of hypopharyngeal defects. Laryngoscope 2006;116:173–181

121. Chang DW, Hussussian C, Lewin JS, Youssef AA, Robb GL, Reece GP. Analysis of pharyngocutaneous fistula following free jejunal transfer for total laryngopharyngectomy. Plast Reconstr Surg 2002;109:1522–1527

122. Wei WI, Lam LK, Yuen PW, Wong J. Current status of pharyngolaryngo-esophagectomy and pharyngogastric anastomosis. Head Neck 1998;20:240–244

123. Silver CE, Cusumano RJ, Fell SC, Strauch B. Replacement of upper esophagus: results with myocutaneous flap and with gastric transposition. Laryngoscope 1989;99:819–821

124. Lam KH, Wong J, Lim ST, Ong GB. Pharyngogastric anastomosis following pharyngolaryngoesophagectomy. Analysis of 157 cases. World J Surg 1981;5:509–516

125. Le Quesne LP, Ranger D. Pharyngolaryngectomy, with immediate pharyngogastric anastomosis. Br J Surg 1966;53:105–109

126. Cahow CE, Sasaki CT. Gastric pull-up reconstruction for pharyngolaryngo-esophagectomy. Arch Surg 1994;129:425–429; discussion 429–430

127. Marmuse JP, Koka VN, Guedon C, Benhamou G. Surgical treatment of carcinoma of the proximal esophagus. Am J Surg 1995;169:386–390

128. Bardini R, Ruol A, Peracchia A. Therapeutic options for cancer of the hypopharynx and cervical oesophagus. Ann Chir Gynaecol 1995;84:202–207

129. Goldberg M, Freeman J, Gullane PJ, Patterson GA, Todd TR, McShane D. Transhiatal esophagectomy with gastric transposition for pharyngolaryngeal malignant disease. J Thorac Cardiovasc Surg 1989;97:327–333

130. Fabian RL. Reconstruction of the laryngopharynx and cervical esophagus. Laryngoscope 1984;94:1334–1350

131. Jones AS, Roland NJ, Husband D, Hamilton JW, Gati I. Free revascularized jejunal loop repair following total pharyngolaryngectomy for carcinoma of the hypopharynx: report of 90 patients. Br J Surg 1996;83:1279–1283

132. Lewin JS, Barringer DA, May AH, et al. Functional outcomes after circumferential pharyngoesophageal reconstruction. Laryngoscope 2005;115:1266–1271

133. Chen HC, Tang YB. Microsurgical reconstruction of the esophagus. Semin Surg Oncol 2000;19:235–245

134. Peters CR, McKee DM, Berry BE. Pharyngoesophageal reconstruction with revascularized jejunal transplants. Am J Surg 1971;121:675–678

135. Gherardini G, Gurlek A, Staley C , Ross DA, Pazmino BP, Miller MJ. Laparoscopic harvesting of jejunal free flaps for esophageal reconstruction. Plast Reconstr Surg 1998;102:473–477

136. Wadsworth JT, Futran N, Eubanks TR. Laparoscopic harvest of the jejunal free flap for reconstruction of hypopharyngeal and cervical esophageal defects. Arch Otolaryngol Head Neck Surg 2002;128:1384–1387

137. Reece GP, Bengtson BP, Schusterman MA. Reconstruction of the pharynx and cervical esophagus using free jejunal transfer. Clin Plast Surg 1994;21:125–136

138. Kerlin P, McCafferty GJ, Robinson DW, Theile D. Function of a free jejunal "conduit" graft in the cervical esophagus. Gastroenterology 1986;90:1956–1963

139. Mendelsohn M, Morris M, Gallagher R. A comparative study of speech after total laryngectomy and total laryngopharyngectomy. Arch Otolaryngol Head Neck Surg 1993;119:508–510

140. Genden EM, Kaufman MR, Katz B, Vine A, Urken ML. Tubed gastro-omental free flap for pharyngoesophageal reconstruction. Arch Otolaryngol Head Neck Surg 2001;127:847–853

141. Righini CA, Bettega G, Lequeux T, Chaffanjeon P, Lebeau J, Reyt E. Use of tubed gastro-omental free flap for hypopharynx and cervical esophagus reconstruction after total laryngo-pharyngectomy. Eur Arch Otorhinolaryngol 2005;262:362–367

142. Yu P. Characteristics of the anterolateral thigh flap in a Western population and its application in head and neck reconstruction. Head Neck 2004;26:759–769

143. Scharpf J, Esclamado RM. Reconstruction with radial forearm flaps after ablative surgery for hypopharyngeal cancer. Head Neck 2003;25:261–266

144. Azizzadeh B, Yafai S, Rawnsley JD, et al. Radial forearm free flap pharyngoesophageal reconstruction. Laryngoscope 2001;111:807–810

145. Anthony JP, Singer MI, Deschler DG, Dougherty ET, Reed CG, Kaplan MJ. Long-term functional results after pharyngoesophageal reconstruction with the radial forearm free flap. Am J Surg 1994;168:441–445

146. Anthony JP, Singer MI, Mathes SJ. Pharyngoesophageal reconstruction using the tubed free radial forearm flap. Clin Plast Surg 1994;21:137–147

147. Deschler DG, Doherty ET, Reed CG, Anthony JP, Singer MI. Tracheoesophageal voice following tubed free radial forearm flap reconstruction of the neopharynx. Ann Otol Rhinol Laryngol 1994;103:929–936

148. Kelly KE, Anthony JP, Singer M. Pharyngoesophageal reconstruction using the radial forearm fasciocutaneous free flap: preliminary results. Otolaryngol Head Neck Surg 1994;111:16–24

149. Kato H, Watanabe H, Iizuka T, et al. Primary esophageal reconstruction after resection of the cancer in the hypopharynx or cervical esophagus: comparison of free forearm skin tube flap, free jejunal transplantation and pull-through esophagectomy. Jpn J Clin Oncol 1987;17:255–261

150. Varvares MA, Cheney ML, Gliklich RE, et al. Use of the radial forearm fasciocutaneous free flap and montgomery salivary bypass tube for pharyngoesophageal reconstruction. Head Neck 2000;22:463–468

151. Ganly I, Kaye SB. Recurrent squamous-cell carcinoma of the head and neck: overview of current therapy and future prospects. Ann Oncol 2000;11:11–16

152. Chmura SJ, Milano MT, Haraf DJ. Reirradiation of recurrent head and neck cancers with curative intent. Semin Oncol 2004;31:816–821

153. Goodwin WJ Jr. Salvage surgery for patients with recurrent squamous cell carcinoma of the upper aerodigestive tract: when do the ends justify the means? Laryngoscope 2000;110:1–18

154. McLaughlin MP, Parsons JT, Fein DA, et al. Salvage surgery after radiotherapy failure in T1–T2 squamous cell carcinoma of the glottic larynx. Head Neck 1996;18:229–235

155. Williams RG. Recurrent head and neck cancer: the results of treatment. Br J Surg 1974;61:691–697

156. Ridge JA. Squamous cancer of the head and neck: surgical treatment of local and regional recurrence. Semin Oncol 1993;20:419–429

157. Stoeckli SJ, Pawlik AB, Lipp M, Huber A, Schmid S. Salvage surgery after failure of nonsurgical therapy for carcinoma of the larynx and hypopharynx. Arch Otolaryngol Head Neck Surg 2000;126:1473–1477

158. Jones AS. The management of early hypopharyngeal cancer: primary radiotherapy and salvage surgery. Clin Otolaryngol Allied Sci 1992;17:545–549

159. Wong LY, Wei WI, Lam LK, Yuen AP. Salvage of recurrent head and neck squamous cell carcinoma after primary curative surgery. Head Neck 2003;25:953–959

160. Johansen LV, Overgaard J, Elbrond O. Pharyngo-cutaneous fistulae after laryngectomy. Influence of previous radiotherapy and prophylactic metronidazole. Cancer 1988;61:673–678

161. Sassler AM, Esclamado RM, Wolf GT. Surgery after organ preservation therapy. Analysis of wound complications. Arch Otolaryngol Head Neck Surg 1995;121:162–165

162. Weber RS, Berkey BA, Forastiere A, et al. Outcome of salvage total laryngectomy following organ preservation therapy: the Radiation Therapy Oncology Group trial 91–11. Arch Otolaryngol Head Neck Surg 2003;129:44–49

163. Garden AS, Morrison WH, Clayman GL, Ang KK, Peters LJ. Early squamous cell carcinoma of the hypopharynx: outcomes of treatment with radiation alone to the primary disease. Head Neck 1996;18:317–322

164. Fein DA, Mendenhall WM, Parsons JT, Stringer SP, Cassisi NJ, Million RR. Pharyngeal wall carcinoma treated with radiotherapy: impact of treatment technique and fractionation. Int J Radiat Oncol Biol Phys 1993;26:751–757

165. Horiot JC, Le Fur R, N'Guyen T, et al. Hyperfractionation versus conventional fractionation in oropharyngeal carcinoma: final analysis of a randomized trial of the EORTC cooperative group of radiotherapy. Radiother Oncol 1992;25:231–241

166. Overgaard J, Hansen HS, Specht L, et al. Five compared with six fractions per week of conventional radiotherapy of squamous-cell carcinoma of head and neck: DAHANCA 6 and 7 randomized controlled trial. Lancet 2003;362:933–940

167. Cummings B, Keane T, O'Sullivan B, et al. 5 year results of 4 week/twice daily radiation schedule—The Toronto Trial. Presented at: The 19th Annual Meeting of the European Society of Radiation Oncology (ESTRO); 2000

168. Brizel DM, Albers ME, Fisher SR, et al. Hyperfractionated irradiation with or without concurrent chemotherapy for locally advanced head and neck cancer. N Engl J Med 1998;338:1798–1804

169. Nguyen LN, Ang KK. Radiotherapy for cancer of the head and neck: altered fractionation regimens. Lancet Oncol 2002;3:693–701

170. Amdur RJ, Mendenhall WM, Stringer SP, Villaret DB, Cassisi NJ. Organ preservation with radiotherapy for T1–T2 carcinoma of the pyriform sinus. Head Neck 2001;23:353–362

171. Mendenhall WM, Million RR, Cassisi NJ. Squamous cell carcinoma of the head and neck treated with radiation therapy: the role of neck dissection for clinically positive neck nodes. Int J Radiat Oncol Biol Phys 1986;12:733–740

172. Bataini P, Brugere J, Bernier J, Jaulerry CH, Picot C, Ghossein NA. Results of radical radiotherapeutic treatment of carcinoma of the pyriform sinus: experience of the Institut Curie. Int J Radiat Oncol Biol Phys 1982;8:1277–1286

173. Mendenhall WM, Parsons JT, Devine JW, Cassisi NJ, Million RR. Squamous cell carcinoma of the pyriform sinus treated with surgery and/or radiotherapy. Head Neck Surg 1987;10:88–92

174. Rosenthal DI, Ang KK. Altered radiation therapy fractionation, chemoradiation, and patient selection for the treatment of head and neck squamous carcinoma. Semin Radiat Oncol 2004;14:153–166

175. Wang CC, Blitzer PH, Suit HD. Twice-a-day radiation therapy for cancer of the head and neck. Cancer 1985;55:2100–2104

176. Waldron JN, O'Sullivan B, Irish J, et al. A phase II study of hyperfractionated accelerated radiation delivered with integrated neck surgery (HARDWINS) for advanced squamous cell carcinoma of the head and neck. Int J Radiat Oncol Biol Phys 2000;48:48

177. Bahadur S, Thakar A, Mohanti BK, Lal P. Results of radiotherapy with, or without, salvage combined surgery and radiotherapy in advanced carcinoma of the hypopharynx. J Laryngol Otol 2002;116:29–32

178. Tombolini V, Santarelli M, Raffetto N, et al. Radiotherapy in the treatment of stage III–IV hypopharyngeal carcinoma. Anticancer Res 2004;24:349–354

179. Vikram B, Strong EW, Shah JP, Spiro R. Failure at the primary site following multimodality treatment in advanced head and neck cancer. Head Neck Surg 1984;6:720–723

180. Kramer S, Gelber RD, Snow JB, et al. Combined radiation therapy and surgery in the management of advanced head and neck cancer: final report of study 73–03 of the Radiation Therapy Oncology Group. Head Neck Surg 1987;10:19–30

181. Cancer Care Ontario Head and Neck Group Guidelines. The role of post-operative chemoradiotherapy for squamous cell carcinoma of the head and neck. Toronto, Canada: Cancer Care Ontario Program in Evidence Based Medicine; 2004

182. Frank JL, Garb JL, Kay S, et al. Postoperative radiotherapy improves survival in squamous cell carcinoma of the hypopharynx. Am J Surg 1994;168:476–480

183. Tupchong L, Scott CB, Blitzer PH, et al. Randomized study of preoperative versus postoperative radiation therapy in advanced head and neck carcinoma: long-term follow-up of RTOG study 73–03. Int J Radiat Oncol Biol Phys 1991;20:21–28

184. Vandenbrouck C, Sancho H, Le Fur R, Richard JM, Cachin Y. Results of a randomized clinical trial of preoperative irradiation versus postoperative in treatment of tumors of the hypopharynx. Cancer 1977;39:1445–1449

185. Lin A, Kim HM, Terrell JE, Dawson LA, Ship JA, Eisbruch A. Quality of life after parotid-sparing IMRT for head-and-neck cancer: a prospective longitudinal study. Int J Radiat Oncol Biol Phys 2003;57:61–70

186. Eisbruch A Marsh LH, Dawson LA, et al. Recurrences near base of skull after IMRT for head-and-neck cancer: implications for target delineation in high neck and for parotid gland sparing. Int J Radiat Oncol Biol Phys 2004;59:28–42

187. Pignon JP, Bourhis J, Domenge C, Designe L. Chemotherapy added to locoregional treatment for head and neck squamous-cell carcinoma: three meta-analyses of updated individual data. MACH-NC Collaborative Group. Meta-Analysis of Chemotherapy on Head and Neck Cancer. Lancet 2000;355:949–955

188. Cohen EE, Lingen MW, Vokes EE. The expanding role of systemic therapy in head and neck cancer. J Clin Oncol 2004;22:1743–1752

189. Induction chemotherapy plus radiation compared with surgery plus radiation in patients with advanced laryngeal cancer. The Department of Veterans Affairs Laryngeal Cancer Study Group. N Engl J Med 1991;324:1685–1690

190. Richard JM, Sancho-Garnier H, Pessey JJ, et al. Randomized trial of induction chemotherapy in larynx carcinoma. Oral Oncol 1998;34:224–228

191. Lefebvre JL, Chevalier D, Luboinski B, Kirkpatrick A, Collette L, Sahmoud T. Larynx preservation in pyriform sinus cancer: preliminary results of a European Organization for Research and Treatment of Cancer phase III trial. EORTC Head and Neck Cancer Cooperative Group. J Natl Cancer Inst 1996;88:890–899

192. Altundag O, Gullu I, Altundag K, et al. Induction chemotherapy with cisplatin and 5-fluorouracil followed by chemoradiotherapy or radiotherapy alone in the treatment of locoregionally advanced resectable cancers of the larynx and hypopharynx: results of single-center study of 45 patients. Head Neck 2005;27:15–21

193. Urba SG, Moon J, Giri PG, et al. Organ preservation for advanced resectable cancer of the base of tongue and hypopharynx: a Southwest Oncology Group Trial. J Clin Oncol 2005;23:88–95

194. Cancer Care Ontario Head and Neck Group Guidelines. The role of neoadjuvant chemotherapy in the treatment of locally advanced squamous cell carcinoma of the head and neck (excluding nasopharynx). Toronto, Canada: Cancer Care Ontario Program in Evidence Based Medicine; 2003

195. Jeremic B, Milicic B, Dagovic A, Vaskovic Z, Tadic L. Radiation therapy with or without concurrent low-dose daily chemotherapy in locally advanced, nonmetastatic squamous cell carcinoma of the head and neck. J Clin Oncol 2004;22:3540–3548

196. Forastiere AA, Goepfert H, Maor M, et al. Concurrent chemotherapy and radiotherapy for organ preservation in advanced laryngeal cancer. N Engl J Med 2003;349:2091–2098

197. El-Sayed S, Nelson N. Adjuvant and adjunctive chemotherapy in the management of squamous cell carcinoma of the head and neck region. A meta-analysis of prospective and randomized trials. J Clin Oncol 1996;14:838–847

198. Munro AJ. An overview of randomised controlled trials of adjuvant chemotherapy in head and neck cancer. Br J Cancer 1995;71:83–91

199. Cancer Care Ontario Head and Neck Group Guidelines. Concomitant chemotherapy and radiotherapy in squamous cell head and neck cancer (excluding nasopharynx). Toronto, Canada: Cancer Care Ontario Program in Evidence Based Medicine; 2000

200. Abitbol AA, Sridhar KS, Lewin AA, et al. Hyperfractionated radiation therapy and 5-fluorouracil, cisplatin, and mitomycin-C (+/- granulocyte-colony stimulating factor) in the treatment of patients with locally advanced head and neck carcinoma. Cancer 1997;80:266–276

201. Eisbruch A, Lyden T, Bradford CR, et al. Objective assessment of swallowing dysfunction and aspiration after radiation concurrent with chemotherapy for head-and-neck cancer. Int J Radiat Oncol Biol Phys 2002;53:23–28

202. Smith RV, Kotz T, Beitler JJ, Wadler S. Long-term swallowing problems after organ preservation therapy with concomitant radiation therapy and intravenous hydroxyurea: initial results. Arch Otolaryngol Head Neck Surg 2000;126:384–389

203. Vokes EE, Kies MS, Haraf DJ, et al. Concomitant chemoradiotherapy as primary therapy for locoregionally advanced head and neck cancer. J Clin Oncol 2000;18:1652–1661

204. Koch WM, Lee DJ, Eisele DW, et al. Chemoradiotherapy for organ preservation in oral and pharyngeal carcinoma. Arch Otolaryngol Head Neck Surg 1995;121:974–980

205. Staton J, Robbins KT, Newman L, Samant S, Sebelik M, Vieira F. Factors predictive of poor functional outcome after chemoradiation for advanced laryngeal cancer. Otolaryngol Head Neck Surg 2002;127:43–47

206. Bernier J, Domenge C, Ozsahin M, et al. Postoperative irradiation with or without concomitant chemotherapy for locally advanced head and neck cancer. N Engl J Med 2004;350:1945–1952

207. Cooper JS, Pajak TF, Forastiere AA, et al. Postoperative concurrent radiotherapy and chemotherapy for high-risk squamous-cell carcinoma of the head and neck. N Engl J Med 2004;350:1937–1944

208. Chan AW, Ancukiewicz M, Carballo N, Montgomery W, Wang CC. The role of postradiotherapy neck dissection in supraglottic carcinoma. Int J Radiat Oncol Biol Phys 2001;50:367–375

209. Clayman GL, Johnson CJ II , Morrison W, Ginsberg L, Lippman SM. The role of neck dissection after chemoradiotherapy for oropharyngeal cancer with advanced nodal disease. Arch Otolaryngol Head Neck Surg 2001;127:135–139

210. Johnson CR, Silverman LN, Clay LB, Schmidt-Ullrich R. Radiotherapeutic management of bulky cervical lymphadenopathy in squamous cell carcinoma of the head and neck: is postradiotherapy neck dissection necessary? Radiat Oncol Investig 1998;6:52–57

211. McHam SA, Adelstein DJ, Rybicki LA, et al. Who merits a neck dissection after definitive chemoradiotherapy for N2–N3 squamous cell head and neck cancer? Head Neck 2003;25:791–798

212. Peters LJ, Weber RS, Morrison WH, Byers RM, Garden AS, Goepfert H. Neck surgery in patients with primary oropharyngeal cancer treated by radiotherapy. Head Neck 1996;18:552–559

213. Corry J, Smith JG, Peters LJ. The concept of a planned neck dissection is obsolete. Cancer J 2001;7:472–474

214. Pitman KT, Bradley PJ. Management of the N3 neck. Curr Opin Otolaryngol Head Neck Surg 2003;11:129–133

215. Bernier J, Bataini JP. Regional outcome in oropharyngeal and pharyngolaryngeal cancer treated with high dose per fraction radiotherapy. Analysis of neck disease response in 1646 cases. Radiother Oncol 1986;6:87–103

216. Bollet MA, Lapeyre M, Marchal C, et al. Cervical lymph node relapses of head-and-neck squamous cell carcinoma: is brachytherapy a therapeutic option? Int J Radiat Oncol Biol Phys 2001;51:1305–1312

217. Mabanta SR, Mendenhall WM, Stringer SP, Cassisi NJ. Salvage treatment for neck recurrence after irradiation alone for head and neck squamous cell carcinoma with clinically positive neck nodes. Head Neck 1999;21:591–594

218. Mendenhall WM, Villaret DB, Amdur RJ, Hinerman RW, Mancuso AA. Planned neck dissection after definitive radiotherapy for squamous cell carcinoma of the head and neck. Head Neck 2002;24:1012–1018

219. Parsons JT, Mendenhall WM, Cassisi NJ, Stringer SP, Million RR. Neck dissection after twice-a-day radiotherapy: morbidity and recurrence rates. Head Neck 1989;11:400–404

220. Ellis ER, Mendenhall WM, Rao PV, et al. Incisional or excisional neck-node biopsy before definitive radiotherapy, alone or followed by neck dissection. Head Neck 1991;13:177–183

221. Yao M, Smith RB, Graham MM, et al. The role of FDG pet in management of neck metastasis from head-and-neck cancer after definitive radiation treatment. Int J Radiat Oncol Biol Phys 2005;63:991–999

222. Yao M, Graham MM, Smith RB, et al. Value of FDG PET in assessment of treatment response and surveillance in head-and-neck cancer patients after intensity modulated radiation treatment: a preliminary report. Int J Radiat Oncol Biol Phys 2004;60:1410–1418

223. Porceddu SV, Jarmolowski E, Hicks RJ, et al. Utility of positron emission tomography for the detection of disease in residual neck nodes after (chemo)radiotherapy in head and neck cancer. Head Neck 2005;27:175–181

224. Creak AL, Harrington K, Nutting C. Treatment of recurrent head and neck cancer: re-irradiation or chemotherapy? Clin Oncol (R Coll Radiol) 2005;17:138–147

225. Forastiere AA, Metch B, Schuller DE, et al. Randomized comparison of cisplatin plus fluorouracil and carboplatin plus fluorouracil versus methotrexate in advanced squamous-cell carcinoma of the head and neck: a Southwest Oncology Group study. J Clin Oncol 1992;10:1245–1251

226. Jacobs C, Lyman G, Velez-Garcia E, et al. A phase III randomized study comparing cisplatin and fluorouracil as single agents and in combination for advanced squamous cell carcinoma of the head and neck. J Clin Oncol 1992;10:257–263

227. Irish JC, Bernstein A. Oncogenes in head and neck cancer. Laryngoscope 1993;103:42–52

228. He Y, Zeng Q, Drenning SD, et al. Inhibition of human squamous cell carcinoma growth in vivo by epidermal growth factor receptor antisense RNA transcribed from the U6 promoter. J Natl Cancer Inst 1998;90:1080–1087

229. Ullrich A, Schlessinger J. Signal transduction by receptors with tyrosine kinase activity. Cell 1990;61:203–212

230. Baselga J, Trigo JM, Bourhis J, et al. Phase II multicenter study of the antiepidermal growth factor receptor monoclonal antibody cetuximab in combination with platinum-based chemotherapy in patients with platinum-refractory metastatic and/or recurrent squamous cell carcinoma of the head and neck. J Clin Oncol 2005;23:5568–5577

231. Cohen EE, Rosen F, Stadler WM, et al. Phase II trial of ZD1839 in recurrent or metastatic squamous cell carcinoma of the head and neck. J Clin Oncol 2003;21:1980–1987

232. Herbst RS, Arquette M, Shin DM, et al. Phase II multicenter study of the epidermal growth factor receptor antibody cetuximab and cisplatin for recurrent and refractory squamous cell carcinoma of the head and neck. J Clin Oncol 2005;23:5578–5587

233. Soulieres D, Senzer NN, Vokes EE, Hidalgo M, Agarwala SS, Siu LL. Multicenter phase II study of erlotinib, an oral epidermal growth factor receptor tyrosine kinase inhibitor, in patients with recurrent or

metastatic squamous cell cancer of the head and neck. J Clin Oncol 2004;22:77–85

234. Bonner JAGJ, Harari PM, Cohen R, et al. Cetuximab prolongs survival in patients with locoregionally advanced squamous cell carcinoma of head and neck: a phase III study of high dose radiation therapy with or without cetuximab. 2004 ASCO Annual Meeting Proceedings (post-meeting edition). J Clin Oncol 2004;22:abstract 5507

235. Terhaard CH, Bongers V, van Rijk PP, Hordijk GJ. F-18-fluoro-deoxy-glucose positron-emission tomography scanning in detection of local recurrence after radiotherapy for laryngeal/ pharyngeal cancer. Head Neck 2001;23:933–941

236. Conessa C, Herve S, Foehrenbach H, Poncet JL. FDG-PET scan in local follow-up of irradiated head and neck squamous cell carcinomas. Ann Otol Rhinol Laryngol 2004;113:628–635

237. Fischbein NJ, Aassar OS, Caputo GR, et al. Clinical utility of positron emission tomography with 18F-fluorodeoxyglucose in detecting residual/recurrent squamous cell carcinoma of the head and neck. AJNR Am J Neuroradiol 1998;19:1189–1196

238. McGuirt WF, Greven K, Williams D, et al. PET scanning in head and neck oncology: a review. Head Neck 1998;20:208–215

239. Rugg T, Saunders MI, Dische S. Smoking and mucosal reactions to radiotherapy. Br J Radiol 1990;63:554–556

240. Som PM, Biller HF. Computed tomography of the neck in the postoperative patient: radical neck dissection and the myocutaneous flap. Radiology 1983;148:157–160

241. Fu KK, Woodhouse RJ, Quivey JM, Phillips TL, Dedo HH. The significance of laryngeal edema following radiotherapy of carcinoma of the vocal cord. Cancer 1982;49:655–658

242. Terhaard CH, Snippe K, Ravasz LA, van der Tweel I, Hordijk GJ. Radiotherapy in T1 laryngeal cancer: prognostic factors for locoregional control and survival, uni- and multivariate analysis. Int J Radiat Oncol Biol Phys 1991;21:1179–1186

243. Lowe VJ, Boyd JH, Dunphy FR, et al. Surveillance for recurrent head and neck cancer using positron emission tomography. J Clin Oncol 2000;18:651–658

244. McGuirt WF, Greven KM, Keyes JW, et al. Positron emission tomography in the evaluation of laryngeal carcinoma. Ann Otol Rhinol Laryngol 1995;104:274–278

245. Bataini JP, Jaulerry C, Brunin F, Ponvert D, Ghossein NA. Significance and therapeutic implications of tumor regression following radiotherapy in patients treated for squamous cell carcinoma of the oropharynx and pharyngolarynx. Head Neck 1990;12:41–49

246. Del Valle-Zapico A, Fernandez FF, Suarez AR, Angulo CM, Quintela JR. Prognostic value of histopathologic parameters and DNA flow cytometry in squamous cell carcinoma of the pyriform sinus. Laryngoscope 1998;108:269–272

247. Hirabayashi H, Koshii K, Uno K, et al. Extracapsular spread of squamous cell carcinoma in neck lymph nodes: prognostic factor of laryngeal cancer. Laryngoscope 1991;101:502–506

248. Raslan WF, Barnes L, Krause JR, Contis L, Killeen R, Kapadia SB. Basaloid squamous cell carcinoma of the head and neck: a clinicopathologic and flow cytometric study of 10 new cases with review of the English literature. Am J Otolaryngol 1994;15:204–211

249. Richard JM, Sancho-Garnier H, Micheau C, Saravane D, Cachin Y. Prognostic factors in cervical lymph node metastasis in upper respiratory and digestive tract carcinomas: study of 1,713 cases during a 15-year period. Laryngoscope 1987;97:97–101

250. Snow GB, Annyas AA, van Slooten EA, Bartelink H, Hart AA. Prognostic factors of neck node metastasis. Clin Otolaryngol Allied Sci 1982;7:185–192

251. Bova R, Goh R, Poulson M, Coman WB. Total pharyngolaryngectomy for squamous cell carcinoma of the hypopharynx: a review. Laryngoscope 2005;115:864–869

252. Peracchia A, Bonavina L, Botturi M, Pagani M, Via A, Saino G. Current status of surgery for carcinoma of the hypopharynx and cervical esophagus. Dis Esophagus 2001;14:95–97

253. Triboulet JP, Mariette C, Chevalier D, Amrouni H. Surgical management of carcinoma of the hypopharynx and cervical esophagus: analysis of 209 cases. Arch Surg 2001;136:1164–1170

254. Dubois JB, Guerrier B, Di Ruggiero JM, Pourquier H. Cancer of the piriform sinus: treatment by radiation therapy alone and with surgery. Radiology 1986;160:831–836

255. Hull MC, Morris CG, Tannehill SP, et al. Definitive radiotherapy alone or combined with a planned neck dissection for squamous cell carcinoma of the pharyngeal wall. Cancer 2003;98:2224–2231

4

Carcinoma of the Larynx

Mark W. El-Deiry, Douglas K. Trask, Henry T. Hoffman, and Kenneth J. Dornfeld

◆ Epidemiology

Laryngeal cancer represents 0.7% of all cancers diagnosed in the United States. The American Cancer Society estimates that 9510 new cases of laryngeal cancer will be diagnosed in the United States in 2006 and estimates that 3740 patients are expected to die of their disease.[1] There is a continuing decrease in the level of tobacco use among male patients; however, this may be partially offset by the increasing tobacco use among young women.[1,2] The National Cancer Database demonstrated that squamous cell carcinoma represents ~95% of all laryngeal cancers diagnosed. This chapter will primarily detail treatment as related to squamous cell cancer unless otherwise specified.[3]

◆ Etiology

Several factors have been implicated in the oncogenesis of laryngeal cancers including smoking, human papilloma virus (HPV) infection, and gastric reflux.[4–7] Tobacco is the most important factor in the carcinogenesis of laryngeal cancer. Both primary and secondhand smoke have been implicated. HPV, particularly type 16, has also been implicated in oncogenesis of head and neck cancer.[8,9] Whereas it is a well-recognized etiologic factor in cancer of the oral cavity and oropharynx, the evidence supporting involvement with laryngeal cancer has been less forthcoming.[10,11] The HPV status of a patient remains a relevant consideration, because HPV-positive cancers demonstrate a better prognosis than HPV-negative cancers.[12]

◆ Anatomy of the Larynx

The larynx is a cartilaginous structure consisting of two main components. The thyroid cartilage, named for its shield-like appearance, is the largest of these forming the primary structure of the larynx. It is a bilaminar structure consisting of an inner and an outer cortex. It connects with the cricoid cartilage immediately inferior to it at the cricothyroid joint. This allows the thyroid cartilage to flex in an anterior-posterior direction via the cricothyroid muscle, which is innervated by the external branch of the superior laryngeal nerve. This allows for shortening and lengthening of the vocal cords to vary pitch. The cricoid is a signet ring–shaped cartilage that forms the only complete cartilaginous ring in the airway. The posterior aspect communicates with the arytenoid cartilages, which are superior to the cricoid forming a synovial joint.

The borders of the larynx extend from the tip of the epiglottis to the inferior border of the cricoid cartilage. It is divided into three separate components embryologically. The superior component, the supraglottis, extends from the tip of the epiglottis to an imaginary horizontal plane bisecting the apex of the laryngeal ventricle. It is made up of the epiglottis, arytenoid cartilages, false vocal cords, as well as the corniculate cartilages, which sit just superiorly to the arytenoid cartilage. The lateral border is formed by the aryepiglottic folds, which connect the arytenoids to the epiglottis. These folds often contain a small cartilage called the cuneiform, which is thought to add rigidity to the cords. The anterior aspect of the supraglottis includes the pre-epiglottic space. The anterior border of this space is the thyrohyoid membrane, which is a fibrous membrane extending from the hyoid to the superior border of the thyroid cartilage. The posterior border is the laryngeal surface of the epiglottis. The superior border is the hyoepiglottic ligament. Immediately above the inferior border is the petiole. The pre-epiglottic space communicates with the paraglottic space below and contains fibrofatty tissue. This connection is an important access for direct extension of cancer. The false vocal cords consist of fibrous tissue that overlies the true vocal cords. The quadrangular membrane, which may serve as a barrier to the spread of cancer, extends from the superior edge of the thyroid cartilage to the apex of the false vocal cord. The supraglottis is primarily innervated by the superior laryngeal nerve. This nerve branches off of the vagus nerve (cranial nerve X) at the level of the carotid bifurcation. It divides into two branches at the thyrohyoid membrane. The external branch innervates the cricothyroid muscle. The internal branch provides sensation to the supraglottis. It is important to preserve this nerve during conservation laryngeal surgery for swallow function postoperatively. The supraglottis is a bilateral structure embryologically. As such, it demonstrates bilateral lymphatic drainage.

The middle component, the glottis, is bounded by the horizontal plane bisecting the ventricle superiorly to include the true vocal cords. It terminates 1 cm below the horizontal plane bisecting the vocal cords. The cover of the true vocal cord (TVC) is made up of nonkeratinizing stratified squamous epithelium with keratinized regions and overlies the lamina propria of the TVC, which is divided into three layers. The superficial layer, which corresponds with Reinke's space, is composed of pliable material giving the overlying epithelium the sliding quality that allows for a fluid mucosal wave. The middle and deep layers combine to form the vocal ligament. The thyroarytenoid (TA) muscle lies deep to the vocal ligament and extends from the vocal process of the arytenoid cartilage and terminates anteriorly on the thyroid cartilage at Broyle's ligament. Broyle's ligament has variably been considered either a path or barrier to cancers involving the anterior commissure to invade through the thyroid cartilage. The vocal cord is abducted by the posterior cricoarytenoid muscle, innervated by the recurrent laryngeal nerve, and is the only abductor of the TVC. The lateral cricoarytenoid muscle, along with the interarytenoid and thyroarytenoid muscles, adducts the vocal cords. These muscles are innervated by the recurrent laryngeal nerve as well. Immobility of the vocal cords can be caused by either invasion of the TA muscle or invasion of the cricoarytenoid joint.

The subglottis extends from a plane 1 cm below the true vocal cords to the lower edge of the cricoid cartilage. This region is innervated by the sensory component of the recurrent laryngeal nerve. Extension of cancer into the subglottis predicts a poorer outcome.

◆ Staging

The American Joint Committee on Cancer (AJCC) *Cancer Staging Manual*, 6th edition, remains the primary source for staging laryngeal cancer in the United States.[13] The anatomic definitions and boundaries between sites as published in the AJCC staging manual have remained constant across the multiple editions and are consistent with the anatomic divisions discussed in this chapter. The definition of the posterior commissure, however, remains vague. It is difficult to discriminate between the glottis, the adjacent supraglottis (arytenoids), and the hypopharynx (postcricoid region) in the region of the posterior commissure.[14] The subglottis extends from the inferior border of the glottis to the inferior border of the cricoid cartilage.

T classification of laryngeal cancers is determined by extension to adjacent structures, cartilage invasion, and im-

paired vocal cord mobility. Supraglottic cancers are classified as T1 cancers if they involve only one subsite, T2 cancers if multiple subsites are involved or extend to the glottis or subglottis, and T3 (stage III) based on paraglottic space invasion, pre-epiglottic space invasion, or minor thyroid cartilage invasion (e.g., inner cortex). The AJCC staging manual indicates that T4 status is based on *"tumor invasion through the thyroid cartilage."* It has been a common error in the past to consider that thyroid cartilage invasion to any extent from a supraglottic or glottic cancer mandates T4 classification. Clinically apparent T1 glottic cancers had been accorded T4 status (T4 N0 M0) when "microscopic invasion of adjacent cartilage" was identified.[13] Revision to the 6th edition of the AJCC staging manual more clearly identifies that *"minor cartilage erosion (e.g., inner cortex)"* should now be classified as T3 instead of T4.

Cancers confined to the glottis with normal mobility are staged T1. Subdivision of T1 vocal cord cancers is based on extension to involve the opposite cord. A tumor limited to one vocal cord is T1a. A horseshoe lesion that extends around the anterior commissure to involve both vocal cords without impairing mobility is T1b. Glottic cancers are classified as T2 based on two separate criteria: impaired vocal cord motion and/or transglottic spread beyond the glottis to involve either the supraglottis or subglottis. T3 classification results from vocal cord fixation and/or invasion into the paraglottic space. This clarification is helpful to resolve controversy in the interpretation of subtle differences between impaired vocal cord motion and fixation. If the arytenoid remains mobile but the membranous vocal cord is tethered by deep infiltration to the paraglottic space, the cancer is considered a T3.

Cancers involving the subglottis are upstaged to T3 (stage III) based on vocal cord immobility. T1 cancers are confined to the subglottis, and T2 cancers demonstrate decreased vocal cord mobility or extension to the glottis. Cricoid or thyroid cartilage invasion by subglottic cancer upstages to a T4a, underscoring the aggressive nature of subglottic cancer.

The borders of the paraglottic space remain confusing despite attempts at clarification by several authors. Berman defined the borders of the paraglottic space as they have been commonly reported by others:

- Anterolateral: the thyroid cartilage

- Inferomedial: the conus elasticus

- Medial: the ventricle and the quadrangular membrane

- Posterior: the piriform sinus[15]

The question then remains whether the thyroarytenoid muscle or the lateral cricoarytenoid muscle are part of the paraglottic space.[16] Using the AJCC criteria, it is prudent to consider the paraglottic space to be involved when there is tumor transgression of the laryngeal musculature into the underlying fat. Tumor extension to this fat would upstage the patient to a T3 carcinoma. Patients with thyroarytenoid muscle or lateral cricoarytenoid muscle involvement without transgression of the laryngeal musculature and only limited mobility may be considered as having a T2 carcinoma.

Evaluating patients with carcinoma in situ remains a difficult endeavor because of a lack of uniformity in classification among pathologists. Many pathologists do not discriminate between high-grade dysplasia and carcinoma in situ (Tis), classifying both as type III neoplasia. Others feel that there is an important distinction.[17-19] Histopathologic studies have shown that severe keratinizing dysplasia may be more common than carcinoma in situ and should be treated accordingly.[20]

◆ Presentation

The early diagnosis of laryngeal cancer requires an understanding of the presenting signs and symptoms of the disease. Often, patients will present with a neck mass and without any other findings consistent with laryngeal cancer. Alternately, the symptom of hoarseness may go untreated or undiagnosed for long periods of time; because smoking plays such a large role in the etiology, worsening symptoms are often attributed to more benign manifestations of tobacco use. Many patients with laryngeal cancer will have been treated for several months with oral antibiotics for hoarseness or sore throat. It is important, therefore, to have a high index of suspicion and a low threshold for laryngoscopy and biopsy of suspicious lesions in the smoking population.

Local Disease

The larynx has three dominant functions. It provides a conduit for breathing, creates the voice, and protects the lungs during swallowing. Any of these three major functions can be disrupted by the presence of a cancer. Patients may also present with refractory odynophagia or referred otalgia due to involvement of the pain fibers in the vagus, which share connections with the tympanic plexus (cranial nerves V, IX, X). Hemoptysis may indicate either an exophytic tumor or synchronous lung primary or lung metastasis. Patients with late-stage laryngeal carcinoma will often have a significant weight loss greater than 10%. Weight loss of this magnitude may portend a worse prognosis or alternatively may lead to surgical complications.

◆ Diagnosis and Workup

The diagnosis of laryngeal cancer requires a biopsy but relies heavily on the physical examination to direct management. Patients presenting with laryngeal cancer are often at high risk for other head and neck tumors. Because referred otalgia is a common presenting symptom, special attention should be placed on examination of the ear and pharynx. Examination of the oral cavity should be carefully performed to rule out synchronous primary tumors of the oral cavity. The base of the tongue should be carefully palpated in the clinic to evaluate for potential involvement. Flexible fiberoptic laryngoscopy provides an excellent and often complementary role to indirect mirror laryngoscopy. Video endoscopy is a useful tool for both resident and patient education. Video endoscopy permits acquisition of permanent recordings and allows the patient to see what the surgeon is describing. When performing flexible laryngoscopy, a systematic approach should be used, starting with the supraglottis and proceeding to the glottis to visualize key involved subsites. Airway patency must be evaluated as some patients may be candidates for tracheotomy in the primary setting. Dynamic examination of the TVC should be performed. If possible, the anterior commissure should be visualized as well as taking care to identify the extent of involvement of the vocal process and intraarytenoid space. Extension into the postcricoid space, piriform sinus, pharyngeal wall, or base of the tongue should be evaluated and correlated at the time of panendoscopy.

Some patients may benefit from the application of flexible transnasal esophagoscopes to evaluate the larynx, trachea, and esophagus.[21-24] Certain lesions are amenable to biopsy via the side-port that exists on the endoscopes. The ability to deliver topical anesthetic through the scope also augments its use in the clinic. In the appropriate setting, the ability to perform a biopsy in the clinic may allow the patient to avoid a trip to the operating room merely to confirm the diagnosis. In most cases, fiberoptic laryngoscopy is not sufficient to replace direct laryngoscopy, which remains the standard approach for the majority of lesions.

Videoendoscopy and videostroboscopy offer further refinement in assessing glottic lesions. It has become standard practice in many institutions to permanently record the appearance of all laryngeal cancers through video recording using rigid or fiberoptic endoscopy. The capacity to refer to these permanent records documenting the extent of the original lesion often improves long-term patient care.[25]

Radiologic imaging is a useful correlate with clinical examination. A chest radiograph may help in the evaluation of patients with laryngeal cancers to assess for concurrent pulmonary disease and to screen for second primary lung cancers. Annual chest radiographs should be obtained in the course of clinic follow-up examinations primarily because of the high incidence of second primary lung cancers in patients managed for laryngeal cancer.[21] Imaging of the primary tumor is best accomplished by computed tomography (CT) scan; however, the role of CT and magnetic resonance imaging (MRI) in early glottic lesions is still being defined.[26] CT and MRI are useful in staging both early- and late-stage laryngeal tumors (**Fig. 4–1**). Tumors of the larynx may demonstrate cartilage invasion as well as paraglottic space invasion that is not readily observable on clinical exam. Tumor volume can be better measured by CT, as well perhaps predicting curability via radiotherapy; however, some investigators have not found any association between tumor volume and radiocurability.[27] Some authors advocate MRI for any patient undergoing less than a total laryngectomy to adequately define tumor extension and thus direct appropriate surgical planning.[28] Currently, positron emission tomography (PET) scan has limited application in evaluation of the primary tumor. The ultimate value of PET scan for evaluation of the primary disease may be in establishing a baseline from which to follow the patient posttreatment. PET is useful in surveying for metastatic disease and synchronous second primary tumors.

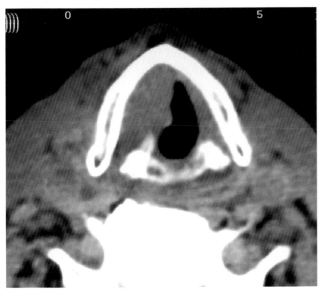

Figure 4–1 Axial CT scan of the larynx demonstrating irregularity of the vocal cord and sclerosis of the arytenoid suggestive of an invasive tumor.

Regional Disease

The rate and location of regional metastasis is subsite dependent. Patients with supraglottic cancers are more likely to have associated metastasis at earlier stages due to the rich lymphatic drainage of the supraglottic (**Fig. 4–2**). The supraglottis has bilateral lymphatic drainage patterns and, therefore, the potential for an increased risk of bilateral metastasis in comparison with glottic or subglottic carcinoma.[29] The bilateral

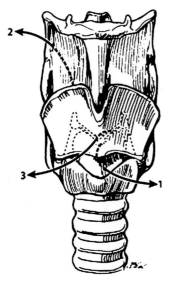

Figure 4–2 Inferior glottic and subglottic tumors commonly gain access to the regional lymphatics via the cricothyroid ligament (*1*) while glottic tumors may also spread by direct cartilage extension (*2*). Supraglottic tumors gain access to the regional lymphatics via the thyrohyoid ligament (*3*).

nature has important implications in directing treatment for supraglottic carcinoma. Kowalski and Medina[30] published a review looking at rates of metastasis for supraglottic carcinoma, finding rates of occult metastasis (clinically N0) around 75% for all T stages with 18% demonstrating bilateral metastasis Byers[29] and Shah[31] independently reported rates of occult metastasis of 34% regardless of T stage for supraglottic cancer with Byers reporting 26% bilateral metastasis.

The glottis embryologically is a unilateral structure. It has a more sparse lymphatic drainage pattern than the supraglottis. Studies have confirmed a much lower rate of regional metastasis for glottic cancer, particularly T1 and T2 cancer where the rate of regional metastasis has been reported as low as 0%.[32] For T3 and T4 glottic cancer, studies have demonstrated at least 20 to 30% rate of regional metastasis.[32,33] The data are less clear for subglottic cancer, but it is generally thought that subglottic cancer behaves more like glottic cancer and should be treated as such.

Unfortunately, the failure rate of clinical examination of the neck ranges from 21 to 51% depending on the examiner, body habitus of the patient, previous treatment, or previous radiation exposure.[34] CT scan has a 95% overall accuracy for patients with known neck disease. This is also somewhat dependent on the size criteria for lymph nodes of the particular institution, although, generally, 10 mm or greater tends to suggest metastasis.[34] Other findings include rounded nodes that have lost their normal oblong shape or nodes with areas of necrosis. Unfortunately, the literature has reported as high as a 67% failure rate for CT in cases of occult metastasis.[35] Currently, PET scan is unable to diagnose disease smaller than 5 mm.[36] As a result, the challenge of detection of clinically occult regional metastasis remains.

The role for PET continues to expand for regional and distant disease. [18F]Fluoro-2-deoxy-D-glucose (FDG) PET scanning has been reported as useful in detecting subclinical recurrent or persistent cancer at a stage when it is highly curable.[37] Some authors suggest that a negative PET scan in the posttreatment setting obviates the need for biopsy.[38] Direct laryngoscopy with directed biopsy, however, remains the gold standard for diagnosis of locally recurrent tumors. Most investigators suggest waiting at least 3 months after treatment to perform PET imaging because false-positive results are common if the imaging is done soon after radiotherapy is completed.[39] False-positives may also result from infection, radionecrosis, or accumulation of saliva in the vallecula.[40] Some of these shortcomings of PET imaging are being addressed by use of pharmaceuticals other than FDG. L-[1-11C] Tyrosine (TYR) PET imaging analyzes protein synthesis activity and may be useful in predicting outcomes in treatment of SCCa of the larynx.[41]

Fine-needle aspiration (FNA) has some use in the diagnosis of neck metastasis for patients with a known laryngeal primary. Patients with neck nodes outside the predicted basins (II to IV) or patients presenting with a neck mass without other symptoms may benefit from FNA. A positive result in either of these situations will usually alter the treatment plan and can aid in patient counseling. In some circumstances, sequential examination with ultrasound and ultrasound-guided FNA is an alternative to elective neck dissection.

◆ Treatment

The management of laryngeal cancer remains controversial. In 1990, the VA Laryngeal Cancer Study Group published their landmark study demonstrating the efficacy of induction chemotherapy and radiation therapy in the treatment of advanced laryngeal cancer.[42] This report ushered in the era of organ-preservation therapy. To this day, no statistically significant survival benefit is conferred by either surgical or nonsurgical therapy for laryngeal cancer. As such, there is no clear answer for the treatment of laryngeal cancer. Most clinicians agree that radiotherapy plays an important role in early-stage cancers of the glottis and supraglottis with outcomes that approach or equal the local regional control rates of surgical therapy. Questions arise in addressing bulky T3 tumors, or T4 tumors with extensive cartilage involvement. Recently, the Radiation Therapy Oncology Group (RTOG) published a study looking at concurrent therapy versus induction therapy and demonstrated that patients in the concurrent group were more likely to keep their larynx than were patients in the induction group.[43] The final conclusion of this study was that concurrent chemoradiation should represent the standard of care for advanced-stage laryngeal cancer. Patients with T4 laryngeal cancer, however, were excluded from the study. Proponents of surgical therapy suggested that there should be a more cooperative approach with each patient being treated individually depending on their particular tumor characteristics.[44] The group at the University of Michigan has continued to expand the use of induction chemotherapy as a predictor of radiosensitivity.[45] This work appears promising with disease-free survival hovering near 90% for bulky T3/T4 disease. The future will likely see even more accurate patient selection as groups continue to look at biologic tumor markers in an attempt to predict treatment response.

Surgical Treatment

There are a wide variety of surgical options for the treatment of laryngeal cancer. Whereas in many cancers the surgical treatment is often tumor based, in laryngeal cancer it is often patient based (i.e., patients with poor pulmonary function may not be candidates for conservation laryngeal approaches, despite the fact their tumors may be amenable to surgical intervention). This creates an interesting paradigm for the surgical treatment of these cancers. Rather than discuss the treatment by subsite, we have chosen to look at each treatment option (endoscopic, laser, open conservation, total laryngectomy) separately with the idea that the reader will be able to apply each modality to the particular tumor in question.

Endoscopic Techniques

In particular, early-stage laryngeal cancer, both supraglottic and glottic, may be amenable to excision via endoscopic routes. Tis tumors of the TVC are ideally suited to endoscopic excision because by definition they are superficial (do

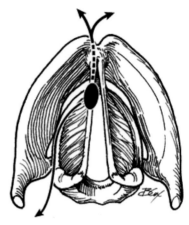

Figure 4–3 Glottic carcinoma. Glottic carcinoma may extend anterior or posterior into the paraglottic space. The findings are often subtle and may best be identified on imaging. Posterior *arrow* represents extralaryngeal spread through the thyroartenoid gap.

not invade the basement membrane). As a result, they can be removed with less damage to the vocal cord. Not all small tumors of the glottis are amenable to superficial resection. With regard to glottic cancer, 20% of T1 tumors have normal mobility despite invasion into the vocal ligament.[46] These tumors may require more aggressive therapy but may still be able to be removed endoscopically. Tumors of the anterior glottic larynx may invade anteriorly; however, they may also extend posteriorly into the paraglottic space (**Fig. 4–3**). More advanced tumors can extend inferiorly along Broyle's ligament or superiorly into the pre-epiglottic space

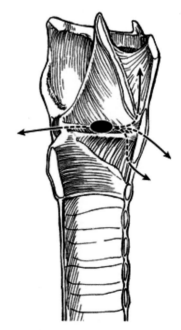

Figure 4–4 Advanced glottic tumors may extend in one or more of four pathways including superior and anterior into the preepiglottic space, anterior through the thyroid cartilage, inferior through the cricothyroid membrane, or posterior.

(**Fig. 4–4**). In both situations, endoscopic resection is often not possible. Careful attention to these areas is essential. CT scan can be helpful because the clinical presentation is often subtle.

Excisional Biopsy

For patients with discrete lesions of the vocal cords, excisional biopsy may provide greater benefit than removal piecemeal. Patients treated with excisional biopsy with the ultimate pathologic diagnosis of high-grade dysplasia or carcinoma in situ may be cured of their disease via the biopsy. Sampling error may be avoided in patients with a small focus of invasive squamous cell carcinoma in a larger field of dysplasia. Excisional biopsy may be accomplished using a microflap technique rather than stripping the vocal cords. This technique allows for sparing of the underlying muscle and can be used if a plane exists between the epithelium and underlying lamina. By removing the lesion in a controlled manner, margins may be taken. For patients with Tis or high-grade dysplasia, resection via this technique can be curative. If the patient is a candidate for radiation, it may be prudent to take a smaller biopsy to avoid significant impairment of the voice prior to radiation treatment. As with all surgical therapy of the larynx, it is important to have a thorough understanding of the patient's wishes prior to beginning treatment.

Laser Excision

The carbon dioxide laser was introduced for resecting laryngeal cancer in 1972 by Strong and Jako.[47] Recently, reports have focused on the successful use of the carbon dioxide laser to manage early glottic lesions.[48] This technique has been reported with cure rates equivalent to those of laryngofissure with cordectomy, classic hemilaryngectomy, and radiotherapy for selected early lesions.[48,49] Endoscopic use of the laser has required a reassessment of the underlying oncologic principle of *en bloc* resection, which has allowed some investigators to extend even further the approach by which cancers are removed endoscopically. Clinical practice has not supported Halstead's principle of "en bloc" resection to avoid tumor spill with regard to endoscopic laser excision. As Bruce Pearson identified: "Halstead did not have a laser."[50] Pearson observed that viable tumor cell implantation is prevented by use of laser as a cutting instrument to sear the cut surfaces. In their book entitled *Endoscopic Laser Surgery of the Upper Aerodigestive Track*,[51] Dr. Steiner and Dr. Ambrosch have stated that adherence to Halstead's "en bloc" resection principle may actually impair the capacity to obtain a tumor-free margin in the process of endoscopic resection. As a result, the key to endoscopic resection of larger tumors is to identify (through microscopic dissection) the interface between the tumor and the normal tissue. To adequately define this interface, often the initial laser cuts are made directly through the tumor, often debulking it in the process as well. This approach to endoscopic cancer surgery has permitted more aggressive resections to be done in a controlled fashion as the depth of the tumor extent

is more readily determined. It is not always necessary to cut through tumors to ensure their complete removal. Steiner and Ambrosch identify that smaller tumors may be removed *en bloc* with a traditional approach to excision. "Cold steel" removal with or without laser assistance can also be used effectively for these smaller lesions.

Supraglottic Laryngectomy

Supraglottic laryngectomy involves removal of that portion of the larynx that lies above the true vocal cords. Extended supraglottic laryngectomy may entail removal of one or both of the arytenoid cartilages. It is ideally suited for patients with T1 or T2 cancers of the supraglottis. In very rare cases, it may be applicable for patients with T3 tumors, but this is limited to patients where the vocal cords are still functional. Since the introduction of endoscopic laser supraglottic laryngectomy, it has remained a useful tool in the oncologic surgeon's armamentarium.

Local control rates with supraglottic laryngectomy are equal to control rates with other treatment modalities including radiation therapy and total laryngectomy.[52] Sessions et al[53] recently examined their series of 653 patients treated for supraglottic cancer since 1955. There was no survival advantage regardless of the type of therapy used, and survival was equivalent to previous reports (65.5% disease-specific survival at 5 years). It is interesting to note, however, with regard to patient-related voice satisfaction that there was no statistical difference between patients treated with supraglottic laryngectomy and patients treated with primary radiation therapy concerning how they rated their voice (83% vs. 85% respectively rated as "good"). Furthermore, patients treated with supraglottic laryngectomy were more likely to keep their larynxes (86.1% vs. 72.7% P = 0.0190). Based on these findings, the authors believe that supraglottic laryngectomy represents the first choice for treatment of patients with supraglottic cancer. This report calls into question the widely held conception that patients treated with radiation generally have much higher voice qualities, despite the retrospective nature.

The role of for salvage of patients failing radiation therapy for early laryngeal cancer remains somewhat unclear. A recent meta-analysis by Motamed et al[54] found local control rates for patients salvaged with external conservation surgical approaches to be 77% with local control rates of 90% for patients ultimately salvaged with total laryngectomy. This would suggest an expanded indication for surgical salvage via conservation laryngeal surgery in selected patients.

Laryngofissure, Cordectomy, and Vertical Partial Laryngectomy

The basic external approach to resection of early glottic cancer is a laryngofissure (or thyrotomy). This procedure involves opening the larynx along the midline like a book. Care is taken to avoid damage to the anterior attachment of the true vocal cords in most cases. If the anterior commissure is involved, the larynx can be entered in a more paramedian position. This is usually the first step in either cordectomy or vertical partial laryngectomy (VPL). Cordectomy is useful for patients who have T1 glottic cancers who are not amenable to endoscopic resection.

VPL is better suited to patients with more advanced T1 and T2 tumors. VPL can be extended to involve resecting either one of the arytenoid cartilages or across the midline to resect the anterior commissure. In performing this procedure, at least two thirds of the contralateral cord must be preserved. If this is not possible, the patient may be better served by a supracricoid partial laryngectomy. Endoscopy immediately prior to the procedure will allow the surgeon to appropriately plan for the amount of thyroid cartilage that needs be removed as well as where to enter the larynx to avoid tumor transgression. Patients undergoing VPL generally require tracheotomy. A keel may also be required to stent the neolarynx. Reconstruction can range from allowing the defect to granulate to requiring a free flap to reconstruct a neolarynx.[55]

Supracricoid Laryngectomy

Supracricoid partial laryngectomy (SPL) extends the option of conservation surgery to patients with more extensive glottic cancers than can be treated with VPL and its extensions. Weinstein and Laccourreye suggest limiting the use of VPL to cases in which the resection is limited to the mid-membranous vocal cord permitting reconstruction with imbrication laryngoplasty to improve the chance for glottic phonation.[56] They identify that the standardized supracricoid laryngectomy offers predictable results without the need to "invent" a new modification of VPL for each case, which then requires further innovation in choosing from a large number of reconstructive options.[56]

SPL is based on the idea the tumor size should not determine the amount of thyroid cartilage resected during the procedure. Instead, the entire thyroid cartilage is removed, not so much for oncologic reasons, but to aid in reconstruction of the neolarynx.[57] By removing the entire thyroid cartilage, the cricoid cartilage can be approximated to the hyoid bringing these two structures together in the design of a functional neolarynx. The procedure includes resection of the thyroid cartilage, the true vocal cords, and can be extended to remove the epiglottis and pre-epiglottic space, false vocal cords, and one but not both arytenoids. Contraindications to supracricoid partial laryngectomy include fixation of an arytenoid cartilage, subglottic extension invading the cricoid cartilage, posterior commissure involvement, and extralaryngeal spread (including outside the outer perichondrium of the thyroid cartilage).

SPL can be defined by the reconstruction after extirpation. Patients in which the superior portion of the epiglottis is preserved are reconstructed via a cricohyoidoepiglottopexy (CHEP) (**Fig. 4–5**). In patients where the entire epiglottis and periepiglottic space is removed, a cricohyoidopexy (CHP) is performed for reconstruction (**Fig. 4–6**). The indications and contraindications are the same for both procedures, and which procedure is performed is mostly a function of the extent and location of the tumor. Patients with cancer that

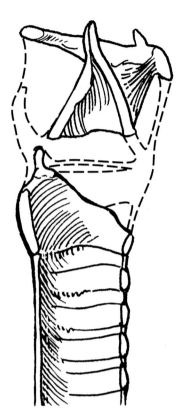

Figure 4–5 Patients in which the superior portion of the epiglottis is preserved are reconstructed via a CHEP.

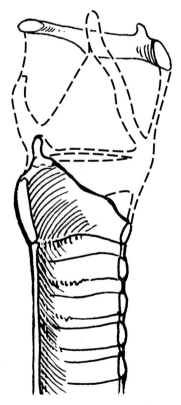

Figure 4–6 In patients where the entire epiglottis and periepiglottic space is removed, a CHP is performed for reconstruction.

involves tissue above the anterior commissure may benefit more from SPL-CHP because of the propensity of these cancers to invade the pre-epiglottic space.[58]

Patients' perception of speech and swallowing are good after SPL. Weinstein et al evaluated the quality of life in patients treated with supracricoid laryngectomy and compared this data with normative data and with patients treated with total laryngectomy with tracheoesophageal puncture (TEP) speech.[59] The outcomes measures of physical functioning, general health, vitality, and physical limitations were significantly better among the 16 patients treated with supracricoid laryngectomy than among 15 matched patients treated with total laryngectomy and TEP. The group treated with supracricoid laryngectomy actually scored higher than the U.S. norms (ages 55 to 64) in every domain within the 36-question short-form health survey (SF-36). The authors attributed this phenomenon to "frame-shifting" wherein a very positive perspective resulted from the outcome of "saving their voice box" in the context of the fear of losing it. The authors also stated that strict adherence to the indications and contraindications for the surgery was required to achieve good results.

Total Laryngectomy/Laryngopharyngectomy

Total laryngectomy (TL) refers to the complete removal of the larynx extending from the tip of the epiglottis to encompass the area below the subglottis, with partial or complete laryngopharyngectomy referring to removal of all or part of the associated pharynx. Total laryngectomy is the gold standard by which all other therapy is judged with regard to local control for laryngeal cancer. Unfortunately, there is a significant amount of social stigma associated with total laryngectomy. Patients' quality of life is significantly affected by the loss of voice as well as placement of a stoma for breathing. This has been the driving force behind the development of organ-sparing protocols for laryngeal cancer. Clinicians are attempting to use alternative surgical as well as nonsurgical means to allow patients to keep their voice and avoid a stoma while maintaining appropriate locoregional control. This has led some authors to suggest that whereas overall survival is important, it may not be the deciding factor in choosing the modality of treatment for any particular patient.

There has been growing controversy regarding the indications for TL over the past 15 years. In 1990, the Department of Veterans Affairs Laryngeal Cancer Study Group published a study looking at the use of induction chemotherapy with radiation therapy to treat advanced-stage cancers. The study compared patients' overall survival as well as the ability to maintain their larynxes. Overall, the larynx was preserved in 64% of patients and overall 5-year survival was the same for both groups.[42] The European Organization for Research and Treatment of Cancer (EORTC) phase III clinical study looking at advanced laryngeal and hypopharyngeal cancer demonstrated an equivalent 5-year survival as well with 42% of patients maintaining their larynxes.[60] Later studies, however, reported contradictory results. The Groupe d'Etudes des Tumeurs de la Tete et du Cou (GETTEC) study, which involved T3 squamous cell carcinoma of the larynx, demonstrated a 2-year survival of 84% for patients in the surgery-radiation therapy group versus 69% in the chemotherapy–radiation therapy group ($P < 0.02$).[61] A fourth study compared induction chemotherapy and radiation versus induction chemotherapy and surgery–radiation therapy to manage advanced-stage hypopharyngeal squamous cell carcinomas.[23] The results demonstrated a significant increase in local control rates as well as overall survival for patients treated with surgery–radiation therapy. The contradictory results led to induction chemotherapy being called into question as a primary modality for treatment of advanced laryngeal cancer.[62]

Most recently, the RTOG 91-11 study demonstrated good laryngeal preservation rates for concurrent radiation therapy when compared with radiation alone or induction chemoradiation with 84% of patients in the concurrent group maintaining their larynxes at 3.8 years versus 72% and 67%, respectively, in the other groups. This study excluded T4 disease as it was generally expected that these patients would do worse than patients with stage III disease.[43] Despite the controversy, TL remains an important tool for the head and neck oncologic surgeon. For patients with advanced-stage T4 carcinoma, TL should be strongly considered as a primary treatment modality. It is a viable option for patients who wish to avoid chemotherapy or for whom swallowing is a more important consideration than maintaining their voice. Current studies at the University of Michigan looking at a single course of induction chemotherapy response as an indicator for radiosensitive tumors demonstrated an 85% overall survival at 3 years and 70% preservation of the larynx.[45] This evidence suggests an important role for total laryngectomy for patients with radioresistant tumors.

As primary radiotherapy and chemoradiation have become more prevalent as primary treatment modalities, the rate of salvage surgery has increased as well. Whereas some authors maintain partial laryngectomy (supraglottic or supracricoid laryngectomy) for select cases of early-stage recurrent laryngeal cancer, most patients with advanced-stage cancers benefit from total laryngectomy for salvage. A recent review of the literature by Motamed et al looking at conservation laryngeal procedures for early-stage laryngeal cancer salvage demonstrated a local control rate of 77% and 65% for external and endolaryngeal laser approaches, respectively, and an overall control rate of 90% and 83%, respectively, for patients in each group who ultimately required total laryngectomy.[54] However, Ganly et al demonstrated that up to 50% of patients with early-stage cancer who fail primary radiotherapy will ultimately require total laryngectomy.[63] Current data out of the RTOG 91-11 study group has demonstrated local regional control to be 90% after total laryngectomy when patients were treated with concurrent chemoradiation for advanced-stage cancer. The 2-year survival data for that group was 76%. Although nearly one third of patients undergoing total laryngectomy after nonsurgical organ-sparing protocols developed a pharyngocutaneous fistula, the authors found that long-term survival was not affected by primary treatment modality, nor did they find that the perioperative morbidity was prohibitive, suggesting that total laryngectomy remains the standard for salvage for patients with advanced-stage cancer.[64] This supports the notion that total laryngectomy remains a valuable tool in the treatment of laryngeal cancer.

Reconstruction

Prior to the advent of microsurgical free tissue transfer, reconstruction of the pharynx was fraught with complications. In 1965, Bakamjian described a two-stage reconstruction of the pharynx that involved creating a pharyngostome, esophagostome, and a tracheostome with the intervening tissue left to granulate for an extended period of time. Once the wound achieved neoepithelialization, a deltopectoral flap would then be lifted and tubed over the newly granulated neopharynx.[65] This flap was labor intensive and risked significant complications. The introduction of the pectoralis myocutaneous pedicle flap provided for an opportunity to create a neopharynx in the primary setting, but unfortunately the skin paddle of a pectoralis flap is difficult to tube and is somewhat bulky, and this often led to postoperative complications. The free flap era has allowed for a fully functional reconstruction of the pharynx in the primary setting. Early work involved the jejunal flap, based on the vessels of the mesenteric arcade. In the mid-1980s, Harii et al[51] and Song et al[66] introduced the radial forearm and anterolateral thigh, respectively, for pharyngeal reconstruction. Since then, the use of the radial forearm free flap (RFFF) has become increasingly common for neopharyngeal reconstruction. More recently, the anterolateral thigh (ALT) flap has begun to replace the radial forearm in patients who are good candidates.

Primary Closure

Primary closure remains the mainstay for patients undergoing total laryngectomy or open conservation laryngeal procedures. Most patients undergoing total laryngectomy are able to retain much of the pharyngeal mucosa. A minimal width of 3 to 3.5 cm of posterior pharyngeal wall mucosa is required for adequate tension-free closure. Although there are several techniques available, we find that using a Connell suture technique modified to stay out of the lumen of the pharynx provides excellent results. It is important to note that the size and shape of the defect may suggest a linear or combined vertical and horizontal closure. As such, the surgeon should be facile with several techniques for primarily closing the pharynx. Questions persist regarding the value in closing the constrictor muscles over the pharynx. Some authors believe that this extra layer of closure can lead to stricture.[67] In previously irradiated patients, meticulous care must be taken in handling the tissues as there is already a high risk of pharyngocutaneous fistula.

Pectoralis Major Myocutaneous Flap

For many years, the pectoralis major myocutaneous flap (PMMF) served as the primary source of hypopharyngeal reconstruction. This flap has several disadvantages related to its bulk, as well as the decreased pliability of the skin paddle; however, despite these limitations, in the era of free tissue transfer, the PMMF remains a useful tool for reconstruction of the neopharynx.

Jejunal Flap

The jejunum has been used for pharyngeal reconstruction since 1959.[68] It provides an excellent reconstruction option based on its enteric properties. The jejunum is self-lubricating and maintains some intrinsic peristaltic function. These factors make it the ideal candidate for pharyngoesophageal reconstruction. A significant disadvantage of this flap is that it requires a laparotomy to harvest. Besides requiring a third team (general surgery) to harvest, all the risks attendant with laparotomy exist with this procedure; however, with the advent of laparoscopic procedures, some of these risks have been minimized. Wadsworth et al described this as the procedure of choice for harvesting the jejunum. They noted several benefits of laparoscopic harvest including a short procedure time (2.4 hours), immediate postoperative enteric feeding, short warm ischemia time (4 minutes), and in 10 of 11 patients, time to discharge was independent of the abdominal procedure. The authors conclude that by using laparoscopic techniques, the use of jejunal free tissue transfer becomes feasible in patients who may have otherwise undergone tubed radial forearm reconstruction due to the risk of laparotomy.[69]

The jejunum may also have other clinical benefits when compared with the RFFF. A recent study by Harri et al compared their 10-year experience in the use of jejunal free tissue transfer and tubed radial forearm reconstruction. They noted a 39% stricture rate with the tubed RFFF versus a 9% rate with the jejunal flap. There was also a significantly higher rate of fistula ($P < 0.0001$) in the immediate postoperative period with the RFFF group. Furthermore, they also noted a higher rate of fistulization on the patients treated with a tubed RFFF who received postoperative radiation of 60 Gy. The authors attributed this risk to the vascular nature of the jejunum being able to tolerate higher doses of radiation. Based on these findings, they suggest that the jejunum may be the flap of choice for pharyngoesophageal reconstruction; however, it is important to note that 4% of the jejunal flaps developed total necrosis, whereas none of the radial forearm flap patients developed this complication.[70] The patients who underwent jejunal flap reconstruction demonstrated more postoperative complications based on their flap harvest.[70] They also noted that the potential for speech seemed greater in the tubed RFFF group.

Radial Forearm Free Flap

In 1985, Harii et al[71] introduced the tubed radial forearm flap for reconstruction of the pharynx (**Fig. 4–7**). This flap had several benefits. It provides for a very thin, pliable piece of skin that could be harvested using a single-team approach. This last point was key in distinguishing it from visceral free

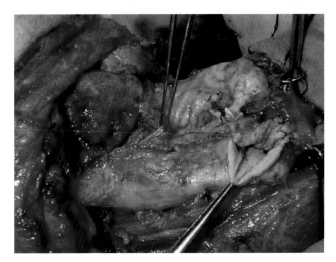

Figure 4–7 Tubed radial forearm free flap reconstruction of the pharynx. It has been tubed on itself and sutured into the base of the tongue and esophagus along the posterior borders.

flaps requiring several teams for harvest. As such, this flap has gained significant popularity replacing the jejunal flap as the primary method of reconstruction at some centers. Patients have demonstrated excellent outcomes with this flap. Blackwell et al[72] in 2001 reported on a series of 20 patients undergoing tubed radial forearm reconstruction. Most patients in this series undergoing tubed radial forearm flap reconstruction demonstrated resumption of oral diets with ~80% of patients able to maintain their weight via oral alimentation. Furthermore, patients in this study rehabilitated with TEP demonstrated functional speech with the prosthesis. There was a high rate of stricture and pharyngocutaneous fistula, particularly with circumferential tubed flaps (27% vs. 11%). They also reported an increased risk of anastomotic stricture when compared with jejunal flaps but stated that patients responded well to dilation and were able to resume an oral diet. The authors concluded that the major disadvantage of this reconstruction was delay in oral feeding, otherwise patients did very well. As such, this flap remains an excellent option for pharyngeal reconstruction for patients undergoing total or near-total laryngopharyngectomy for advanced laryngeal or hypopharyngeal cancer.

Anterolateral Thigh Free Flap

Over the past decade, the radial forearm flap and jejunal flap have been the mainstays for pharyngeal reconstruction. Recently, however, microvascular surgeons have rediscovered the ALT flap for reconstruction of the pharynx. Initially introduced by Song[66] in 1984, the ALT flap has several distinct advantages over the radial forearm flap. The primary advantage lies specifically with the donor site, however, as the ALT flap does not require a split-thickness skin graft for coverage. Unlike the radial forearm, the donor site can be closed primarily. Other advantages include the ease of raising the flap, the size of the skin paddle that can be raised, and the fact that muscle can be harvested with the flap. The largest series

looked at 672 ALT flaps, suggested that it may be the "ideal soft tissue flap."[73] Perhaps the only real disadvantage is that in overweight patients, the amount of fat required to harvest the flap may be prohibitive. Genden et al recently published their experience comparing the ALT flap with the RFFF for pharyngeal reconstruction. They found that the biggest advantage of this flap was the absence of donor site morbidity. They also noted a decreased rate of stenosis with the ALT flap, but the authors observed that because of the limited number of patients in the study (N = 23), the significance was unknown but may be related to the conical structure of the flap, thus allowing for a wider opening at each anastomosis site. They also noted that 10 of 11 patients were able to achieve speech with TEP.[74]

Radiation Therapy

Early Glottic Cancer

T1 glottic cancers can be readily treated with radiotherapy. Treatment fields are typically limited to the region between the superior border of the thyroid cartilage extending inferiorly to the cricoid. The posterior edge of the field is the anterior portion of the vertebral bodies, and the anterior portion of the field extends beyond the neck. Several dose schedules have been employed, 2 Gy per fraction to a total of 66 to 70 Gy, 2.25 to 63 Gy, and others. Schedules with daily dosing below 2 Gy appear to be less effective, and indeed recent evidence suggests that 2 Gy per day is inferior to 2.25 Gy per day.[75] High dose per fraction may increase late-term toxicity. Wedges are used to compensate for the difference in tissue thickness from anterior to posterior. Use of CT-based planning can avoid inadvertent shielding of the anterior commissure, which may have led to increased failures in the past. Local control with radiotherapy alone is 80 to 90%, with most relapses ultimately controlled with surgical salvage.

T2 glottic cancers are treated similarly to T1 lesions, with slightly larger fields, as the risk of nodal involvement remains low and treatment of the neck is not indicated. Dose guidelines for T2 lesions are similar for T1 lesions. The outcome for T2 lesions is slightly lower than T1 lesions, prompting investigational use of more aggressive treatment. The RTOG recently completed a phase III study examining the use of twice daily fractionation of 1.2 Gy to a total of 79.2 Gy versus 2 Gy single fraction per day to a total of 70 Gy. The results are pending. Retrospective results from M.D. Anderson suggest a nominal improvement from twice daily dosing.[76] They also find doses lower than 2 Gy result in inferior outcome. Local control of 70 to 80% with radiotherapy alone or more than 90% with surgical salvage has been reported by several institutions.

Advanced Glottic Cancer

Potentially Resectable Disease A major goal for radiotherapeutic management of larynx cancer is preservation of laryngeal structure and function while maintaining high cure rates. T3 or T4 disease and/or patients with nodal disease have lower locoregional control rates than for T1 or T2 disease. T3 or T4 cancers invariably involve structures within or adjacent to the larynx that contain lymphatic drainage, and therefore lymphatic involvement is much more common than for T1 or T2 lesions. Therefore, uninvolved nodal regions at risk, particularly levels II, III, and IV and the Delphian nodal region, require prophylactic treatment. Standard radiotherapy for these lesions include treatment to the primary site and grossly involved lymph nodes to 70 Gy in 2-Gy fractions, with high-risk but clinically negative lymph node levels receiving 56 to 60 Gy and low-risk nodal regions receiving 50 to 54 Gy. For the uninvolved neck, the superior portion of the field is designed to cover the jugulodigastric node. In most patients, this results in shielding at least a portion of the parotid gland. Conventional radiotherapy, using 2 Gy per day to a total of 70 Gy, results in 50 to 60% locoregional control for locally advanced yet still resectable lesions.

Maneuvers to increase the efficacy of radiotherapy for this group of patients include use of radiosensitizing systemic agents and altered fractionation. Radiosensitizers include cisplatin and the epidermal growth factor receptor (EGFR) blocking agent cetuximab. Many other radiosensitizing agents such as Taxol (paclitaxel), 5-fluorouracil, and hydroxyurea have also been used. The optimal agent(s), schedule of delivery with radiation, and patient selection all remain under investigation. A landmark phase III study by the RTOG[43] compared radiation alone, radiation with concurrent cisplatin, and radiation or laryngectomy based on response to induction cisplatin and 5-fluorouracil (RTOG 91-11). The induction arm of this trial was shown to result in similar overall survival to total laryngectomy in the Veterans Administration Larynx Preservation Study. Overall survival was similar for all three arms of RTOG 91-11. Locoregional control was superior in the treatment arm receiving concurrent cisplatin and 70 Gy. As for most concurrent chemoradiation schemes, morbidity was also increased. Meta-analyses examining the use of chemotherapy and radiation therapy for squamous cell cancer of the head and neck also support the concurrent use of platinum-based regimens as the most effective combination of radiation and sensitizers.[62]

A recent study by Urba and colleagues at the University of Michigan[45] reported a phase II trial using one cycle of induction cisplatinum and fluorouracil to assign definitive treatment. Patients with a partial response (50% or greater) went on to receive concurrent chemoradiotherapy, whereas nonresponders underwent resection and postoperative radiation therapy. This approach combines the attractiveness of induction therapy as a way to identify responders together with the effectiveness of concurrent chemoradiation. Of note, the Michigan study included patients with advanced T4 lesions with cartilage and soft tissue invasion but still resulted in laryngeal preservation and overall survival rates similar to those reported for RTOG 91-11.

Other options to enhance the efficacy of radiotherapy for locally advanced disease include the use of cetuximab. This EGFR blocking agent was shown to add improvements in local control and overall survival compared with radiotherapy alone in the treatment of squamous cell cancer of the head and neck, including laryngeal cancers.[77] Whether cisplatinum or cetuximab is the more effective radiation sensitizer is a question that will require careful investigation. These different agents have significantly different systemic toxicities and sensitize tissues to radiation by distinct mechanisms. Careful attention to efficacy and toxicity will be required to determine which sensitizer is able to produce the greatest therapeutic ratio (greatest anticancer effect and least normal tissue toxicity). Cetuximab and radiotherapy is an option for those patients with medical contraindications to platinum (renal insufficiency or hearing impairment).

As mentioned above, RTOG 91-11 included a radiotherapy-only arm. Overall survival was comparable with the two arms containing chemotherapy. Disease-free survival was greater for the concurrent arm (2-year disease-free survival of 61% for concurrent chemoradiotherapy vs. 44% for radiotherapy alone); however, toxicity was also greater. Given the comparable overall survival, radiation monotherapy remains a treatment option, though one best reserved for patients who are not candidates for either surgery or chemotherapy. Monotherapy radiation treatment can be improved by use of altered fractionation. Delivery of 70 Gy in 2-Gy fractions over 7 weeks is considered standard treatment. Total radiation dose can be increased while maintaining equivalent long-term toxicity by dividing the total dose into even smaller doses per fraction. This strategy, called *hyperfractionation*, was shown to result in superior locoregional control for locally advanced squamous cell cancers of the head and neck in RTOG 90-03. Fu et al[78] reported that 1.2 Gy delivered twice daily to a total of 81.6 Gy resulted in improved locoregional control compared with 70 Gy delivered in daily 2-Gy fractions. Another maneuver to increase the effectiveness of radiotherapy, termed *accelerated fractionation*, is to shorten the overall treatment time. RTOG 90-03 also examined the benefit of two schedules that used twice-daily dosing for a portion of the overall treatment course to shorten treatment time from 7 weeks to 6 weeks. These schedules also produced a modest improvement in locoregional control and a trend toward improvement in overall survival. Locoregional control at 2 years from RTOG 90-03 using hyperfractionation is 54%.

For patients with locoregionally advanced disease treated with resection, certain clinical or pathologic findings are correlated with increased risk of recurrence. These findings include involvement of two or more nodes or one node with extracapsular extension (ECE). Disease present at the ultimate resection margin is also a risk factor for recurrence. Other features, such as perineural invasion, large tumor bulk, extension into soft tissues or through cartilage, and lymphovascular invasion, decrease the certainty of complete resection and increase the potential recurrence rate. In these situations, adjuvant radiotherapy can be used to decrease the risk of recurrence. Of all these features, extracapsular extension appears to carry the worst prognosis. Based on size, nodes greater than 3 cm have a very high rate of extracapsular extension and should be treated as such until proved otherwise. Postoperative treatment should commence within 6 weeks of resection. Postresection dosing is typically 60 to 66 Gy to areas of preresection gross disease, with a minimum of 63 Gy for nodal stations that harbored nodal disease with ECE. Resected nodal stations adjacent to involved regions should receive 56 to 60 Gy, and uninvolved and unresected nodal regions (often supraclavicular or level IV region) should receive 50 to 54 Gy.

Recently, RTOG[79] and EORTC[80] have both reported large phase III studies supporting the postoperative use of chemoradiotherapy for patients with high-risk squamous cell cancers of the head and neck including laryngeal cancer. The EORTC trial showed a benefit in terms of locoregional control and overall survival, whereas the RTOG study showed improved locoregional control without improvement in overall survival. Both studies showed a significant increase in treatment-related morbidity, including treatment-related deaths, in the chemoradiotherapy arms. The greatest benefit from adjuvant chemoradiotherapy may be in those patients with positive surgical margins or in those patients with ECE.

Unresectable Disease Tumor invasion into normal tissues such as the carotid artery or vertebral bodies render some cancers surgically unresectable. In addition, comorbid illness may render the patient medically unresectable. Patients with locoregionally advanced disease who are not operative candidates may be treated with radiotherapy. Treatment with radiation alone for locoregionally advanced, unresectable disease is associated with a 20 to 25% local control rate. The measures listed above for enhancing the activity of radiotherapy should be considered, including concurrent platinum-based chemotherapy, concurrent cetuximab, and hyperfractionation. Each of these measures improves locoregional control compared with conventional fractionation of 2 Gy per day to a total of 70 Gy; however, they have not been compared directly with each other. The choice of either conventional treatment or more aggressive nonsurgical therapy using one of these approaches is best made by considering the individual patient and their comorbidities. All efforts to improve the efficacy of radiotherapy for laryngeal cancers also increase the morbidity of treatment.

Early Supraglottic Cancer

For T1 and T2 lesions, both radiotherapy and surgery offer high rates of local control and overall survival. Surgical options able to achieve cure and maintain laryngeal function are available. Surgery is often the preferred treatment for early-stage lesions that are amenable to laryngeal-preserving resection. T1 lesions not amenable to laryngeal-preserving resection either because of disease location or comorbid ill-

ness can be treated with radiotherapy. The risk of nodal metastasis warrants prophylactic nodal irradiation, even for T1 disease. Prophylactic neck irradiation should address levels II to IV. CT treatment planning allows the upper treatment border to be the jugulodigastric (JD) node. Eisbruch et al[81] have described very low failure rates for the N0 neck treated using this upper border in squamous cell cancers from a variety of head and neck sites. Using the JD node as the superior border of the treatment fields allows the dose to the parotid gland to remain low, as most patients have their JD node at a level of the very inferior portion of the parotid gland. Similar dose guidelines for glottic cancer apply to supraglottic cancer. Conventional fractionation consists of 2 Gy per day to a total of 70 Gy, with high-risk nodal stations, levels II and III, receiving 56 to 60 Gy. Nodal stations at lower risk, for example supraclavicular nodes, may be treated to 50 to 54 Gy.

Tumor bulk and decreased cord mobility have been described as poor prognostic features for supraglottic cancers treated with radiation therapy alone. For bulky lesions, greater than 6 cm³ in volume, hyperfractionation appears to offer benefit.[82]

Advanced Supraglottic Cancer

Potentially Resectable Disease Concurrent chemoradiotherapy for locoregionally advanced disease is a treatment option for supraglottic laryngeal cancers, similar to this option for glottic cancers. Indeed, RTOG 91-11 had a larger number of supraglottic compared with glottic cancers. Patients not eligible for chemotherapy or resection may be treated with cetuximab concurrently with radiation or radiotherapy alone, as described for glottic cancers. Hyperfractionation or accelerated fractionation should be considered for those patients undergoing radiotherapy only.

For cancers with cartilage destruction, airway compromise, and large bulk, laryngectomy likely represents the optimal treatment. Although a direct comparison has not been made between resection and chemoradiotherapy for this group, retrospective data from several institutions report poor local control. In addition, laryngeal function in this group is often compromised when treated nonsurgically.

Unresectable Disease Concurrent chemotherapy and radiation therapy should be considered. For patients not eligible to receive chemotherapy, use of cetuximab or hyperfractionation can improve standard radiotherapy.

Subglottic Cancer

Subglottic tumors are rare. Transglottic extension of supraglottic lesions is an ominous finding. If a tracheostomy was performed because of airway compromise resulting from subglottic extension, this area should be boosted.

Complications

Side effects of therapy for comprehensive radiotherapy of the larynx and lymph node regions include skin and mucosal surface reactions, decreased amount of and thickened saliva, dysphagia, and fatigue. Long-term complications include permanent xerostomia, hypothyroidism, and necrosis involving cartilage or bone and new second cancers. Decreased saliva decreases protection for teeth and increases the rate of dental decay. Tooth extraction after radiation to the underlying mandible may precipitate osteoradionecrosis, even years after treatment. Consultation with a dentist experienced in head and neck cancer should be sought prior to radiotherapy for all patients, and consideration should be given to dental extraction for teeth at risk before starting treatment.

Treatment of Recurrence

Reirradiation for recurrent disease or for a new larynx cancer in the setting of prior radiotherapy for head and neck cancer presents a challenge. Reirradiation is possible, and several institutions have reported their experiences with a second full course of radiotherapy[83]; however, a second course of therapy increases the likelihood of normal tissue necrosis. Osteoradionecrosis, skin necrosis, even vascular injury and carotid disruption have been reported for patients receiving two full courses of radiotherapy. For these reasons, reirradiation should be carefully considered and used when other treatment options have been exhausted. Because the treatment field size and amount of tissue irradiated for T1 and T2 N0 glottic cancers is so small, the relative risk of reirradiation is smaller than for patients who have had comprehensive head and neck irradiation.

Management of the Neck

The predicted nodal basins for spread of laryngeal cancer, regardless of subsite, are usually regarded as level II (posterior belly of the digastric) to level IV.[29,33] Lymph node metastasis is a poor prognostic factor in head and neck cancer, holding true for laryngeal cancer as well. Positive nodal disease confers at least a 50% decrease in 5-year survival for all sites of the head and neck. Patients with N1 disease can be managed by single-modality therapy. Survival data from RTOG 91-11 is based on the premise patients with N2 or greater disease received a scheduled neck dissection 8 weeks after the culmination of radiotherapy.[43] Advent of the PET scan has allowed us to look for metabolically active disease usually 3 months after completion of therapy. Current studies out of Iowa have demonstrated no cancer in patients with PET−/CT+ necks after radiotherapy. This may suggest that these patients may be able to avoid posttreatment neck dissection and be treated by observation instead.[84]

Some controversy, however, arises in the treatment of the N0 neck. Options for treatment of the N0 neck include observation, staging neck dissection, or radiotherapy. The controversy arises when considering that only 30% of patients with a head and neck primary cancer will develop regional metastasis. This would imply that 70% of patients are undergoing an unnecessary neck dissection or radiation therapy. Unfortunately, imaging modalities are limited in the ability to diagnose occult metastasis. Although it is certainly beneficial to treat 30% of patients with regional nodal disease, it becomes concerning when considering the morbidity of

radiotherapy or the rare but associated shoulder dysfunction of neck dissection.

Currently, there is a limited role of observation in patients with laryngeal cancer. Occult metastasis rates for early-stage (T1 or T2) glottic or subglottic cancer are believed to be sufficiently low to warrant this therapeutic approach, particularly for patients undergoing endoscopic resection of the tumor. Patients without poor prognostic indicators on pathologic examination (perineural invasion, angiolymphatic invasion) and who are pN0 can avoid postoperative radiotherapy; however, this is becoming an increasingly rare occurrence as early supraglottic and glottic tumors are more commonly being treated with nonsurgical modalities. Patients with T3 or T4 lesions of the glottis or subglottis should have a neck dissection performed.[33]

Treatment of the N0 neck is divided into surgical and nonsurgical treatment. It is generally accepted that the neck should be treated for tumors that are T2 of the supraglottis or greater, or T3/T4 of the glottis. This is based on the concept that if the rate of occult metastasis is greater than 20%, then the neck should be treated. In the case of supraglottic carcinoma, it is generally accepted that the rate of bilateral metastasis (18 to 26%) is high enough to warrant bilateral neck dissection. Although there is some growing controversy in regard to this with certain authors pointing out that bilateral neck dissection has not had any effect on overall survival nor on local/regional control,[85] bilateral treatment of the neck remains the standard of care for supraglottic carcinoma. Patients with the above tumors undergoing radiotherapy should have the neck addressed at the time of their therapies.

Elective neck dissection (ELND) has several advantages over radiotherapy. It represents the gold standard for staging of the neck at this time. Also, as stated previously, patients undergoing ELND may avoid radiotherapy if they are pN0 without perineural invasion or capillary-lymphatic invasion. The indications for ELND remain somewhat controversial, although it is generally accepted that patients whose necks will be exposed during the tumor removal or for reconstructive purposes should undergo ELND. Furthermore, it may be indicated in patients who wish to avoid radiotherapy for potentially borderline tumors.

There have been several advances in an attempt to limit the morbidity of radical neck dissection. It is accepted that patients undergoing ELND for laryngeal cancer should selectively have levels II to IV removed at the time of their surgery leaving the sternocleidomastoid (SCM), eighth cranial nerve, and jugular vein in place. Other studies have demonstrated extremely low rates of metastasis to level IIb thus allowing surgeons to limit damage to the ninth cranial nerve by avoiding intensive dissection in this area.[86,87] This has allowed surgeons to obtain adequate staging information while maintaining decrease morbidity for these patients.

◆ Clinical Cases

Case 1 T2 supraglottic carcinoma.

Presentation The patient is a 45-year-old man with a 4-month history of hoarseness. He is a 25 pack-year smoker who drinks socially. He is currently self-employed as a trial lawyer. During his initial visit, he is interrupted constantly by cellular phone calls and states that "It's all just part of the job."

Physical Examination   On examination, the patient demonstrates normal laryngeal crepitus and elevation with swallow. The patient demonstrated an overly vigorous gag on indirect laryngoscopy. Flexible fiberoptic laryngoscopy reveals a 2-cm lesion on the laryngeal surface of the epiglottis extending to involve the anterior aspect of the left TVC. The airway appears widely patent with normal TVC motion and an otherwise unremarkable exam. Cranial nerves II to XII are intact.

Diagnosis and Workup   Based on clinical examination, this patient has a T2 (two subsites starting in the supraglottis) N0 tumor of the supraglottis, most likely squamous cell. Initial workup should include a CT scan to evaluate the extent of the primary tumor as well as for lymphadenopathy not detected on the initial clinical exam. The CT should be carefully examined for pre-epiglottic involvement as well as extension along Broyle's ligament. Because this is a T2 carcinoma of the supraglottis, it has a reasonably high propensity for regional and distant metastasis and may warrant a PET scan. A screening chest x-ray because of the patient's smoking history is indicated. Furthermore, should the patient be considering conservation laryngeal surgery, he should be seen by a pulmonologist for pulmonary function testing. This is important as patients undergoing SPL–CHP/CHEP will need to tolerate some aspiration postoperatively.

Panendoscopy plays an extremely important role in the care of this patient. First of all, it allows for biopsy of the lesion to confirm the diagnosis. Furthermore, it allows for evaluation of the tumor in an adynamic setting. Special attention should be placed on the anterior commissure, intraarytenoid space, and vocal process. Also, the patient needs to be evaluated for subglottic extension. Knowing this information allows for accurate counseling of the patient as well as accurate surgical planning should the patient desire a conservation procedure.

Options for Treatment   This patient has several options for therapy. He is a candidate for both endoscopic laser resection as well as a conservation open procedure most likely supracricoid laryngectomy with CHP. This would be the procedure of choice as the tumor has no subglottic extension and spares both of the arytenoid complexes. Furthermore, with excision of the epiglottis, the patient would require CHP. This is also an ideal tumor to be treated with radiation therapy. The choice of therapy should depend on the patients' wishes with regard to his quality of life. Most likely, a high-functioning patient like this would benefit from either a conservation open procedure or external beam radiotherapy. Both options should be explained, and the choice should be made in a multidisciplinary manner. The patient should be discussed at tumor board and should meet individually with both the surgeon and the radiation oncologist. This allows the best therapy to be chosen for this particular patient.

Treatment of the Primary Tumor   This tumor represents a typical T2 tumor presenting to the otolaryngologist. This patient is an ideal candidate for radiotherapy, particularly if the anterior commissure is spared and the contralateral cord is not involved. Radiotherapy would allow this patient to continue to work as a high-functioning lawyer while providing similar control rates as conservational laryngeal surgery. Most patients tolerate the side effects of localized radiation well. It may be beneficial to have the patient seen by speech pathology to help maintain swallowing throughout the course of therapy. Endoscopic laser resection is an excellent option, but one might expect the voicing to be less adequate without reconstruction.

This case represents the ideal case for the dialogue that the surgeon, radiation oncologist, and patient should have regarding the treatment of this tumor. At the University of Iowa, this patient would be evaluated in a multidisciplinary clinic run by both a head and neck surgeon and a radiation oncologist. Both physicians see the patient together and discuss the benefits and alternatives of each therapy allowing the patient to choose the therapy best suited for his or her needs after tumor board review.

Treatment of the Neck   Case 1 demonstrates several controversies in the treatment of the neck as well. Because this is a T2 carcinoma of the supraglottis with what appears to be a mostly midline distribution, this patient requires treatment of the neck bilaterally. How the neck is treated is wholly dependent on what kind of treatment modality is used. Should the patient ultimately proceed with radiation, then it would be prudent to radiate both necks during the course of therapy (56 to 60 Gy [II to III]). Alternatively, should a SPL-CHP be performed, then the patient should undergo bilateral selective neck dissection with dissection of levels II to IV potentially sparing level IIb.[86,87] There is a growing body of literature suggesting that dissection here may be unnecessary. Should the patient undergo endoscopic surgical excision, then a neck dissection would still be indicated. This should be done at the time of primary resection.

Treatment of Distant Sites   There is a small risk of distant metastasis with this tumor. Management of synchronous primary lung tumors will be discussed in a later section.

Summary of Treatment   T1 and T2 tumors of the larynx are well managed by radiation therapy. Locoregional control approaches that of conservational laryngeal procedures, and voicing is generally better. Conservational laryngeal procedures may provide excellent local control rates and may actually be better for T1b glottic (subgroup that "horseshoes" the anterior commissure) tumors. Furthermore, this may allow the patient to avoid radiotherapy, which may be beneficial. A patient without negative findings on open procedure and N1 or less without extracapsular spread could avoid radiotherapy through this course of therapy.

Case 2   T4 glottic with neck disease and pharyngeal involvement.

Presentation   The patient is a 65-year-old man with a 6-month history of neck and ear pain. The patient states that it is very difficult for him to swallow and he has lost ~40 lb in the past 3 months. He states that he has been seen by his local family doctor and was treated with multiple courses of antibiotics. He states his family doctor became extremely worried and referred him on when he developed a rapidly enlarging neck mass 2 weeks ago. His voice is extremely weak but it does not seem to bother him overly much. The patient is accompanied by his wife and states that he is retired. He is a 80 pack-year smoker but does not drink alcohol.

Physical Examination On examination, the patient presents with normal otoscopy and rhinoscopy. Examination of the oral cavity reveals no abnormal lesions. Palpation of the base of the tongue reveals no palpable mass. Palpation of the neck reveals a 4-cm mass in the right neck. The mass is firm, fixed, and not tender to palpation. The larynx itself seems to be fixed as well, and attempting to move it causes the patient a significant amount of pain. Flexible fiberoptic laryngoscopy reveals a large right-sided exophytic lesion nearly obstructing the airway. The lesion appears to involve the entire right cord and extends onto the left vocal cord. Neither cord appears to be mobile. The mass also extends laterally to obliterate the entire piriform sinus as well as encroach on the posterior pharyngeal wall. The patient appears to be aspirating his secretions with significant pooling in the contralateral piriform sinus. The base of the tongue is soft to palpation.

Diagnosis and Workup This patient has what is at least a T3 carcinoma of the larynx. A CT scan is indicated to evaluate the extent of the tumor. In this patient with fixed cords and bulky disease, it is important to discern whether there is cartilage involvement or whether the tumor extends into the soft tissues of the neck. Glottic tumors involving the paraglottic space can spread posteriorly through the thyroarytenoid gap and involve the hypopharynx. This becomes more important when considering a conservation surgery for a small T3 glottic carcinoma. It is also important to attempt to evaluate the extent of pharyngeal involvement in this patient, although the CT scan will tend to underestimate the extent of the tumor. In this case, we would expect that the cartilage would be eroded with tumor extending into the soft tissue of the neck, automatically upstaging the patient to T4a. Attention should also be paid to the extent of lymphadenopathy in the neck. This patient will most likely require at least a modified radical neck dissection, and it is important to understand the extent of disease to adequately counsel the patient.

A PET scan is warranted as well. The PET confers several benefits here. It is excellent in determining if there are any distant metastasis greater than 5 mm in size. Second, this allows the PET scan to be used in the surveillance of the patient postoperatively. Also, a patient with this significant history of a smoking has a reasonable likelihood of a synchronous primary of the lung.

The key step in this patient's workup is the panendoscopy and possible tracheotomy. In the ideal situation, the patient would be taken for primary surgery to perform the stoma and relieve the airway obstruction at the same time; however, this is rare, and these patients often require an interim tracheotomy. The panendoscopy in this situation serves several purposes. First, it allows confirmation of the diagnosis via biopsy. Second, it is extremely important for surgical planning. Most likely, this patient will require a laryngopharyngectomy. It is extremely important to understand the extent of postcricoid or esophageal involvement as this will have a significant bearing on the patient's reconstruction and prognosis. As discussed in an earlier section, patients with cervical esophageal involvement requiring resection below the thoracic inlet almost universally require gastric pull-up for reconstruction. Patients whose defect extends above the thoracic inlet can be reconstructed with a free flap or less ideally with a tubed pedicled flap, specifically the pectoralis major flap. Patients who are candidates for free flap reconstruction should undergo color-flow Doppler of the upper extremities to evaluate for potential radial forearm free flap reconstruction.

Options for Treatment This patient has multiple options for treatment and highlights the role of the tumor board in offering recommendations to the patient. The options include (1) total laryngectomy with postoperative radiation therapy ± neck dissection; (2) total laryngectomy without postoperative radiation therapy; (3) chemotherapy/radiation therapy; (4) radiation therapy + cetuximab; (5) radiation therapy alone; and (6) no treatment. Because not all of the options are equivalent, the tumor board may recommend the best options in descending order. Although the less ideal options are not advised, the final decision still rests with the patient. Option no. 6 does not represent a legitimate treatment option, but by offering no treatment to the patient, it enforces the fact that the decision lies with the patient.

Based on the findings of RTOG 91-11, this patient should not be considered a candidate for concurrent chemoradiation or radiation alone. The fact that the cartilage is involved would suggest that this patient would benefit from primary surgical therapy. Patients who undergo concurrent chemoradiation in this setting tend to develop significant side effects of the therapy including chronic aspiration, chondronecrosis, and tracheotomy tube and G-tube dependence. This patient would most likely benefit from total laryngectomy with partial pharyngectomy. He will require pharyngeal reconstruction either via a radial forearm or ALT flap. Based on the characteristics of the primary tumor and the extent of neck disease, the patient will require postoperative radiotherapy.

Should extracapsular spread be noted in the neck, as suggested by the size of adenopathy, this patient may benefit from concurrent postoperative chemoradiotherapy. Given his significant weight loss and the toxicity of postoperative chemoradiotherapy, a percutaneous endoscopic gastrostomy (PEG) tube should be placed as soon as possible.

Treatment of the Primary Tumor Based on the extent of the tumor, this patient should undergo laryngopharyngectomy. Because the tumor is through the thyroid cartilage as well as into the pharynx, organ preservation is contraindicated. Because of the extent of the tumor, the resecting surgeon should be facile at entering the pharynx with either an anterior or lateral pharyngotomy. Preservation of mucosa is important but should not compromise tumor resection; however, patients in whom a strip of mucosa can be preserved posteriorly may have decreased stenosis of the neopharynx after postoperative radiotherapy. Margins should be taken and confirmed with more extensive resection required for findings on frozen section of severe dysplasia or worse. For patients requiring tracheotomy, the tracheotomy should be placed as high as possible to facilitate formation of the stoma and adequate inferior margins. Of note, it is important to widen the stoma as much as possible to prevent stenosis during chemoradiation.

Treatment of the Neck   The neck management in this situation is less controversial. This patient has N2 disease and should undergo at least a modified radical neck dissection. Contraindications to surgery would be if the tumor completely encompassed the carotid artery or had invaded deep into the prevertebral musculature.

Reconstruction of the Neopharynx   Several reconstruction options are available to this patient depending on the extent of the surgical defect. For patients with defects above the thoracic inlet, microvascular reconstruction of the hypopharynx remains the mainstay of treatment. Depending on the patient's comorbidities and personal preference, he can be either reconstructed with a jejunal, radial forearm, or ALT graft. Should the resection involve the cervical esophagus, the patient will require gastric pull-up or colonic interposition graft depending again on the patient's comorbidity.

Treatment of Distant Sites   This patient is at high risk for a synchronous or metachronous primary in the lungs or elsewhere in the head and neck. The combined PET scan and CT of the chest, abdomen, and pelvis provides an excellent tool to evaluate these patients for distant metastasis. For patients who do have positive findings on the PET scan in the lungs, often the pulmonology team can obtain a biopsy via bronchoscopy. For patients with isolated lung tumors, surgery provides the best chance of cure. Patients who have extensive lung metastasis or extensive primary lung disease should undergo palliative chemoradiation for tumor control at the primary site in the neck as well as the chest.

Summary of Treatment   This patient has several negative prognostic factors, and aggressive multimodality treatment with surgery and radiation therapy is indicated. Regardless of therapy, the patient's prognosis is poor. That being said, surgery with adjuvant therapy provides for excellent locoregional control in these patients. Patients at high risk of distant metastasis will benefit from a postoperative course of chemoradiation. These patients can usually be predicted by the presence of extracapsular spread on pathologic examination of the regional neck disease. Chemoradiotherapy as a primary modality is relatively contraindicated but may have use in patients unable to undergo surgery or patients requiring palliative therapy. This patient will also require close surveillance. A PET scan at 3 months and again at 1 year after treatment can be highly effective in detecting tumor recurrence or the appearance of metastatic disease.

Case 3   T1b glottic.

Presentation   The patient is a 45-year-old woman with a 25 pack-year history of smoking. She presents to the clinic with a 4-month history of hoarseness that has not improved on antibiotics. She does note that her mother underwent chemoradiation for a lung cancer and she wishes to avoid radiation at all costs.

Physical Examination   On exam, this patient demonstrates normal otoscopy and rhinoscopy. Examination of the oral cavity reveals no masses or lesions. The neck feels benign with no lesions noted in the thyroid or along the jugulodigastric chain. Flexible fiberoptic examination reveals a 1.5-cm mass involving the anterior commissure as well as the anterior two thirds of both true vocal cords. Both vocal cords demonstrated normal motion with both arytenoids appearing normal as well. The interarytenoid space appeared clear, and there did not appear to be any significant subglottic extension.

Diagnosis and Workup   Based on clinical exam, this patient is a good candidate for conservation laryngeal surgery, namely a supracricoid laryngectomy. She most likely has a T1b (involving the anterior commissure) N0 glottic carcinoma. The patient should undergo a preoperative panendoscopy. Care should be taken to document the extent of subglottic involvement. Also, the piriform sinus and postcricoid area must be clear of disease. There should also be no involvement of the vocal process of the arytenoids. It is important to note that the arytenoids remain mobile with no involvement of the interarytenoid space. A CT with contrast must be done to evaluate for cartilage involvement. Transcartilage spread is a contraindication for conservation laryngeal surgery, and its absence must be confirmed to proceed. The presence of nodal disease should be noted as well to plan for treatment of the neck. A PET scan may be warranted to screen for distant disease as well or synchronous primary in the lungs. Because this patient is a candidate for a supracricoid or other conservation laryngeal surgery, a thorough pulmonary history must be performed. Pulmonary function tests may be necessary as well to confirm a good forced expiratory volume in one second (FEV1) and normal flow volume loops.

Options for Treatment   Until the advent of conservation laryngeal surgery, the only surgical therapy available to this patient would have been a total laryngectomy. Since then, we have become much more sophisticated with regard to treatment. Whereas total laryngectomy remains an option for patients wishing to avoid radiation as a primary modality with poor lung function, it is certainly not the first choice for a young otherwise healthy patient with excellent lung function. This patient should be treated by either a supracricoid laryngectomy or primary radiation therapy. Based on her exam and wish to avoid radiation, she is an excellent candidate for supracricoid laryngectomy. Contraindications for this procedure would be poor pulmonary function, inability to preserve one complete functional arytenoids unit (arytenoid, superior laryngeal nerve, recurrent laryngeal nerve, etc.), bilateral fixed arytenoids, transcartilaginous spread or subglottic extension greater than 1 cm below the TVC. Radiotherapy remains an excellent option for this patient. The toxicity of treatment for early glottic cancer is significantly less than aggressive chemoradiotherapy for unresectable lung cancer where treatment can affect lung, esophageal, and cardiac function. She should be offered consultation with a radiation oncologist to review this option.

Treatment of the Primary Tumor   This tumor was managed via supracricoid laryngectomy. When performing this surgery, several considerations come into play. For patients with a single involved arytenoid, an extended supracricoid laryngectomy may be performed allowing for preservation of a single arytenoid unit. Involvement of the epiglottis should also be evaluated as it will affect whether the patient is closed via a CHP, where the cricoid is sutured directly to the hyoid, or a CHEP, where the tip of the epiglottis it preserved to aid with swallow and this entire complex is sutured to the hyoid. Special care must be taken when dividing the cricothyroid joint as the recurrent laryngeal nerve travels only a few millimeters posterior to this. Damage to the nerve in this location can lead to intractable aspiration and need for total laryngectomy.

Treatment of the Neck   The risk of neck metastasis is low in patients with T1 glottic cancer. An argument could be made for observing the neck in this situation. Although selective neck dissection is a safe procedure, it is not without risk. Therefore, in patients with T1 cancers of the glottis, where the risk of regional metastasis is less than 20%, the recommendation would be to not perform a neck dissection. Alternatively, should postoperative radiation be indicated for poor primary tumor characteristics, there may be indications to radiate the neck.

Treatment of Distant Sites   The risk of distant metastasis is low in this patient.

Summary of Treatment   This patient is the ideal patient for conservation laryngeal surgery. She is young, healthy, and clearly able to tolerate this procedure. Local control for this procedure is probably above 90%. Patients who are radiated may have a higher voice quality, but patients undergoing supracricoid laryngectomy develop functional voices that are easily intelligible. In any patient who is a candidate for multiple-modality therapy, a long discussion must be undertaken with the patient such that both the patient and surgeon enter into the procedure with reasonable expectations. This is especially true for patients opting out of primary radiation for tumors where it is indicated.

Case 4   Large-volume T3 disease (fixed TVC).

Presentation   Case 4 is a 55-year-old man who presents with severe hoarseness that has become progressively worse over the past year. He is a 45 pack-year smoker. The patient states that he has had increasing ear and throat pain over the past 6 months. He feels that this is a cold that he cannot get over and points to the multiple nodes in his left neck as proof.

Physical Examination   On examination, the patient presents with a 5-cm mass involving the left vocal cord.

The airway is precarious at best with significant difficulty visualizing the airway, although the patient does not appear to be in distress. The arytenoid on the left appears fixed with no mobility of that cord. Furthermore, the mass appears to be extending up onto the aryepiglottic fold and involving the interarytenoid space. Exam of the neck reveals a 2.5-cm mass in level III and a 2-cm mass in level IIa. These are fixed, nontender, and firm to palpation. The contralateral neck appears free of disease.

Diagnosis and Workup   Based on clinical exam, this patient has what appears to be a T3 (fixed TVC) N2b cancer of the glottis. There appears to be supraglottic extension as well. Panendoscopy should be performed, as in all cases, to evaluate the extent of tumor spread and to confirm diagnosis. The patient will also require a contrast CT of the larynx and neck. This should be done to further elucidate the extent of the neck disease, confirm the lack of disease in the contralateral neck, and evaluate the submucosal extent of the tumor. Important findings would be whether or not the cartilage is involved and what the total volume of the disease is. Whereas inner cortex involvement would not upstage the patient, through-and-through involvement of the cartilage would upstage this patient to T4. This is important because it will affect counseling of the patient prior to therapy. Because of his smoking history and presence of regional disease, this patient is at higher risk of distant metastasis. He should undergo a PET scan or at least a chest x-ray and lactate dehydrogenase (LDH) to evaluate for distant disease. PET-CT is an excellent modality for confirming positive uptake on PET scan. Furthermore, this allows for PET to be used to follow response to therapy. For these reasons, PET-CT is the diagnostic method of choice at the University of Iowa.

Options for Treatment   Much of the debate regarding the treatment of advanced-stage laryngeal cancer revolves around the treatment of bulky T3 disease. Although a very select few of these patients are candidates for conservation laryngeal surgery and, in select institutions, laser resection, in most situations total laryngectomy is the surgical option available to this patient. The RTOG study group would suggest that concurrent chemoradiation should be the treatment of choice for this patient at the current juncture. This is not without risk, however, as nine patients experienced grade V toxicity (death) as a result of their treatment. Ultimately, most patients were able to keep their larynx with only 16% requiring salvage total laryngectomy (28% and 31%, respectively, for the induction and radiation-alone groups). This did not affect the overall survival, with 90% of the patients who were salvaged being alive at 2 years.[43] It is clear, however, that a subset of these patients do not do well with concurrent chemoradiation. The question becomes how to select for these patients and target them for primary surgical therapy. Response to induction chemotherapy may represent a novel attempt to segregate patients who will not do well with concurrent chemoradiation and to provide them with optimum therapy.[51] The role of cetuximab in enhancing the efficacy of radiotherapy or cisplatin-based chemoradiotherapy is currently under investigation.

Treatment of the Primary Tumor This patient was ultimately managed via nonsurgical means. He required a tracheostomy to secure the airway prior to beginning therapy and ultimately a G-tube to maintain alimentation during therapy. Patients undergoing concurrent chemoradiation should be required to meet with a speech pathologist prior to beginning therapy to receive counseling regarding maintaining swallowing throughout the course of therapy. This can be instrumental in keeping patients swallowing through therapy and theoretically may help to prevent or at least limit G-tube dependence. During the course of therapy, the patient should be monitored by the head and neck surgeon primarily to aid with toxicity associated with therapy but also to help monitor response. Maintaining adequate caloric intake, hydration, and pain control is essential not only in terms of patient safety but also to avoid treatment breaks or termination of therapy before reaching 70 Gy. Both treatment breaks and lower radiation dose lead to increased failure rates.

Treatment of the Neck Management of the neck for patients undergoing primary chemoradiation is increasingly controversial. Patients in the RTOG study underwent scheduled neck dissection for N2 or greater disease 8 weeks after the completion of therapy regardless of response.[43] Unfortunately, significant evidence to support scheduled neck dissection is lacking. Recently, a multicenter international group attempted to define the state of the art with regard to planned neck dissection in the setting of concurrent chemoradiation therapy.[62] They argue there is no controversy regarding dissecting clinically positive necks; the controversy lies with patients who have complete response after therapy. Several of the studies reviewed demonstrated that patients with complete response demonstrated pathologically negative necks. Furthermore, several other reviewed studies showed patients with incomplete response demonstrated pathologically negative necks. Certainly, the challenge becomes how to predict which patients actually need neck dissection versus which patients can be safely observed. The literature appears to be somewhat split on the effect of scheduled neck dissection on overall survival and locoregional control. Currently, it is believed that PET scan will play an important role in the determination of whether patients require neck dissection. Currently, there are groups who suggest that observation or serial PET may allow avoidance of scheduled neck dissection including patients who are PET−/CT+. Recent studies out of the University of Iowa demonstrated the potential to observe patients basing the likelihood of recurrence on the standardized uptake value (SUV).[84] Although this may not be a widely accepted approach, it certainly opens the door for a more surgically conservative approach in the treatment of N2 disease for patients undergoing concurrent therapy.

Treatment of Distant Sites See previous discussion in Case 2.

Summary of Treatment Concurrent chemoradiation is becoming a more common treatment modality for laryngeal cancer. Unfortunately, recent publications have illus-

trated that we are currently not winning the battle in the treatment of advanced laryngeal cancer. Data out of the National Cancer Database has suggested that survival for laryngeal cancer has gradually decreased or at best stabilized between the 1980s and 1990s. Among other factors, this seems to correspond with an increase in the incidence of nonsurgical management of laryngeal cancer.[88] Although there are several possible reasons to explain this phenomenon, it serves to illustrate the importance of an organized team-based approach to the treatment of this complicated cancer. It is incumbent on surgeons, medical oncologists, and radiation oncologists to work together to develop successful treatment algorithms for this complicated disease. Until a definitive answer is found either in the form of tumor markers or via treatment selection, all options must be explained equally to the patient. In the end, the ultimate treatment should be patient specific until a definitive answer can be found.

References

1. American Cancer Society Facts and Figures 2006. Available at http://documents.cancer.org/148.00/148.00.pdf
2. Coleman MP, Esteve J, Damiecki P, Arslan A, Renard H. Trends in cancer incidence and mortality 1993. IARC Sci Publ 1993;121:1–806
3. Ferlito A. Histological classification of larynx and hypopharynx cancers and their clinical implications: pathologic aspects of 2052 malignant neoplasms diagnosed at the ORL department of Padua University from 1966 to 1976. Acta Otolaryngol Suppl 1976;342:1–88
4. Bradford CR, Hoffman HT, Wolf GT, et al. Squamous carcinoma of the head and neck in organ transplant recipients: possible role of oncogenic viruses. Laryngoscope 1990;100:190–194
5. Harrison DFN. Laryngeal cancer: a preventable disease. In Ferlito A, ed. Neoplasms of the Larynx. Edinburgh, UK: Churchill Livingstone; 1993
6. Hoshikawa T, Nakajima T, Uhara H, et al. Detection of human papillomavirus DNA in laryngeal squamous cell carcinomas by polymerase chain reaction. Laryngoscope 1990;100:647–650
7. Ward PH, Hanson DG. Reflux as an etiological factor of carcinoma of the laryngopharynx. Laryngoscope 1988;98:1195–1199
8. Gillison ML, Koch WM, Capone RB, et al. Evidence for casual association between human papillomavirus and a subset of head and neck cancers. J Natl Cancer Inst 2000;92:709–720
9. Smith EM, Hoffman HT, Summersgill KS, Kirchner HL, Turek LP, Haugen TH. Human papillomavirus and risk of oral cancer. Laryngoscope 1998;108(7):1098–1103
10. Almadoria G, Galli J, Cadoni G, Bussu F, Maurizi M. Human papilloma virus infection dn cyclin D1 gene amplification in laryngeal squamous cell carcinoma: biologic function and clinical significance. Head Neck 2002;24(6):597–604
11. Smith EM, Summersgill KF, Allen J, et al. Human papillomavirus and risk of laryngeal cancer. Ann Otol Rhinol Laryngol 2000;109(11):1069–1076
12. Ritchie JM, Smith EM, Summergill KF, et al. Human papillomavirus infection as a prognostic factor in carcinomas of the oral cavity and oropharynx. Int J Cancer 2003;104:336–344
13. Greene F, Page D, Fleming I, et al, eds. Cancer Staging Manual. 6th ed. New York, NY: Springer-Verlag; 2002
14. Ferlito A, Carbone A, DeSanto L, et al. "Early" cancer of the larynx: the concept as defined by clinicians, pathologists, and biologists. Ann Otol Rhinol Laryngol 1996;105:245–250
15. Belafsky PC, Postma GN, Daniel E, Koufman JA. Transnasal esophagoscopy. Otolaryngol Head Neck Surg 2001;125(6):588–589
16. Silver C. Surgical anatomy. In: Silver CE, Ferlito A, eds. Surgery for Cancer of the Larynx and Related Structures. 2nd ed. Philadelphia, PA: W.B. Saunders; 1996:25
17. Crissman JD, Zarbo RJ, Drozdowicz S, et al. Carcinoma in situ and microinvasive squamous cell carcinoma of the laryngeal glottis. Arch Otolaryngol Head Neck Surg 1988;114:299–307

18. Miller AH. Premalignant laryngeal lesions, carcinoma in situ, superficial carcinoma: definition and management. Can J Otolaryngol 1974;3:573–575

19. Flint PW. Minimally invasive techniques for management of early glottic cancer. Otolaryngol Clin North Am 2002;35:1055–1066

20. Blackwell KE, Fu YS, Calcaterra TC. Laryngeal dysplasia. A clinicopathologic study. Cancer 1995;75:457–463

21. Postma GN, Bch KK, Belafsky PC, Koufman JA. The role of transnasal esophagoscopy in head and neck oncology. Laryngoscope 2002;112(12):2242–2243

22. Aviv JE, Takoudes TG, Ma G, Close LG. Office-based esophagoscopy: a preliminary report. Otolaryngol Head Neck Surg 2001;125(3):170–175

23. Beauvillian C, Mahe M, Bourdin S, et al. Final results of a randomized trial comparing chemotherapy plus radiotherapy with chemotherapy plus surgery plus radiotherapy in locally advanced respectable hypopharyngeal carcinomas. Laryngoscope 1997;107:648–653

24. Belafsky PC, Postma GN, Koufman JA. Normal transnasal esophagoscopy. (comment) Ear Nose Throat J 2001;80(7):438

25. Colden D, Zeitels SM, Hillman RE, Jarboe J, Bunting G, Spanou K. Stroboscopic assessment of vocal fold keratosis and glottic cancer. Ann Otol Rhinol Laryngol 2001;110:293–298

26. Weber RS, Hankins P, Wolf P, et al. CT versus MRI for staging carcinoma of the larynx (L) and hypopharynx (HP). Presented at: American Laryngological Association; May 4, 1996; Orlando, FL

27. Mukherji SK, Mancuso AA, Mendenhall W, et al. Can pretreatment CT predict local control of T2 glottic carcinomas treated with radiation therapy alone? AJNR Am J Neuroradiol 1995;16:655–662

28. Wenig BL, Ziffra KL, Mafee MF, et al. MR imaging of squamous cell carcinoma of the larynx and hypopharynx. Otolaryngol Clin North Am 1995;28:609–619

29. Byers RM, Wolf PF, Ballantyne AJ. Rationale for elective modified neck dissection. Head Neck Surg 1988;10:160–167

30. Kowalski LP, Medina JE. Nodal metastasis: predictive factors. management of the neck in head and neck cancer. Otolaryngol Clin North Am 1998;31(5):803–814

31. Shah JP, Tollefsen HR. Epidermoid carcinoma of the supraglottic larynx. Am J Surg 1974;128(4):494–499

32. Yang CY, Andersen PE, Everts EC, Cohen JI. Nodal disease in purely glottic carcinoma: is elective neck treatment worthwhile? Laryngoscope 1998;108(7):1006–1008

33. Johnson JT. Carcinoma of the larynx: selective approach to the management of cervical lymphatics. Ear Nose Throat J 1994;73:303–305

34. Medina J. Neck dissection. In: Bailey B, Calhoun K, Healy G, Johnson JT, eds. Head and Neck Surgery – Otolaryngology. Vol. II. Philadelphia: Lippincott Williams & Wilkins; 2001:1346–1365

35. Madison MT, Remley KB, Latchaw RE, et al. Radiologic diagnosis and staging of head and neck squamous cell carcinoma. Otolaryngol Clin North Am 1998;31(4):727–754

36. Myers LL, Wax MK, Nabi H, et al. Positron emission tomography in the evaluation of the N0 neck. Laryngoscope 1998;108:232–236

37. Austin JR, Wong FC, Kim EE. Positron emission tomograph in the detection of residual laryngeal carcinoma. Otolaryngol Head Neck Surg 1995;113:404–407

38. Terhaard CH, Bongers V, Van Rijk P, Hordijk G. F-18-Fluoro-deoxy-glucose positron-emission tomography scanning in detection of local recurrence after radiotherapy for laryngeal/pharyngeal cancer. Head Neck 2001;23(11):933–941

39. McGuirt WF, Keyes JW, Geising KR, et al. Positron emission tomography in the evaluation of laryngeal carcinoma. Ann Otol Rhinol Laryngol 1995;104:274–278

40. Uematsu H, Sadato N, Yonekura Y, et al. Coregistration of FDB PET and MRI of the head and neck using normal distribution of FDG. J Nucl Med 1998;39:2121–2127

41. De Boer JR, Pruim J, Burlage F, et al. Therapy evaluation of laryngeal carcinomas by tyrosine-pet. Head Neck 2003;25(8):634–644

42. The Department of Veterans Affairs Laryngeal Cancer Study Group. Induction chemotherapy plus radiation compared with surgery plus radiation in patients with advanced laryngeal cancer. N Engl J Med 1991;324:1685–1690

43. Forastiere AA, Goepfert H, Maor M, et al. Concurrent chemotherapy and radiotherapy for organ preservation in advanced laryngeal cancer. N Engl J Med 2003;349(22):2091–2098

44. Weinstein GS, Myers E, Shapshay SN, et al. Nonsurgical treatment of laryngeal cancer. N Engl J Med 2004;350:1049–1053

45. Urba S, Wolf G, Eisbruch A, et al. Single-cycle induction chemotherapy selects patients with advanced laryngeal cancer for combined chemoradiation: a new treatment paradigm. J Clin Oncol 2006;24:593–598

46. DeSanto LW, Olsen KD. Early glottic cancer. Am J Otolaryngol 1994;15:242–249

47. Strong MS, Jako GJ. Laser surgery in the larynx: early clinical experience with continuous CO2 laser. Ann Otol Rhinol Laryngol 1972;81:791–798

48. Cragle SP, Brandenburg J. Laser cordectomy or radiotherapy: cure rates, communication, and cost. Otolaryngol Head Neck Surg 1993;108:648–654

49. Eckel HE, Thumfart WF. Laser surgery for the treatment of larynx carcinomas: indications, techniques, and preliminary results. Ann Otol Rhinol Laryngol 1992;101:113–118

50. Pearson B. Foreword. In: Steiner W, Abrosch P. Endoscopic Laser Surgery of the Upper Aerodigestive Tract. New York, NY: Thieme Medical Publishers; 2000;viii

51. Steiner W, Ambrosch P. Endoscopic Laser Surgery of the Upper Aerodigestive Tract. New York, NY: Thieme Medical Publishers; 2000

52. Lefebvre JL. What is the role of primary surgery in the treatment of laryngeal and hypopharyngeal cancer. Hayes Martin Lecture. Arch Otolaryngol Head Neck Surg 2000;126:285–288

53. Sessions DG, Lenox J, Spector GJ. Supraglottic laryngeal cancer: analysis of treatment results. Laryngoscope 2005;115(8):1402–1410

54. Motamed M, Laccourreye O, Bradley PJ. Salvage conservation laryngeal surgery after irradiation failure for early laryngeal cancer. Laryngoscope 2006;116(3):451–455

55. Burgess LP. Laryngeal reconstruction following vertical partial laryngectomy. Laryngoscope 1993;103:109–132

56. Weinstein GS, Laccourreye O. Vertical parital larygnsocmties. In: Weinstein GS, Laccourreye O, Brasnu D, Laccourreye H, eds. Organ Preservation Surgery for Laryngeal Cancer. San Diego, CA: Thomson Learning; 2000:59–71

57. Laccourreye O, Laccourreye H, El-Sawy M, Weinstein G. Supracricoid partial laryngecotmy with cricohyoidoepiglottopexy. In: Weinstein GS, Laccourreye O, Brasnu D, Laccourreye H, eds. Organ Preservation Surgery for Laryngeal Cancer. San Diego, CA: Thomson Learning; 2000

58. Kim MS, Sun D, Park K, Cho K, Park Y, Cho S. Paraglottic space in supracricoid larygnecotmy. Arch Otolaryngol Head Neck Surg 2002;128:304–307

59. Weinstein GS, El-Sawy MM, Ruiz C, et al. Laryngeal preservation with supracricoid partial laryngectomy results in improved quality of life when compared with total laryngectomy. Laryngoscope 2001;111:191–199

60. Lefebvre JL, Chevalier D, Luboinski B, et al. Larynx preservation in pyriform sinus cancer: preliminary results of a European Organization for Research and Treatment of Cancer phase III trial. J Natl Cancer Inst 1996;88:890–899

61. Richard JM, Sancho-Garnier H, Pessey JJ, et al. Randomized trial of induction chemotherapy in larynx carcinoma. Oral Oncol 1998;34:224–228

62. Pignon JP, Bourhis J, Domenge C, Designe L. Chemotherapy added to locoregional treatment for head and neck squamous-cell carcinoma: three meta-analyses of updated individual data. MACH-NC Collaborative Group. Meta-Analysis of Chemotherapy on Head and Neck Cancer. Lancet 2000;355(9208):949–955

63. Ganly I, Patel SG, Matsuo J, et al. Results of surgical salvage after failure of definitive radiation therapy for early-stage squamous cell carcinoma of the glottic larynx. Arch Otolaryngol Head Neck Surg 2006;132(1):59–66

64. Weber RS, Berkey BA, Forastiere A, et al. Outcome of salvage total laryngectomy following organ preservation therapy: the Radiation Therapy Oncology Group trial 91-11. Arch Otolaryngol Head Neck Surg 2003;129(1):44–49

65. Bakamjian VY. A two stage method for pharyngoesophageal reconstruction with a primary pectoral skin flap. Plast Reconstr Surg 1965;36:173–184

66. Song YG, Chen GZ, Song YL. The free thigh flap: a new free flap concept based on the septocutaneous artery. Br J Plast Surg 1984;37(2):149–159

67. Eibling D. Surgery for glottic carcinoma. In: Myers E, ed. Operative Otolaryngology–Head and Neck Surgery. Philadelphia, PA: W.B. Saunders; 1997:416–444

68. Seidenberg B, Rosenak SS, Hurwitt ES, Som ML. Immediate reconstruction of the cervical esophagus by a revascularized isolated jejunal segment. Ann Surg 1959;149(2):162–171

69. Wadsworth JT, Futran N, Eubanks TR. Laparoscopic harvest of the jejunal free flap for reconstruction of hypopharyngeal and cervical esophageal defects. Arch Otolaryngol Head Neck Surg 2002;128(12):1384–1387

70. Nakatsuka T, Harii K, Asato H, Ebihara S, Yoshizumi T, Saikawa M. Comparative evaluation in pharyngo-oesophageal reconstruction: radial forearm flap compared with jejunal flap. A 10-year experience. Scand J Plast Reconstr Surg Hand Surg 1998;32(3):307–310

71. Harii K, Ebihara S, Ono I, Saito H, Terui S, Takato T. Pharyngoesophageal reconstruction using a fabricated forearm free flap. Plast Reconstr Surg 1985;75(4):463–476

72. Azizzadeh B, Yafai S, Rawnsley JD, et al. Radial forearm free flap pharyngoesophageal reconstruction. Laryngoscope 2001;111(5):807–810

73. Wei FC, Jain V, Celik N, Chen HC, Chuang DC, Lin CH. Have we found an ideal soft-tissue flap? An experience with 672 anterolateral thigh flaps. Plast Reconstr Surg 2002;109(7):2219–2226

74. Genden EM, Jacobson AS. The role of the anterolateral thigh flap for pharyngoesophageal reconstruction. Arch Otolaryngol Head Neck Surg 2005;131(9):796–799

75. Yamazaki H, Nishiyama K, Tanaka E, Koizumi M, Chatani M. Radiotherapy for early glottic carcinoma (T1N0M0): results of prospective randomized study of radiation fraction size and overall treatment time. Int J Radiat Oncol Biol Phys 2006;64:77–82

76. Garden AS, Forster K, Wong PF, et al. Results of radiotherapy for T2N0 grottic carcinoma: does the "2" stand for twice-daily treatment? Int J Radiat Oncol Biol Phys 2003;55:322–328

77. Bonner JA, Harai PM, Giralt J, et al. Radiotherapy plus cetuximab for squamous-cell carcinoma of the head and neck. N Engl J Med 2006;354:567–578

78. Fu KK, Pajak TF, Trotti A, et al. A Radiation Therapy Oncology Group (RTOG) phase III randomized study to compare hyperfractionation and two variants of accelerated fractionation to standard fractionation radiotherapy for head and neck squamous cell carcinomas: First report of RTOG 9003. Int J Radiat Oncol Biol Phys 2000;48(1):7–16

79. Cooper JS, Pajak TF, Forstiere AA, et al. Postoperative concurrent radiotherapy and chemotherapy for high-risk squamous cell carcinoma of the head and neck. N Engl J Med 2004;350:1937–1944

80. Bernier J, Domenge C, Ozsahin M, et al. Postoperative irradiation with or without concomitant chemotherapy for locally advanced head and neck cancer. N Engl J Med 2004;350:1945–1952

81. Eisbruch A, Marsh LH, Dawson LA, et al. Recurrences near base of skull after IMRT for head and neck cancer: implications for target delineation in high neck and for parotid gland sparing. Int J Radiat Oncol Biol Phys 2004;59(1):28–42

82. Hinerman RW, Mendenhall WM, Amdur RJ, Stringer SP, Villaret DB, Robbins KT. Carcinoma of the supraglottic larynx: treatment results with radiotherapy alone or with planned neck dissection. Head Neck 2002;24:456–467

83. Dawson LA, Meyers LL, Bradford CR, et al. Conformal re-irradiation of recurrent and new primary head and neck cancer. Int J Radiat Oncol Biol Phys 2001;50(2):377–385

84. Yao M, Smith RB, Graham MM, et al. The role of FDG PET in management of neck metastasis from head-and-neck cancer after definitive radiation treatment. Int J Radiat Oncol Biol Phys 2005;63(4):991–999

85. Rodrigo JP, Cabanillas R, Franco V, Suarez C. Efficacy of routine bilateral neck dissection in the management of the N0 neck in T1–T2 unilateral supraglottic cancer. Head Neck 2006;28(6):534–539

86. Lim YC, Lee JS, Koo BS, Choi EC. Level IIb lymph node metastasis in laryngeal squamous cell carcinoma. Laryngoscope 2006;116(2):268–272

87. Silverman DA, El-Hajj M, Strome S, Esclamado RM. Prevalence of nodal metastases in the submuscular recess (level IIb) during selective neck dissection. Arch Otolaryngol Head Neck Surg 2003;129(7):724–728

88. Hoffman HT, Porter K, Karnell LH, et al. Laryngeal cancer in the United States: changes in demographics, patterns of care, and survival. Laryngoscope 2006;116:1–13

5

Carcinoma of the Thyroid

Eric M. Genden and Elise M. Brett

◆ Etiology

Thyroid carcinoma is a result of a poorly understood cascade of molecular events that has been linked to activation of protooncogenes or defects related to a tumor suppressor gene. All thyroid tumors are derived from defects that occur in either the follicular cells or the parafollicular cells. Malignant transformation occurs most commonly in the follicular cell population resulting in well-differentiated carcinoma or less commonly in the parafollicular cell or c-cell population resulting in poorly differentiated carcinoma.

Thyroid cancer is relatively uncommon although the incidence has increased by 82% over the past decade making thyroid cancer the fastest growing cancer nationwide.[1] Although this may suggest that there is an environmental exposure associated with cancer, the dramatic increase in the rate of newly diagnosed thyroid cancers is more likely a result of the improvement in imaging. Advances in imaging technology and the more common use of high-resolution ultrasound (HUS), positron emission tomography (PET), magnetic resonance imaging (MRI), and computed tomography (CT) has led to an increase in the number of incidentally found thyroid nodules, often referred to as "incidentalomas." Although more than 25,000 people in the United States will be diagnosed with thyroid cancer next year, only 1500 will die from the disease. This highlights the fact that whereas well-differentiated thyroid cancer is common, it is rarely fatal. Recent data suggest that the female to male ratio has increased to 3:1 and that this may be due to growth-promoting effects of female estradiol.[2]

◆ Epidemiology

The thyroid gland is composed of two lobes, a right and a left lobe that are connected by a narrow isthmus that traverses the anterior trachea. The thyroid gland lies deep to the anterior cervical strap muscles, and the size of the gland varies greatly weighing ~25 g and tending to be larger in women.

The pretracheal fascia, derived from the deep cervical fascia, surrounds the thyroid gland. The vascular supply to the thyroid gland is derived from the superior and inferior thyroid arteries. There is a rich vascular anastomotic network within the parenchyma of the gland. The superior thyroid artery is the first branch of the external carotid artery and descends to supply the superior thyroid pole. The inferior thyroid artery is a branch of the thyrocervical trunk, and it provides vascular supply to the inferior thyroid pole and the parathyroid glands. The inferior thyroid artery has an intimate relationship with the parathyroid glands and the recurrent laryngeal nerve (RLN); however, the relationship between the artery and the recurrent nerve is inconsistent. The RLN may run superficial or deep to the inferior thyroid artery. Therefore, when performing a thyroidectomy, it is essential to identify the nerve prior to ligating the inferior thyroid artery to avoid injury to the nerve. The usual course of the RLN differs in the two sides of the neck. The right RLN travels on the undersurface of the right subclavian artery and ascends in the neck along the right tracheoesophageal groove (**Fig. 5–1**). It may pass superficially or deep to the inferior thyroid artery or between its distal branches. The left RLN passes around the arch of the aorta and ascends in the left tracheoesophageal groove. Both nerves enter the larynx at the cricothyroid articulation through the fibers of the inferior constrictor muscles of the pharynx. A thorough understanding of the anatomy and an appreciation for meticulous dissection is essential to prevent injury to the RLN or parathyroid glands.

The lymphatics of the thyroid gland follow two major pathways (**Fig. 5–2**). The first is adjacent to the inferior thyroid vein, and the second is along the path of the middle thyroid

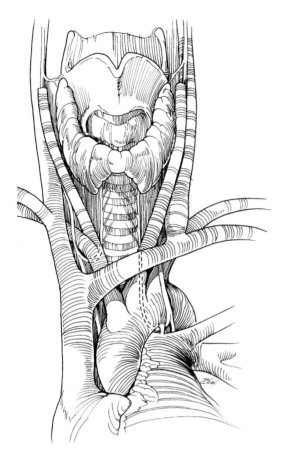

Figure 5–1 The course of the RLN. The right RLN travels on the undersurface of the right subclavian artery and ascends in the neck along the right tracheoesophageal groove. The left RLN passes around the arch of the aorta and ascends in the left tracheoesophageal groove.

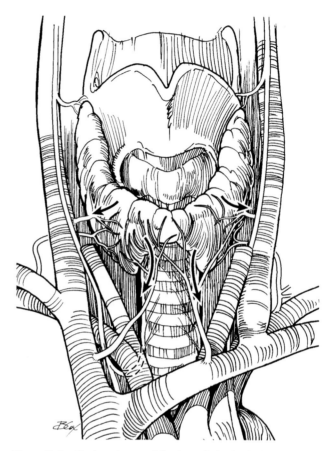

Figure 5–2 The lymphatics of the thyroid gland. The lymphatics of the thyroid gland travel adjacent to the inferior thyroid vein and along the path of the middle thyroid vein (*arrows*).

vein. Occasionally, the prelaryngeal lymph nodes may be involved in superior medial, or isthmus tumors (**Fig. 5–3**). In spite of these pathways, the site of regional disease does not always correlate with the site of the tumor within the gland. Noguchi first defined the pattern of thyroid metastasis and found that the paratracheal lymph nodes were most commonly affected regardless of the site of the primary tumor; however, when the disease progressed laterally, the lower jugular chain was most commonly affected.[3]

◆ Presentation

Thyroid carcinoma usually presents as a palpable thyroid nodule or a nodule that is discovered incidentally on neck imaging for evaluation of the cervical spine, carotid arteries, or other diagnoses. Less commonly it may present as a lateral neck mass.[4] Thyroid nodules are common; however, in most studies, the rate of malignancy is only 4 to 5%.[5,6] The prevalence of thyroid nodules increases with age and is estimated to occur in roughly 50% of the U.S. population 50 years of age and older.[7] Thyroid cancer may present as a dominant nodule in a multinodular gland or as a solitary nodule. It was previously thought that the risk of malignancy was lower in a multinodular gland, but it is now recognized that the risk per gland is equivalent[8] and that incidentally discovered nodules carry a similar risk of malignancy.[9] What this suggests is that any nodule may represent a cancer and that every nodule should be evaluated.

Upon initial presentation, a careful history is essential because it can reveal information that immediately stratifies a patient into a high-risk category. High-risk factors include a prior history of head and neck radiation including radiation for Hodgkin's disease,[10] radiation exposure from the Chernobyl accident,[11] and a family history of thyroid cancer. The risk of thyroid cancer in first-degree relatives of patients with differentiated thyroid cancer has been shown to be 6 times that of the general population.[12] Other important high-risk factors include a history of rapid growth of a solid nodule, pain, dysphagia, or dysphonia. Although less than 20% of patients with thyroid carcinoma will present with a regional metastasis, a neck mass in the presence of a thyroid nodule raises the likelihood of malignancy. Young age (<20 years), older age (>70 years), and male gender may also represent an increased risk.[13] To most accurately determine the risk of malignancy, it is essential to consider a variety of factors (**Table 5–1**).

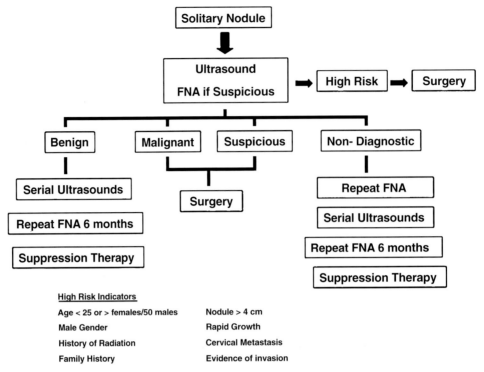

High Risk Indicators

Age < 25 or > females/50 males	Nodule > 4 cm
Male Gender	Rapid Growth
History of Radiation	Cervical Metastasis
Family History	Evidence of invasion

Figure 5–3 Algorithm for evaluation of a solitary thyroid nodule.

Table 5–1 Risk Factors for Thyroid Carcinoma

History of radiation exposure
Family history of papillary thyroid carcinoma
Single dominant solid nodule greater than 4 cm
Male gender
Rapid growth of a nodule
Younger than 20 years
Older than 70 years
Cervical metastasis
Evidence of invasion on imaging

◆ Diagnosis and Workup

There is no single laboratory study that is able to determine the presence of thyroid malignancy. Although elevated baseline calcitonin levels represent occult medullary carcinoma in 10 to 40% of cases, the presence of false-positive elevations, the low incidence of medullary carcinoma, and the high cost of testing have led to recommendations against routine testing in the United States.[14] Calcitonin levels are usually reserved for high-risk patients and those with a family history of medullary thyroid carcinoma or multiple endocrine neoplasia (MEN). Thyroglobulin is not useful in the workup because there are a variety of conditions that can lead to elevated levels including thyroid inflammation, glandular stimulation, or injury after radiation, surgery, or even a biopsy. Thyroid stimulating hormone should be measured to exclude a toxic nodule, as toxic nodules are almost never malignant and generally do not require fine-needle aspiration. If the TSH is suppressed, then radioisotope imaging should be performed to confirm and localize the toxic nodule(s).

Ultrasound

In contrast with other malignancies of the head and neck, the physical exam may not always be a strong predictor of malignancy.[15] Rare characteristics such as attachment to overlying skin and muscle, vocal cord paralysis, firmness to palpation, and the presence of lymphadenopathy may raise the suspicion of a malignancy; however, the majority of well-differentiated thyroid cancers will present with subtle findings that may only be identified on imaging or cytology. HUS offers the most sensitive and cost-effective method for detecting a thyroid carcinoma.[16–18] Using a 10- to 13-MHz transducer, nodules as small as 2 mm can be clearly identified and evaluated (**Table 5–2**). Ultrasonographic characteristics suggestive of malignancy include hypoechogenicity, ill-defined margins, irregular borders, heterogeneity, and

Table 5–2 Findings on Ultrasonography That Suggest Malignancy

Absence of a "halo" sign
Solid/hypoechogenic nodule
Heterogeneous echogenic structure
Irregular margins
Extraglandular extension
Fine punctuate internal calcifications

presence of calcification, particularly microcalcifications. Using these criteria, the sensitivity of ultrasound has been demonstrated as high as 86.5% and specificity 92.3% for nonfollicular neoplasms.[19] Doppler ultrasound has recently been shown to have a sensitivity of 92% and specificity of 87.5% in distinguishing follicular adenoma from follicular carcinoma.[20] Generally, no additional imaging is required although CT and MRI scanning can sometimes be helpful in assessing presence of a substernal component of the gland or in preoperative planning in cases where there is suspicion of laryngeal, tracheal, or esophageal invasion.

Ultrasound-Guided Fine-Needle Aspiration

Once a suspicious nodule has been identified, ultrasound-guided fine-needle aspiration should be performed (**Fig. 5–3**). Determining which nodules should be aspirated and whether there should be a size cutoff has been a heavily debated topic largely because microscopic tumors are generally less aggressive.[21] The American Thyroid Association and the American Association of Clinical Endocrinologist recommended against routine aspiration of nodules <1 cm unless there are suspicious ultrasound characteristics, a family history of thyroid cancer, or history of head or neck irradiation.[22]

Fine-needle aspiration (FNA) has been demonstrated as a highly sensitive method for identifying malignancy,[23] and the diagnostic information that FNA provides has been successful in decreasing the number of thyroidectomies while increasing the yield of malignancies in patients who undergo thyroidectomy.[24] Several studies have demonstrated that FNA is extremely reliable yielding a false-positive rate less than 1% and a false-negative rate less than 2%,[25,26] although other studies have shown substantially higher false-negative rates.[24,27]

The FNA may yield one of four possible diagnoses: malignant disease, benign disease, suspicious for malignancy, or nondiagnostic. Malignant lesions on FNA should prompt a hemithyroidectomy with frozen-section examination; in most cases this will result in total thyroidectomy. In the event that the FNA reveals a benign diagnosis, observation with repeat ultrasound in 6 months is generally appropriate. Levothyroxine suppression therapy is no longer routinely recommended. In the event that there is an increase in size of the nodule, the FNA should be repeated or the patient should be managed with a hemithyroidectomy. A single repeat FNA for a previously benign aspirate will increase the sensitivity for malignancy from 81.7 to 90.4% and decrease the false-negative rate from 17.1 to 11.4%.

In the event that the FNA reveals a suspicious diagnosis, a hemithyroidectomy with frozen-section pathologic analysis is recommended. Based on the intraoperative frozen section, the decision to complete the thyroidectomy or terminate the operation can be made. We offer patients with bilateral nodules and a suspicious aspirate the option of total thyroidectomy initially to avoid the possibility of requiring completion thyroidectomy or continued monitoring of the contralateral lobe.

In some cases, a FNA may yield the diagnosis of "follicular neoplasm, cannot rule out carcinoma" or "Hürthle cell neoplasm." In these cases, the decision making is more difficult. The FNA cannot differentiate a follicular carcinoma or Hurtle cell carcinoma from an adenoma because angioinvasion and invasion of the capsule cannot be detected on cytology. The patient's risk factors, the size of the nodule, and the patient's preference should be considered in the decision-making process. If observation is elected, the nodule should be followed closely with ultrasound. Cytology specimens that reveal predominately Hürthle cells should prompt hemithyroidectomy because up to two thirds represent neoplastic disease with a 16% malignancy rate.[28] If the FNA yields a nondiagnostic result, a repeat of the FNA is warranted.[29]

Preoperative Evaluation

The preoperative evaluation of a patient with suspected thyroid cancer should include a complete physical examination and a direct examination of the larynx to assess vocal fold motion. Preoperative ultrasound of the neck for patients with cytology suspicious for malignancy can be useful in identifying nonpalpable lymph nodes and should routinely be performed. In one recent study, ultrasound detection of nodes altered the surgical procedure in 40.5% of patients undergoing an initial procedure.[30] Ultrasound has also been shown to be highly sensitive and specific for detecting tracheal invasion by papillary thyroid cancer, which may be important in preoperative planning.[31]

◆ Staging

To effectively treat a malignancy of the thyroid gland, it is essential to understand and document the behavior of the tumor. Clinical staging and risk group classification is particularly important in the management of thyroid cancer because it often will direct management, in particular the decision to treat the patient with radioactive iodine, external beam radiation, or combination therapy. The lack of prospective randomized studies assessing the relationships between tumor stage, treatment, and outcome means that the majority of data that is used to create risk-group classifications is derived from retrospective reviews. As a result, there is a variety of classification systems that are based on factors such as age, tumor size, gender, tumor grade, multicentricity, metastatic disease, and other variables. The AGES system[32] is based on factors including age, grade, extent, and size of the tumor (**Table 5–3**). In the AGES system, those patients with an aggregate score 4+ are high risk and those with a score less than 4 are low risk. The AMES system[33] considers age of the patient when the tumor was discovered, distant metastasis, extent of primary tumor, and size of tumor (**Table 5–4**). Additionally, there are systems devised by the European Organization for Research on Treatment of Cancer (EORTC),[34] the National Thyroid Cancer Treatment Cooperative Study,[35] and others.[33,36] Most of these classification systems utilize similar information with minor variations. Irrespective of the classification system that is used, it is important to consider risk-group stratification during the management of a patient with thyroid cancer. Separate from these stratification

Table 5–3 AGES Classification System

Prognostic Score = 0.05 × Age (if Age ≥40 Years)
+1 (if grade 2)
+3 (if grade 3 or 4)
+1 (if extrathyroidal)
+3 (if distant spread)
+0.2 × tumor size (cm maximum diameter)

Survival by AGES Score
≤3.99 = 99%
4–4.99 = 80%
5–5.99 = 67%
≥6 = 13%

systems is the TNM (tumor, node, metastasis) tumor staging system endorsed by the American Joint Committee on Cancer (AJCC) (**Table 5–5**), which serves to provide a uniform language when evaluating management and outcome.

◆ Classification

Papillary Thyroid Carcinoma

Papillary thyroid carcinoma (PTC) is the most common form of the follicular cell–derived carcinomas and comprises three quarters of all newly diagnosed thyroid cancers.[37] PTC is derived from the follicular cells. These cells tend to concentrate iodine and secrete thyroglobulin. As a result, surveillance and detection of recurrence can be relatively straightforward. The prognosis for PTC is usually excellent.

Treatment of Papillary Thyroid Carcinoma

Surgery is the primary treatment for papillary thyroid cancer, and a complete resection offers the best chance of cure.[13,38]

Table 5–4 AMES Classification System

Low Risk
Young patients (men ≤41 years old, women ≤51 years old) without distant metastasis
Older patients (intrathyroidal papillary thyroid cancer, minor capsular invasion for follicular lesion)
Primary cancers <5 cm in diameter
No distant metastasis

High Risk
All patients with distant metastasis
Extrathyroidal papillary
Major capsular invasion for follicular
All older patients with extrathyroidal spread
All older patients with primary cancer >5 cm in diameter (men >40 years, women >50 years)

Survival by AMES Score
Low risk = 99%
High risk = 61%

Table 5–5 TNM Classification System for Differentiated Thyroid Carcinoma

T1	Tumor diameter 2 cm or smaller
T2	Primary tumor diameter >2 to 4 cm
T3	Primary tumor diameter >4 cm limited to the thyroid or with minimal extracapsular extension
T4a	Tumor of any size extending beyond the thyroid capsule to invade the subcutaneous soft tissues, larynx, trachea, esophagus, or recurrent laryngeal nerve
T4b	Tumor invades prevertebral fascia or encases carotid artery or mediastinal nerves
TX	Primary tumor size unknown, but without extrathyroid extension
N0	No metastatic nodes
N1a	Metastasis to level VI (pretracheal, paratracheal, prelaryngeal)
N1b	Metastasis to unilateral or bilateral or contralateral cervical or superior mediastinum
NX	Nodes not assessed at surgery
M0	No distant metastasis
M1	Distant metastasis

Stages for Differentiated Thyroid Cancer

	Patient Age <45 Years	Patient Age >45 Years
Stage I	Any T, any N, M0	T1, N0, M0
Stage II	Any T, any N, M1	T2, N0, M0
Stage III	T3, N0, M0	T3, N0, M0
	T1, N1a, M0	T1, N1a, M0
	T2, N1a, M0	T2, N1a, M0
	T3, N1a, M0	T3, N1a, M0
Stage IVA	T4a, N0, M0	T4a, N0, M0
	T4a, N1a, M0	T4a, N1a, M0
	T2, N1b, M0	T2, N1b, M0
	T3, N1b, M0	T3, N1b, M0
	T4a, N1b, M0	T4a, N1b, M0
Stage IVB	Any T4b, any N, M0	Any T4b, any N, M0
Stage IVC	Any T, Any N, M1	Any T, Any N, M1

Although the role of a complete surgical resection is indisputable, the extent of the initial surgical resection has been a topic of controversy. Primary management of thyroid malignancy has included nodulectomy, hemithyroidectomy with and without isthmusectomy, subtotal thyroidectomy, and total thyroidectomy. The high rate of recurrence associated with nodulectomy has confirmed that this approach is inadequate. Although there has been a trend toward more aggressive surgical resection based on the well-documented multicentric nature of the disease, there are still some who insist that a partial thyroidectomy is sufficient.[39] Proponents of total thyroidectomy point to data that demonstrate a rate of multicentric bilateral disease ranging from 18 to 46%.[40,41] Opponents of total thyroidectomy suggest that multicentric bilateral disease is often microscopic and not clinically significant. This is further supported by the observation that several large studies have failed to demonstrate a survival advantage to total thyroidectomy when compared with hemithyroidectomy.[42,43] In spite of these findings, most clinicians agree that there is a subset of patients who benefit from total thyroidectomy and there is another distinct subset of patients that may be treated more conservatively. The concern regarding "overtreating" a patient by performing a total thyroidectomy instead of a hemithyroidectomy relates to the surgical risk including an increased risk of vocal cord paralysis and a risk of permanent hypoparathyroidism.

In an effort to guide surgical management, the AGES and the AMES classification systems represent two commonly used systems that are utilized to classify patients into either a "high-risk" group or a "low-risk" group. It has been suggested that "low-risk" patients can be managed with a thyroid lobectomy and isthmusectomy, whereas "high-risk" patients are better managed with a total thyroidectomy. Most surgeons agree with the recommendation to perform a total thyroidectomy when faced with a high-risk patient; however, the controversy exists in the low-risk patient subgroup. Several studies have failed to demonstrate that low-risk patients experience an improvement in cause-specific mortality after undergoing a total thyroidectomy,[32,44] and several large studies have demonstrated that there is a benefit to total thyroidectomy.[43,45] The conflicting data can make the decision-making process a difficult one. As a result, not all surgeons favor such guidelines, and many prefer to perform a total thyroidectomy in spite of the risk stratification suggesting that the rate of morbidity in the hands of an experienced surgeon is exceedingly low.[46] To support this contention, a recent study found that surgeons who perform more than 100 thyroidectomies per year reported complication rates of 4.3%, whereas those surgeons who performed less than 10 thyroidectomies per year reported a fourfold increase in complication rate. In spite of the complication rate, when a subtotal thyroidectomy is performed for the management of thyroid carcinoma, it becomes difficult to follow thyroglobulin levels for surveillance.[47] This may represent the most compelling argument to perform a total thyroidectomy for malignancy. Finally, the American Thyroid Association recently recommended that a total thyroidectomy should be performed for the management of well-differentiated thyroid carcinoma.[22]

Follicular Thyroid Carcinoma

Follicular carcinoma is less common than papillary thyroid carcinoma[37] and typically behaves more aggressively than papillary thyroid carcinoma. The aggressive nature of follicular thyroid carcinoma is largely a result of its propensity for hematogenous dissemination. Unlike papillary thyroid carcinoma, which spreads through the lymphatics, follicular carcinoma has a tendency to metastasize hematogenously to the lung and bones. The incidence of distant metastasis at presentation is not uncommon occurring between 10 and 20% of new cases.[48-50] As a result, a bony lesion or pathologic fracture may represent the initial presentation. The key to effective management of follicular carcinoma is making an early diagnosis and total thyroidectomy.

Treatment of Follicular Thyroid Carcinoma

In contrast with papillary thyroid cancer, the frozen-section pathologic analysis is not helpful in making the diagnosis of follicular carcinoma because capsular and vascular invasion must be identified, and this requires fine-section analysis that cannot be completed with FNA or at the time of frozen section.[51] The definitive diagnosis of follicular thyroid carcinoma can be made only on permanent section. Once the diagnosis of follicular carcinoma has been confirmed, the decision to proceed with a completion thyroidectomy or to follow the patient is based on a variety of factors including risk-group analysis. Most agree that high-risk patients require a total thyroidectomy. Not only does a total thyroidectomy improve prognosis, but also it is very helpful in achieving accurate surveillance by facilitating radioactive iodine (RAI) administration and thyroglobulin monitoring. There is controversy regarding the low-risk group patients who present with minimally invasive lesions. The decision to perform a completion thyroidectomy is often based on age of the patient and invasiveness of the tumor. In patients greater than 50 years old or those with extensive invasion, we recommend a completion thyroidectomy.

Patients with low-grade tumors, tumors that demonstrate minimal invasion, can be managed conservatively with observation and serial ultrasound examination. Minimally invasive follicular thyroid carcinoma tends to behave like a follicular adenoma. There is a very low incidence of metastasis in low-grade follicular carcinoma,[52,53] and unlike papillary thyroid carcinoma, minimally invasive lesions are rarely multifocal. As follicular lesions grow larger than 3 cm, however, nearly 30% will demonstrate malignant conversion.[54] Although some have advocated suppressive therapy for low-risk patients, this approach has failed to demonstrate the benefit of suppressive therapy.

Treatment of Regional Disease Unlike squamous cell carcinoma, the impact of lymph node metastasis from thyroid cancer on survival is negligible, at least in the younger population. Several studies have suggested that lymph node metastasis may not impact survival[55,56]; however, when adjusted for age, it is clear that although regional disease does not significantly impact survival in young patients, it does decrease survival in patients over the age of 45 years.[57] Long-term studies have confirmed these observations and identified that in the population of patients greater than 45 years old, regional metastasis does impact survival.[41] As a result, most experts agree that clinically involved regional lymph nodes should be managed with a lymph node dissection. There is, however, controversy regarding the impact of elective neck dissection on survival. This is largely a result of the paucity of controlled randomized studies.

Thyroid cancer commonly progresses in a defined pathway from the first-echelon lymph nodes of the paratracheal region to the lateral compartment (levels III and IV); however, it has been documented that regional disease may occur in the jugular chain without evidence of disease in the paratracheal basin in as many as 18% of cases.[55] In spite of this rather high rate of "skip metastasis," most surgeons do not advocate a lateral neck dissection unless there is clinical evidence of disease in the lateral compartment. The rate of occult regional metastasis in papillary thyroid carcinoma is relatively high; however, occult metastasis in follicular carcinoma is rare. Hence, in patients with follicular carcinoma, an elective lymph node dissection is not commonly performed in the N0 neck. If lymphadenopathy is detected, a paratracheal and pretracheal central compartment neck dissection should be performed. In papillary thyroid carcinoma, the high rate of paratracheal disease constitutes an ipsilateral paratracheal neck dissection when there is clinical evidence of disease. Node plucking is not acceptable as the rate likelihood of recurrence is exceedingly high.[58]

Management of the N0 Neck The approach to management of the N0 neck in papillary carcinoma has been a topic of controversy largely because there are few randomized, controlled, long-term studies that demonstrate the impact of surgical treatment of the N0 neck. Currently, most surgeons perform a pretracheal and ipsilateral paratracheal lymph node dissection on high-risk patients (those patients aged 45 years or older or patients with tumors greater than 4 cm or invasive disease). Only when the thyroid tumor crosses the midline is a contralateral lymph node dissection warranted. When a contralateral lymph node dissection is performed, the patient must be informed of the increased risk related to transient and permanent hypoparathyroidism.[59]

As discussed earlier, in spite of the relatively high rate of documented skip metastasis, most surgeons do not advocate a lateral neck dissection. The rationale for this approach stems from the lack of data demonstrating the benefit of a lateral neck dissection for subclinical disease and the prevailing belief that ^{131}I can be used to manage microscopic lateral metastasis.

Management of the N+ Neck Unlike follicular carcinoma in which lymph nodes metastases are rare, metastasis in papillary thyroid carcinoma is common. Whereas only a small proportion of patients will initially present with a neck mass,[60] a significant number of patients will harbor subclinical paratracheal disease at the time of diagnosis. The size of the primary thyroid tumor has little bearing on the extent or location of regional disease. Several groups including our own have found that whereas large cancers of the thyroid may remain localized, microcarcinoma may present with extensive regional disease.[61] As a result, it is difficult to predict the risk of regional disease based on the size of the tumor, and therefore every patient must be evaluated for regional metastasis.

When lymph node metastasis is identified, a neck dissection is warranted. [131]I has not been demonstrated to be effective for management of gross regional disease.[62] In the past, there was controversy regarding the extent of the dissection; however, most surgeons now advocate a selective neck dissection (levels III, IV, and VI) in which the jugular vein, sternocleidomastoid muscle, and the accessory nerve are preserved. Although rare, when invasion of the surrounding structures occurs, a modified neck dissection may be warranted.

Radioiodine Therapy Remnant ablation with ^{131}I is routinely performed in all patients except for very low risk patients after total thyroidectomy to decrease the risk of recurrence and facilitate monitoring of thyroglobulin. Thyroid replacement is discontinued and a low iodine diet instituted in an effort to increase the avidity of the residual thyroid tissue. Once the TSH has risen above 25 to 30 mU/L, the patient is given radioiodine in doses ranging from 30 mCi to 100 mCi. Patients in whom residual microscopic disease is suspected and those with more aggressive tumor histology or known distant metastasis are administered higher doses of I[131] in the range of 100 to 300 mCi. Younger patients with iodine-avid tumors tend to have a favorable response to [131]I. The response of pulmonary metastasis to ^{131}I is predicated on the size of the lesion, the age of the patient, and its ability to concentrate [131]I.[63,64] In contrast, bone metastases, which occur more commonly in follicular thyroid carcinoma, are less responsive to therapy. The use of recombinant human TSH (rhTSH) for remnant ablation and in the treatment of metastatic disease is now being studied and has the advantage of avoiding symptomatic hypothyroidism.[65]

Thyroid Hormone Suppression Thyroid hormone suppression is routinely used after total thyroidectomy for differentiated thyroid cancer. Although randomized controlled trials are lacking, benefit was suggested in a large meta-analysis.[66] Higher-risk patients are initially treated with a greater degree of suppression. Because of the risk of osteoporosis, many clinicians will now reduce the levothyroxine dose once the patient has been free of disease for several years.

External Beam Radiotherapy Although prospective controlled trials are lacking, several studies have shown excellent locoregional control of disease with external beam radiotherapy (EBRT) in patients with locally advanced differentiated thyroid cancer after the primary surgery and before or after radioiodine.[67–69] Several groups have suggested that EBRT be considered in patients greater than 45 years old with suspect persistent local disease after surgery, which is unlikely to respond to radioiodine.[69,70]

Treatment of Recurrence and Distant Disease Recurrent or persistent well-differentiated thyroid cancer is not uncommon. After total thyroidectomy, as many as 15% of patients will have neck disease 0 to 5 years after initial therapy.[61,71] Because the volume of recurrent or distant metastatic disease correlates relatively well with the prognosis, early diagnosis and management is essential. Whole-body ^{131}I scanning should be performed in high-risk patients 6 to 12 months after the primary surgery. Low-risk patients can usually be evaluated by recombinant TSH (Thyrogen) stimulated thyroglobulin levels avoiding the need for an iodine scan. Because the majority of recurrences occur in the thyroid bed, neck ultrasonography represents the most sensitive means for detecting recurrence in the presence of elevated thyroglobulin. For those patients with elevated thyroglobulin and a negative iodine scan, PET-CT is exceptionally helpful in identifying recurrent and distant disease and has been shown to provide important prognostic information. Jadvar et al evaluated 10 patients with suspected recurrent papillary thyroid cancer using PET and concluded in this small series that PET was useful in the evaluation of patients with suspected recurrent papillary thyroid cancer when the ^{131}I scan is negative.[72] In a more recent study, eight patients underwent combined PET-CT scanning for suspected recurrence. Four (50%) of eight patients underwent PET-CT indicating recurrence in the head and neck. A total of 11 lesions in these four patients were suspicious for recurrence on combined PET-CT imaging. Three patients with eight lesions suspicious for recurrence on PET-CT underwent surgical removal of disease. All three patients had pathologic confirmation of recurrence, with 75.0% of the eight lesions being positive. The authors concluded that combined PET-CT imaging is a valuable tool for the diagnosis and localization of recurrent thyroid cancer.[73] Recent evidence suggests that PET-positive disease is unlikely to take up ^{131}I and may be associated with a more biologically aggressive tumor.[74]

The management of recurrent or metastatic disease largely depends on the extent of the disease. When there is microscopic persistent or recurrent disease, ^{131}I dosing should be repeated. When palpable gross tumor is identified, however, surgical management is the treatment of choice. When distant disease is identified, adjuvant ^{131}I is usually preferred. [131]I scanning is the most accurate method for assessment of distant disease.[74] Non–iodine-avid tumors represent a challenge and may indicate a poorly differentiated tumor that is often associated with a more aggressive behavior and a poor prognosis.[75] EBRT may be used for gross residual disease unresponsive to radioiodine and not amenable to further surgery. External beam radiation or surgical resection can also be used for the management of pain or to decompress nerve root compression in the vertebrae; however, neither therapy has an impact on prognosis. There are few studies demonstrating the efficacy of systemic chemotherapy; however, there is data to suggest that doxorubicin may be effective in some patients (60 to 75 mg/m² every 3 weeks).[75] Currently, systemic chemotherapy is used only in clinical trials.

Hürthle Cell Carcinoma

Hürthle cell carcinoma (HCC) is a relatively rare form of thyroid cancer that is generally considered to be a more aggressive variant of follicular carcinoma. Similar to follicular carcinoma, the distinction between a benign Hürthle cell adenoma and an HCC is determined on the presence of vascular or capsular invasion. Similar to follicular cell carcinoma, the diagnosis cannot be made on FNA or frozen-section analysis. Patients with HCC tend to be older. In one review series, it was found that the median age of presentation for patients with follicular cell carcinoma was 55 years, whereas the HCC patients presented at a mean age of 62 years. Patients presenting with HCC have

a lower risk of regional metastasis at presentation when compared with follicular carcinoma but a slightly increased risk of distant metastasis.[60] When followed long-term, the number of patients that eventually develop distant metastasis is higher in HCC patients (30%) than in papillary or follicular thyroid carcinoma patients. When distant metastasis occurs, 40% occur in the bone and as many as 30% occur in the lung.[76]

Treatment of Hürthle Cell Carcinoma

The management of HCC is not significantly different from follicular cell carcinoma. HCC with minimal capsular invasion (<1 mm) can be safely managed with a thyroid lobectomy and isthmusectomy. However, because it has been demonstrated that patients treated with a total thyroidectomy have a lower risk of recurrence,[77,78] a total thyroidectomy is recommended. All high-risk patients or patients with more extensive capsular invasion are managed with a total thyroidectomy. After surgery, ^{131}I is administered to achieve ablation and facilitate surveillance with thyroglobulin.

Prognosis of Hürthle Cell Carcinoma

Less that 200 new cases of HCC carcinoma are diagnosed in the United States each year. As a result, there are few long-term outcome studies; however, Evans and Vassilopoulou-Sellin found no difference in outcome between HCC and follicular cell carcinoma when cases are stratified by extent of invasion.[79] Like follicular cell carcinoma, the most important factor in assessing the prognosis seems to be the extent of capsular invasion. When tumors invade less than 1.0 mm, the rate of recurrence in exceedingly small; however, as the extent of capsular invasion increases, the likelihood of regional and distant metastasis increases.[79]

Medullary Thyroid Carcinoma

Medullary thyroid carcinoma (MTC) is derived from the nonepithelial parafollicular cells (c-cells), which produce the peptide calcitonin. Because the parafollicular cells of the embryo logically develop from the neural crest or diffuse neuroendocrine system, they commonly produce neuropeptides and catecholamines. Tumors deriving from diffuse neuroendocrine system, such as carcinoid tumors, pancreatic islet tumors, and pheochromocytomas, are cytologically and functionally similar.

MTC exists in a sporadic and familial forms. Whereas the gender distribution is roughly equivalent, the sporadic form of the disease occurs in 80 to 90% of newly diagnosed cases. The familial form of the disease occurs as an autosomal dominant trait as either isolated familial medullary thyroid carcinoma (FMTC), multiple endocrine neoplasia type IIA (MEN IIA), or multiple endocrine neoplasia type IIB (MEN IIB) (**Table 5–6**). Each of these familial forms of the disease is associated with a *ret* oncogene mutation located on chromosome 10. This provides a reliable screening tool to identify affected family members. Because the penetrance of medullary thyroid cancer is >90% in people with the *ret* gene mutation, prophylactic thyroidectomy is recommended at a young age.[80]

Table 5–6 Familial Medullary Thyroid Carcinoma

MEN IIA (Sipple syndrome)	
	Medullary thyroid cancer
	Parathyroid adenoma
	Pheochromocytoma
MEN IIB	
	Medullary thyroid carcinoma
	Pheochromocytoma
	Ganglioneuromatosis
	Marfanoid habitus

Clinical Presentation of Medullary Thyroid Carcinoma

Not unlike other forms of thyroid carcinoma, sporadic MTC typically presents as a thyroid nodule with or without an associated neck mass. Because MTC is derived from the diffuse neuroendocrine system, patients may present with a paraneoplastic syndrome resulting in diarrhea and abdominal cramping as a result of prostaglandin and vasoactive peptide release. The biological behavior and clinical presentation of MTC can be variable. Most tumors present as a well-circumscribed encapsulated nodule within the thyroid gland. More aggressive tumors may present with a neck mass or in rare cases distant metastasis to the lungs, liver, or adrenal glands. In some cases, tumors may remain stable or quiescent, whereas other tumors may progress rapidly. There has been little data to help predict the biological aggressiveness of MTC.

Diagnosis of Medullary Thyroid Cancer

The most accurate method for diagnosis of MTC is a FNA of the thyroid nodule or neck mass. Although cytodiagnostic features are recognized,[81] immunostaining for calcitonin in the presence of negative thyroglobulin staining is the most accurate method of diagnosis. When the calcitonin polymerizes, amyloid deposits can be found on histologic analysis. There are no histologic differences between the sporadic and familial forms of the disease. It is interesting to note, however, that familial MTC has a predilection for presenting as a thyroid nodule at the junction of the upper third and lower two-thirds of the thyroid gland because this is the area of the gland in which the density of c-cells is the highest. Sporadic disease usually presents as a unilateral nodule, whereas familial disease is more commonly bilateral and multifocal. Familial disease is considered more aggressive and commonly presents in the second or third decades, whereas sporadic disease presents later, in the sixth or seventh decades.

Treatment of Medullary Thyroid Carcinoma

MTC requires a total thyroidectomy and paratracheal lymph node dissection. Larger thyroid tumors are associated with an increased risk of neck disease, and therefore tumors greater than 2 cm should be treated with an ipsilateral selective neck dissection in addition to a bilateral paratracheal lymph node dissection.[82] Some have suggested that all patients should be treated with bilateral selective neck dissections because in patients with unilateral intrathyroidal tumors, as many as 81% of patients have lymph node metastasis in levels II to V and 44% have disease in the contralateral lymph node levels II to V.[83] Aggressive surgical therapy is warranted because occult metastases are common and surgery is the only effective method of therapy.

There is no evidence that medical therapy has any role in the primary management of MTC, and there is little evidence to suggest that adjuvant medical therapy will impact outcome. There is no role for radioiodine or thyroid hormone suppression in the treatment of medullary cancer. Brierley et al treated a series of 40 patients at high risk for recurrence with external beam radiation and demonstrated an improvement in locoregional control (86% vs. 52%) at 10 years[84,85]; however, several other studies have failed to demonstrate an improvement in survival with EBRT.[86,87] Systemic chemotherapy has little impact on the natural course of the disease, and although Schlumberger et al demonstrated 20% response rate in patients treated with doxorubicin, there is little data to support the use of systemic chemotherapy in MTC.[88] A new therapy using pretargeted anticarcinoembryonic antigen radioimmune therapy (RIT) has shown a survival benefit in a small clinical trial.[89]

Treatment of Regional Disease When faced with regional recurrence, surgery is the treatment of choice. Regional metastasis mandates a neck dissection. Unlike well-differentiated thyroid cancer, radioactive iodine uptake is negligible in MTC, and therefore aggressive surgical management of regional disease is justified. If a bilateral neck dissection was not performed at the time of initial therapy, bilateral neck dissections should be considered, even in the face of unilateral recurrence.

Treatment of Distant Disease Distant disease represents a significant dilemma. As discussed, conventional adjuvant therapy offers little for patients with regional or distant disease. Clinical trials are often offered at tertiary-care medical centers.

Treatment of Recurrence When patients demonstrate a persistently elevated calcitonin level after surgery, it is because there is residual or recurrent disease. Identifying the location of the residual disease is often a challenge. CT, MRI, and PET have all been used with little success unless there is gross disease remaining in the neck or thyroid bed. The management of a patient with a persistently elevated calcitonin level and no radiographic evidence of disease is controversial. This is because there is evidence to suggest that this patient group does not necessarily have a compromised outcome,[90] and when reoperation is pursued, the rate of success is low.[91] We recommend bilateral selective neck dissections for those patients that have not already undergone a neck dissection.

Prognosis of Medullary Thyroid Carcinoma

Prognosis is better in younger patients, female gender, familial disease, and those with disease confined to the thyroid gland. The overall 5-year survival rate ranges from 25 to 75%.[92,93] When nodal disease is present at the time of diagnosis, which occurs in 50% of patients, the 5-year survival rate drops to less than 50%.[94] A recent series suggests that the 5- and 10-year survival rates are as high as 90% and 80%.[82]

Anaplastic Thyroid Carcinoma

Although less than 2% of all thyroid carcinomas are anaplastic thyroid carcinoma, it accounts for 14 to 39% of thyroid carcinoma deaths.[37,95] The diagnosis of anaplastic thyroid carcinoma can be elusive. Not uncommonly, a FNA will be repeatedly interpreted as "undifferentiated carcinoma" until an open biopsy provides enough tissue to reveal the anaplastic nature of the carcinoma. Unlike other forms of thyroid cancer, anaplastic is characteristically aggressive and unrelenting. Accounting for less than 5% of malignant thyroid cancers, anaplastic thyroid cancer is often heralded by a rapidly growing thyroid mass with destruction of the adjacent cartilage, nerve, and infiltrating muscles.

Presentation of Anaplastic Thyroid Carcinoma

Anaplastic thyroid carcinoma typically presents in the elderly population with a history of thyroid goiter.[96] Up to 20% of patients will have a history of well-differentiated thyroid cancer or coexisting well-differentiated thyroid cancer present within the thyroid specimen.[97,98] Patients usually present with a rapidly growing neck mass, true vocal cord paralysis, and/or dysphagia.[96] The mass tends to present as a fixed neck mass invading the surrounding structures. Direct invasion of the airway and larynx can lead to hoarseness or airway obstruction. As the lesion becomes more advanced, esophageal invasion can result in dysphagia. Anaplastic carcinoma may arise de novo or as a "conversion tumor" arising in the presence of a preexisting papillary or follicular carcinoma. When anaplastic carcinoma arises de novo, the tumor may progress rapidly metastasizing to the lungs, liver, and bones within weeks of presentation.

Diagnosis of Anaplastic Thyroid Cancer

A FNA is often the first approach to diagnosis; however, necrosis and degeneration of the tumor may occur as the tumor rapidly outgrows its blood supply. A FNA aspiration may yield necrotic material. Alternatively, the FNA may yield poorly differentiated cells suggestive of either lymphoma, anaplastic thyroid cancer, or poorly differentiated carcinoma of unknown origin. Flow cytometry is useful to rule out lymphoma; however, immunohistochemistry and electron microscopy may be necessary to confirm the diagnosis of anaplastic thyroid carcinoma.

Treatment of Anaplastic Thyroid Carcinoma

There is controversy regarding the ideal management of anaplastic carcinoma largely because it is rapidly progressing and poorly responsive to therapy.[99] Defining the goals of management is essential. The options for therapy range from multimodal therapy, surgical resection, debulking, radiotherapy, chemotherapy, and palliative therapy.[96,100,101] Early disease, disease confined to the thyroid gland, is poorly responsive to unimodality therapy; however, in a recent study, investigators reviewed a cohort of 516 patients with anaplastic thyroid carcinoma reported to 12 population-based cancer registries between 1973 and 2000. They found that patients less than 60 years old with intrathyroidal anaplastic thyroid cancer appear to have a better prognosis than older patients with extrathyroidal spread after total thyroidectomy and external beam radiation.[102] Long-term survivors are few; however, in those that do survive the disease, they commonly have only a small focus of anaplastic tumor arising within a preexisting well-differentiated thyroid cancer.[37,103]

Adjuvant therapy has also been controversial. Standard fractionated radiation therapy has not been demonstrated to significantly change the clinical course.[104] Hyperfractionated therapy has resulted in a marginal improvement in response rates; however, the side effects, including esophagitis, can be debilitating.[105] Tennvall et al reported using preoperative hyperfractionated radiation (30 Gy), doxorubicin, and surgical resection followed by postoperative radiation (46 Gy). They demonstrated promising results with this regimen, controlling local recurrence in 48% of patients and disease-free survival in 12%.[106]

In advanced disease, the goals include establishing an airway, a source of nutrition, and an acceptable quality of life. Surgery is warranted for the control or prevention of airway obstruction or extensive skin ulceration.

Prognosis of Anaplastic Thyroid Carcinoma

Anaplastic thyroid carcinoma is one of the most aggressive human malignancies. It is associated with an almost uniformly rapid and lethal clinical course.[1] Several studies have confirmed the universal lethal course associated with anaplastic thyroid cancer. Patient age, gender, tumor size, extent of disease, leukocytosis, presence of acute local symptoms, coexisting multinodular goiter and well-differentiated thyroid carcinoma, surgical resection, and multimodal therapy all reportedly influence patient survival according to some studies[107–109]; however, there are few interventions that have improved survival.

Pediatric Thyroid Cancer

Pediatric thyroid cancer is rare and comprises less than 10% of all newly diagnosed thyroid cancers.[110] The prognosis, even in advanced cases, is thankfully excellent. In contrast with adults, pediatric patients commonly present with advanced disease with regional and, in some cases, distant metastasis at the time of diagnosis.

Etiology of Pediatric Thyroid Cancer

In most cases, the etiology of pediatric thyroid cancer is unclear. There is little debate, however, that ionizing radiation represents a risk factor. In the early to middle part of the 20th century, external beam irradiation was used to treat acne, adenoidal hypertrophy, thymic enlargement, and several dermatologic diseases. This resulted in a generation of patients at risk for the development of thyroid cancer.[111] A similar exposure occurred in 1986 after the Chernobyl disaster where ^{131}I was released over Ukraine, Belarus, and Russia. After this event, the incidence of pediatric thyroid cancer increased 10-fold in the affected areas. In pediatric patients with no history of radiation exposure, thyroid cancer comprises 6% of all pediatric thyroid nodules. Thyroid nodules in the pediatric patient is rare; however, thyroid nodules in the pediatric patient should be evaluated and considered a malignancy until proved otherwise.

Presentation of Pediatric Thyroid Cancer

The most common type of thyroid cancer in the patient under 21 years old is papillary thyroid cancer. Most commonly, a thyroid carcinoma presents as a thyroid mass although a neck mass is not uncommon at presentation. Pediatric thyroid cancer is more common in males by a ratio of 2:1, and males tend to present with more advanced disease than their female counterparts.[112,113] Unlike adults, nearly 50% of children will harbor regional metastasis and 15% will have distant metastasis at the time of diagnosis.[114] The most common site for regional metastasis is level VI (90%), and metastases to levels II, III, and IV occur in greater than 30% of patients.

Diagnosis of Pediatric Thyroid Cancer

Because children with thyroid carcinoma have a high propensity for regional and distant metastasis, a thorough exam including fiberoptic laryngoscopy is warranted. Although hoarseness as a result of a vocal cord paralysis is rare, preoperative documentation is essential. Similar to adults, the HUS is ideal for evaluating both local and regional disease. FNA is ideal to confirm the diagnosis of thyroid cancer; however, because this is often difficult to achieve in a child and most thyroidologists consider a thyroid nodule malignant until definitively proved otherwise, we will often plan on a hemithyroidectomy with frozen-section analysis in lieu of an FNA. In those cases where an FNA is obtained, a "benign" or "indeterminate" diagnosis aspirate can be managed with close observation, serial ultrasound examinations, and repeat FNA. Because thyroid nodules in this age group require intensive follow-up and the false-negative rate is not insignificant,[115] we recommend hemithyroidectomy.

There is no role for radionuclide scanning in the initial workup. Similarly, MRI and CT are not indicated unless a patient presents with hoarseness or signs of airway compromise. A chest x-ray is recommended because of the high incidence of distant pulmonary metastasis. When pediatric patients manifest pulmonary metastasis, the chest x-ray will often demonstrate a diffuse miliary appearance.

Treatment of Pediatric Thyroid Carcinoma

The prognosis for pediatric patients with thyroid cancer is excellent. A combination of surgery and postoperative ra-

dioactive iodine yields 10-year cure rates approaching 100% even in patients with disseminated disease.[112] Surgery should be focused on complete excision of the thyroid gland and all metastatic neck disease. This can be accomplished with minimal morbidity and will allow for careful postoperative surveillance.[114]

Elective neck dissection has not been recommended in patients with well-differentiated thyroid cancer; however, a selective neck dissection for the management of the demonstrable neck disease is essential. Rarely is a modified neck dissection required as the rate of invasion into adjacent structures is rare.

◆ Clinical Cases

Case 1 A dominant nodule in a male patient.

Presentation A 34-year-old man was referred by his primary care physician for a right-sided thyroid nodule. The patient had no family history of thyroid disease or radiation exposure.

Physical Examination On examination, there was a 2 × 3 cm right thyroid nodule located at the inferior pole of the thyroid gland. There was no evidence of palpable adenopathy.

Diagnosis and Workup The patient was referred for an ultrasound-guided FNA of the nodule and ultrasound of the neck. Serum TSH and T4 levels were evaluated. The ultrasound demonstrated a 2.3 × 3.4 × 3.6 cm dominant solid hypoechogenic nodule in the inferior portion of the right thyroid lobe, and there was no evidence of paratracheal or lateral neck adenopathy. The FNA cytology was read as "atypical," and the thyroid function studies and free T4 were normal.

Options for Treatment Indeterminate or "atypical" cytology is not uncommon and may occur in as many as 30% of FNA specimens. The options for therapy include observation with serial ultrasound evaluation or a thyroid lobectomy with frozen-section analysis. In the euthyroid patient, a thyroid lobectomy with frozen-section analysis should be offered to the patient as an option. In contrast, if a thyroid lobectomy with frozen-section analysis is performed, the decision to perform a total thyroidectomy will be predicated on the frozen-section analysis. Unless the pathologist can confirm the presence of papillary thyroid carcinoma, surgery is limited to a hemithyroidectomy.

Treatment Given the high-risk characteristics including male gender, size of the nodule, and the presence of a single dominant solid hypoechogenic nodule, a hemithyroidectomy was performed. The frozen-section analysis demonstrated a papillary thyroid carcinoma. Therefore, a total thyroidectomy and central compartment (level VI) neck dissection was performed. The final pathology demonstrated a "follicular variant" of papillary thyroid carcinoma. The patient was started on levothyroxine therapy after surgery.

Adjuvant Therapy One month after surgery, serum TSH and thyroglobulin were assessed, and an ultrasound was performed demonstrating no evidence of residual disease. The patient was withdrawn from levothyroxine, and diagnostic whole-body scintigraphy was performed, followed by administration of 100 mCi [131]I. Five to eight days after the ablative ^{131}I treatment, a posttreatment whole-body scan was performed.

Summary of Treatment Risk stratification is an essential part of the decision-making process. In addition to the clinical presentation, the findings on ultrasound can contribute important information that may impact the treatment plan. In the absence of demonstrable regional metastasis, a central compartment (level VI) dissection should be performed. The morbidity associated with the neck dissection is minimal in experienced hands and, although controversial, it may improve outcome.

Case 2 Thyroid carcinoma during pregnancy.

Presentation A 24-year-old woman in her third trimester of pregnancy presented with a new thyroid nodule that the patient related had grown significantly over the past month causing dysphagia to solid food.

Physical Examination On examination, there was a 3.5 × 3.5 cm firm nodule in the central portion of the left thyroid lobe with no evidence of tracheal deviation. There was no evidence of adenopathy.

Diagnosis and Workup An ultrasound demonstrated a 3.2 × 2.6 × 3.5 cm single dominant solid hypoechogenic thyroid nodule in the midportion of the left thyroid lobe. Small calcifications were identified, and an FNA was performed. The patient was euthyroid and otherwise in good health. The FNA demonstrated papillary thyroid carcinoma.

Options for Treatment Thyroid carcinoma during pregnancy can be managed with careful observation and sonographic surveillance until after delivery or with surgical thyroidectomy. If the patient elects for observation, it should be understood that in the event that there is an appreciable growth of the nodule, surgery is indicated.

Treatment This patient was monitored sonographically throughout the remainder of her pregnancy, and though there was moderate growth in the nodule, surgery was delayed until 3 weeks after her delivery. A total thyroidectomy and central compartment neck dissection was performed.

Summary of Treatment There is no evidence to demonstrate that thyroid nodules in pregnant women possess a higher risk of malignancy; however, the workup for a pregnant woman is the same for a nonpregnant adult. There is debate regarding the timing of surgery; however, it has been recommended that thyroid nodules found during pregnancy may be monitored and only in the event of substantial growth should surgery be performed. If surgery is performed, it should be done before 24 weeks to reduce the risk of miscarriage.[116] In most cases, surgical therapy can be delayed until after delivery without compromising recurrence rate or survival.[117] There is no evidence to suggest that the biological behavior of thyroid malignancy is affected by pregnancy. Additionally, retrospective data suggests that a delay in treatment of less than 1 year has no adverse impact on survival.[41]

Case 3 A follicular variant of papillary thyroid cancer.

Presentation A 47-year-old woman presented with a right-sided level IV neck mass 7 years after undergoing a total thyroidectomy for a multifocal follicular variant of papillary thyroid carcinoma. The patient was treated with postoperative [131]I 7 years ago and has not been followed since then.

Physical Examination On exam, there are two palpable masses on right lateral aspect of the neck at level IV. The masses are firm but not fixed. They measure 3 × 3.5 cm and 2 × 2 cm. No thyroid gland is palpated.

Diagnosis and Workup An ultrasound and FNA confirmed the presence of recurrent disease in two lymph nodes. Prior records suggested that the tumor was non–iodine avid and the patient had evidence of antithyroglobulin antibodies. A new thyroid scan was performed, and serology confirmed the presence of persistent antithyroglobulin antibodies.

Options for Treatment Gross metastatic disease should be managed surgically unless the tumor is unresectable. EBRT may be considered in unresectable disease or in patients that are not surgical candidates. Elderly patients and poor surgical candidates with minimal disease may be observed if the patient is vigilant about follow-up surveillance. In such cases, surgery is warranted if there is demonstrable evidence of progression of disease.

Surgical Treatment of the Neck A right-sided selective neck dissection including levels II to IV was performed.

Adjuvant Therapy In spite of the non–iodine avidity, most would consider readministration of ^{131}I; however, if the patient experiences recurrence, EBRT may be considered.

Summary of Treatment Recurrent papillary thyroid carcinoma may present as a neck mass or a rise in thyroglobulin. Clinically identifiable disease should be managed surgically with postoperative [131]I. When recurrent disease presents as a progressive rise in thyroglobulin (>2 ng/mL), a thorough metastatic workup should be performed including a diagnostic radioiodine scan, ultrasound of the neck, and high-resolution CT scan of the neck and chest. Not uncommonly, the workup may not reveal the recurrence. In such cases, empiric therapy with 100 to 200 mCi radioactive iodine should be administered. In as many as 50% of cases, this approach may identify the metastatic lesion.[118]

There are several variants of papillary thyroid carcinoma including follicular variant, tall cell variant, and columnar variant. In general, these subtypes are more aggressive and have a higher metastatic potential. Not uncommonly, they do not concentrate iodine well and therefore may be less responsive to [131]I. In non–iodine-avid papillary variant, one may consider EBRT for the management of recurrent disease.

Case 4 Thyroid carcinoma in a pediatric patient.

Presentation An 8-year-old boy was referred for a 2-month history of a right-sided neck mass and "wheezing." The patient had been seen by his pediatrician and treated with a 2-week course of antibiotics. A workup for asthma demonstrated a flow-volume loop consistent with a fixed obstruction. The patient had no history of weight loss, fevers, or night sweats.

Physical Examination On examination, the patient had a right-sided thyroid mass and bilateral lymphadenopathy in levels III and IV, V and VI. The adenopathy was firm but not fixed.

Diagnosis and Workup Complete blood count (CBC) and SMA-12 were normal. A CT scan of the neck demonstrated bilateral adenopathy and a right-sided thyroid nodule with compression of the tracheal airway (**Fig. 5–3**). A chest x-ray demonstrated diffuse bilateral nodules. FNA was attempted twice; however, the patient was unable to tolerate the procedure.

Options for Treatment A tissue diagnosis is ideal; however, the clinical presentation of lymphadenopathy in the presence of a thyroid nodule should be considered thyroid carcinoma until proved otherwise. The options include an FNA under sedation or an open neck biopsy with frozen-section examination under general anesthesia. In this case, we elected to proceed with an open neck biopsy. Consent was obtained to proceed with a total thyroidectomy and bilateral neck dissection in the event that the frozen-section analysis confirmed the diagnosis of papillary thyroid carcinoma.

Surgical Treatment of the Neck The frozen-section analysis confirmed the diagnosis of papillary thyroid carcinoma. A thyroidectomy was performed, and bilateral selective neck dissections were performed (levels II to VI).

Adjuvant Treatment Five weeks after surgery, a radioactive scan demonstrated minimal uptake in the thyroid bed and lung fields bilaterally.

Summary of Treatment Management of pediatric thyroid carcinoma depends on meticulous surgery to remove the thyroid gland and any regional disease. In spite of distant disease, pediatric patients tend to do very well.

References

1. Libutti SK. Understanding the role of gender in the incidence of thyroid cancer. Cancer J 2005;11(2):104–105
2. Lee ML, Chen GG, Vlantis AC, et al. Induction of thyroid papillary carcinoma cell proliferation by estrogen is associated with an altered expression of Bcl-xL. Cancer J 2005;11(2):113–121
3. Noguchi S, Noguchi A, Murakami N. Papillary carcinoma of the thyroid. I. Developing pattern of metastasis. Cancer 1970;26(5):1053–1060
4. Hay ID. Papillary thyroid carcinoma. Endocrinol Metab Clin North Am 1990;19(3):545–576
5. Lin JD, Chao TC, Huang BY, et al. Thyroid cancer in the thyroid nodules evaluated by ultrasonography and fine-needle aspiration cytology. Thyroid 2005;15(7):708–717
6. Rojeski MT, Gharib H. Nodular thyroid disease. Evaluation and management. N Engl J Med 1985;313(7):428–436
7. Mazzaferri EL. Management of a solitary thyroid nodule. N Engl J Med 1993;328(8):553–559
8. Tollin SR, Mery GM, Jelveh N, et al. The use of fine-needle aspiration biopsy under ultrasound guidance to assess the risk of malignancy in patients with a multinodular goiter. Thyroid 2000;10(3):235–241
9. Liebeskind A, Sikora AG, Komisar A, et al. Rates of malignancy in incidentally discovered thyroid nodules evaluated with sonography and fine-needle aspiration. J Ultrasound Med 2005;24(5):629–634
10. Sklar C, Whitton J, Mertens A, et al. Abnormalities of the thyroid in survivors of Hodgkin's disease: data from the Childhood Cancer Survivor Study. J Clin Endocrinol Metab 2000;85(9):3227–3232
11. Tronko MD, Howe GR, Bogdanova TI, et al. A cohort study of thyroid cancer and other thyroid diseases after the Chernobyl accident: thyroid cancer in Ukraine detected during first screening. J Natl Cancer Inst 2006;98(13):897–903
12. Handkiewcz-Junak D, Banasik T, Kolosza Z, et al. Risk of malignant tumors in first-degree relatives of patients with differentiated thyroid cancer–a hospital based study. Neoplasma 2006;53(1):67–72
13. Thyroid Carcinoma Task Force. AACE/AAES medical/surgical guidelines for clinical practice: management of thyroid carcinoma. American Association of Clinical Endocrinologists. American College of Endocrinology. Endocr Pract 2001;7(3):202–220
14. Hodak SP, Burman KD. The calcitonin conundrum–is it time for routine measurement of serum calcitonin in patients with thyroid nodules? J Clin Endocrinol Metab 2004;89(2):511–514
15. Hay ID, Klee GG. Thyroid cancer diagnosis and management. Clin Lab Med 1993;13(3):725–734
16. Krishnamurthy S, Bedi DG, Caraway NP. Ultrasound-guided fine-needle aspiration biopsy of the thyroid bed. Cancer 2001;93(3):199–205
17. Grebe SK, Hay ID. Follicular cell-derived thyroid carcinomas. Cancer Treat Res 1997;89:91–140
18. Reading CC, Gorman CA. Thyroid imaging techniques. Clin Lab Med 1993;13(3):711–724
19. Koike E, Noguchi S, Yamashita H, et al. Ultrasonographic characteristics of thyroid nodules: prediction of malignancy. Arch Surg 2001;136(3):334–337
20. Miyakawa M, Onoda N, Etoh M, et al. Diagnosis of thyroid follicular carcinoma by the vascular pattern and velocimetric parameters using high resolution pulsed and power Doppler ultrasonography. Endocr J 2005;52(2):207–212
21. Burman KD. Micropapillary thyroid cancer: should we aspirate all nodules regardless of size? J Clin Endocrinol Metab 2006;91(6):2043–2046
22. Cooper DS, Doherty GM, Haugen BR, et al. Management guidelines for patients with thyroid nodules and differentiated thyroid cancer. Thyroid 2006;16(2):109–142
23. Mandell DL, Genden EM, Mechanick JI, et al. Diagnostic accuracy of fine-needle aspiration and frozen section in nodular thyroid disease. Otolaryngol Head Neck Surg 2001;124(5):531–536
24. Sidawy MK, Del Vecchio DM, Knoll SM. Fine-needle aspiration of thyroid nodules: correlation between cytology and histology and evaluation of discrepant cases. Cancer 1997;81(4):253–259
25. Gharib H, Goellner JR, Johnson DA. Fine-needle aspiration cytology of the thyroid. A 12-year experience with 11,000 biopsies. Clin Lab Med 1993;13(3):699–709
26. Haber RS. Ultrasound-guided fine-needle aspiration of thyroid nodules. Endocr Pract 2002;8(1):70–71
27. Flanagan MB, Ohori NP, Carty SE, et al. Repeat thyroid nodule fine-needle aspiration in patients with initial benign cytologic results. Am J Clin Pathol 2006;125(5):698–702
28. Alaedeen DI, Khiyami A, McHenry CR. Fine-needle aspiration biopsy specimen with a predominance of Hurthle cells: a dilemma in the management of nodular thyroid disease. Surgery 2005;138(4):650–656; discussion 656–657
29. Orijal B, Hamrahian AH, Reddy SS. Management of nondiagnostic thyroid fine-needle aspiration biopsy: survey of endocrinologists. Endocr Pract 2004;10(4):317–323
30. Stulak JM, Grant CS, Farley DR, et al. Value of preoperative ultrasonography in the surgical management of initial and reoperative papillary thyroid cancer. Arch Surg 2006;141(5):489–496
31. Tomoda C, Uruno T, Takamura Y, et al. Ultrasonography as a method of screening for tracheal invasion by papillary thyroid cancer. Surg Today 2005;35(10):819–822

32. Hay ID, Grant CS, Taylor WF, et al. Ipsilateral lobectomy versus bilateral lobar resection in papillary thyroid carcinoma: a retrospective analysis of surgical outcome using a novel prognostic scoring system. Surgery 1987;102(6):1088–1095

33. Cady B, Rossi R. An expanded view of risk-group definition in differentiated thyroid carcinoma. Surgery 1988;104(6):947–953

34. Byar DP, Green SB, Dor P, et al. A prognostic index for thyroid carcinoma. A study of the E.O.R.T.C. Thyroid Cancer Cooperative Group. Eur J Cancer 1979;15(8):1033–1041

35. Sherman SI, Brierley JD, Sperling M, et al. Prospective multicenter study of thyrois]carcinoma treatment: initial analysis of staging and outcome. National Thyroid Cancer Treatment Cooperative Study Registry Group. Cancer 1998;83(5):1012–1021

36. Hay ID, Bergstralh EJ, Goellner JR, et al. Predicting outcome in papillary thyroid carcinoma: development of a reliable prognostic scoring system in a cohort of 1779 patients surgically treated at one institution during 1940 through 1989. Surgery 1993;114(6):1050–1057

37. Hundahl SA, Fleming ID, Fremgen AM, et al. A National Cancer Data Base report on 53,856 cases of thyroid carcinoma treated in the U.S., 1985–1995. [see comments] Cancer 1998;83(12):2638–2648

38. Nishida T, Nakao K, Hashimoto T. Local control in differentiated carcinoma with extrathyroidal invasion. Am J Surg 2000;179(2):86–91

39. Shah JP, Loree TR, Dharker D, et al. Lobectomy versus total thyroidectomy for differentiated carcinoma of the thyroid: a matched-pair analysis. Am J Surg 1993;166(4):331–335

40. Shah JP, Loree TR, Dharker D, et al. Prognostic factors in differentiated carcinoma of the thyroid gland. Am J Surg 1992;164(6):658–661

41. Mazzaferri EL, Jhiang SM. Long-term impact of initial surgical and medical therapy on papillary and follicular thyroid cancer. Am J Med 1994;97(5):418–428

42. Rossi RL, Loree TR, Dharker D, et al. Current results of conservative surgery for differentiated thyroid carcinoma. World J Surg 1986;10(4):612–622

43. Sanders LE, Cady B. Differentiated thyroid cancer: reexamination of risk groups and outcome of treatment. Arch Surg 1998;133(4):419–425

44. Hay ID, Grant CS, Bergstralh EJ, et al. Unilateral total lobectomy: is it sufficient surgical treatment for patients with AMES low-risk papillary thyroid carcinoma? Surgery 1998;124(6):958–966

45. Hay ID, Grant CS, van Heerden JA, et al. Papillary thyroid microcarcinoma: a study of 535 cases observed in a 50-year period. Surgery 1992;112(6):1139–1147

46. Clark OH, Levin K, Zeng QH, et al. Thyroid cancer: the case for total thyroidectomy. Eur J Cancer Clin Oncol 1988;24(2):305–313

47. Inabnet WB. Surgical management of thyroid cancer. Endocr Pract 2000;6(6):465–468

48. Shaha AR, Shah JP, Loree TR. Differentiated thyroid cancer presenting initially with distant metastasis. Am J Surg 1997;174(5):474–476

49. Eichhorn W, Tabler H, Lippold R, et al. Prognostic factors determining long-term survival in well-differentiated thyroid cancer: an analysis of four hundred eighty-four patients undergoing therapy and aftercare at the same institution. Thyroid 2003;13(10):949–958

50. Lin JD, Huang MJ, Juang JH, et al. Factors related to the survival of papillary and follicular thyroid carcinoma patients with distant metastases. Thyroid 1999;9(12):1227–1235

51. LiVolsi VA, Baloch ZW. Use and abuse of frozen section in the diagnosis of follicular thyroid lesions. Endocr Pathol 2005;16(4):285–293

52. van Heerden JA, Hay ID, Goellner JR, et al. Follicular thyroid carcinoma with capsular invasion alone: a nonthreatening malignancy. Surgery 1992;112(6):1130–1138

53. Young RL, Mazzaferri EL, Rahe AJ, et al. Pure follicular thyroid carcinoma: impact of therapy in 214 patients. J Nucl Med 1980;21(8):733–737

54. Bell B, Mazzaferri EL. Familial adenomatous polyposis (Gardner's syndrome) and thyroid carcinoma. A case report and review of the literature. Dig Dis Sci 1993;38(1):185–190

55. Noguchi M, Kumaki T, Taniya T, et al. Regional lymph node metastases in well-differentiated thyroid carcinoma. Int Surg 1987;72(2):100–103

56. Carcangiu ML, Zampi G, Pupi A, et al. Papillary carcinoma of the thyroid. A clinicopathologic study of 241 cases treated at the University of Florence, Italy. Cancer 1985;55(4):805–828

57. Harwood J, Clark OH, Dunphy JE. Significance of lymph node metastasis in differentiated thyroid cancer. Am J Surg 1978;136(1):107–112

58. Goldman ND, Coniglio JU, Falk SA. Thyroid cancers. I. Papillary, follicular, and Hurthle cell. Otolaryngol Clin North Am 1996;29(4):593–609

59. Henry JF, Gramatica L, Denizot A, et al. Morbidity of prophylactic lymph node dissection in the central neck area in patients with papillary thyroid carcinoma. Langenbecks Arch Surg 1998;383(2):167–169

60. Shaha AR, Shah JP, Loree TR. Patterns of nodal and distant metastasis based on histologic varieties in differentiated carcinoma of the thyroid. Am J Surg 1996;172(6):692–694

61. McConahey WM, Hay ID, Woolner LB, et al. Papillary thyroid cancer treated at the Mayo Clinic, 1946 through 1970: initial manifestations, pathologic findings, therapy, and outcome. Mayo Clin Proc 1986;61(12):978–996

62. Wilson SM, Bock GE. Carcinoma of the thyroid metastatic to lymph nodes of the neck. Arch Surg 1971;102(4):285–291

63. Casara D, Rubello D, Saladini G, et al. Different features of pulmonary metastases in differentiated thyroid cancer: natural history and multivariate statistical analysis of prognostic variables. J Nucl Med 1993;34(10):1626–1631

64. Schlumberger M, Challeton C, De Vathaire F, et al. Radioactive iodine treatment and external radiotherapy for lung and bone metastases from thyroid carcinoma. J Nucl Med 1996;37(4):598–605

65. Luster M, Lippi F, Jarzab B, et al. rhTSH-aided radioiodine ablation and treatment of differentiated thyroid carcinoma: a comprehensive review. Endocr Relat Cancer 2005;12(1):49–64

66. McGriff JN, Csako G, Gourgiotis L, et al. Effects of thyroid hormone suppression therapy on adverse clinical outcomes in thyroid cancer. Ann Med 2002;34(7-8):554–564

67. Tsang RW, Brierley JD, Simpson WJ, et al. The effects of surgery, radioiodine, and external radiation therapy on the clinical outcome of patients with differentiated thyroid carcinoma. Cancer 1998;82(2):375–388

68. Meadows KM, Amdur RJ, Morris CG, et al. External beam radiotherapy for differentiated thyroid cancer. Am J Otolaryngol 2006;27(1):24–28

69. Kim TH, Yang DS, Jung KY, et al. Value of external irradiation for locally advanced papillary thyroid cancer. Int J Radiat Oncol Biol Phys 2003;55(4):1006–1012

70. Brierley JD, Tsang RW. External-beam radiation therapy in the treatment of differentiated thyroid cancer. Semin Surg Oncol 1999;16(1):42–49

71. Mazzaferri EL, Kloos RT. Clinical review 128: current approaches to primary therapy for papillary and follicular thyroid cancer. J Clin Endocrinol Metab 2001;86(4):1447–1463

72. Jadvar H, McDougall IR, Segall GM. Evaluation of suspected recurrent papillary thyroid carcinoma with [18F]fluorodeoxyglucose positron emission tomography. Nucl Med Commun 1998;19(6):547–554

73. Zimmer LA, McCook B, Meltzer C, et al. Combined positron emission tomography/computed tomography imaging of recurrent thyroid cancer. Otolaryngol Head Neck Surg 2003;128(2):178–184

74. Maheshwari YK, Hill CS Jr, Haynie TP III, et al. 131I therapy in differentiated thyroid carcinoma: M. D. Anderson Hospital experience. Cancer 1981;47(4):664–671

75. Gottlieb JA, Hill CS, Ibanez ML, et al. Chemotherapy of thyroid cancer. An evaluation of experience with 37 patients. Cancer 1972;30(3):848–853

76. Ruegemer JJ, Hay ID, Bergstralh EJ, et al. Distant metastases in differentiated thyroid carcinoma: a multivariate analysis of prognostic variables. J Clin Endocrinol Metab 1988;67(3):501–508

77. McDonald MP, Sanders LE, Silverman ML, et al. Hurthle cell carcinoma of the thyroid gland: prognostic factors and results of surgical treatment. Surgery 1996;120(6):1000–1005

78. Carcangiu ML, Bianchi S, Savino D, et al. Follicular Hurthle cell tumors of the thyroid gland. Cancer 1991;68(9):1944–1953

79. Evans HL, Vassilopoulou-Sellin R. Follicular and Hurthle cell carcinomas of the thyroid: a comparative study. Am J Surg Pathol 1998;22(12):1512–1520

80. Moore FD, Dluhy RG. Prophylactic thyroidectomy in MEN-2A—a stitch in time? N Engl J Med 2005;353(11):1162–1164

81. Forrest CH, Frost FA, de Boer WB, et al. Medullary carcinoma of the thyroid: accuracy of diagnosis of fine-needle aspiration cytology. Cancer 1998;84(5):295–302

82. Duh QY, Sancho JJ, Greenspan FS, et al. Medullary thyroid carcinoma. The need for early diagnosis and total thyroidectomy. Arch Surg 1989;124(10):1206–1210

83. Moley JF, DeBenedetti MK. Patterns of nodal metastases in palpable medullary thyroid carcinoma: recommendations for extent of node dissection. Ann Surg 1999;229(6):880–887; discussion 887–888

84. Brierley JD, Tsang RW. External radiation therapy in the treatment of thyroid malignancy. Endocrinol Metab Clin North Am 1996;25(1):141–157

85. Brierley J, Tsang R, Simpson WJ, et al. Medullary thyroid cancer: analyses of survival and prognostic factors and the role of radiation therapy in local control. Thyroid 1996;6(4):305–310

86. Saad MF, Ordonez NG, Rashid RK, et al. Medullary carcinoma of the thyroid. A study of the clinical features and prognostic factors in 161 patients. Medicine (Baltimore) 1984;63(6):319–342

87. Rosenbluth BD, Serrano V, Happersett L, et al. Intensity-modulated radiation therapy for the treatment of nonanaplastic thyroid cancer. Int J Radiat Oncol Biol Phys 2005;63(5):1419–1426

88. Schlumberger M, Abdelmoumene N, Delisle MJ, et al. Treatment of advanced medullary thyroid cancer with an alternating combination of 5 FU-streptozocin and 5 FU-dacarbazine. The Groupe d'Etude des Tumeurs a Calcitonine (GETC). Br J Cancer 1995;71(2):363–365

89. Chatal JF, Campion L, Kraeber-Bodere F, et al. Survival improvement in patients with medullary thyroid carcinoma who undergo pretargeted anti-carcinoembryonic-antigen radioimmunotherapy: a collaborative study with the French Endocrine Tumor Group. J Clin Oncol 2006;24(11):1705–1711

90. van Heerden JA, Grant CS, Gharib H, et al. Long-term course of patients with persistent hypercalcitoninemia after apparent curative primary surgery for medullary thyroid carcinoma. Ann Surg 1990;212(4):395–401

91. Tisell LE, Hansson G, Jansson S, et al. Reoperation in the treatment of asymptomatic metastasizing medullary thyroid carcinoma. Surgery 1986;99(1):60–66

92. Raue F, Frank-Raue K, Grauer A. Multiple endocrine neoplasia type 2. Clinical features and screening. Endocrinol Metab Clin North Am 1994;23(1):137–156

93. Gordon PR, Huvos AG, Strong EW. Medullary carcinoma of the thyroid gland. A clinicopathologic study of 40 cases. Cancer 1973;31(4):915–924

94. Brandi ML, Gagel RF, Angeli A, et al. Guidelines for diagnosis and therapy of MEN type 1 and type 2. J Clin Endocrinol Metab 2001;86(12):5658–5671

95. Kitamura Y, Shimizu K, Nagahama M, et al. Immediate causes of death in thyroid carcinoma: clinicopathological analysis of 161 fatal cases. J Clin Endocrinol Metab 1999;84(11):4043–4049

96. Aldinger KA, Samaan NA, Ibanez M, et al. Anaplastic carcinoma of the thyroid: a review of 84 cases of spindle and giant cell carcinoma of the thyroid. Cancer 1978;41(6):2267–2275

97. Venkatesh YS, Ordonez NG, Schultz PN, et al. Anaplastic carcinoma of the thyroid. A clinicopathologic study of 121 cases. Cancer 1990;66(2):321–330

98. Spires JR, Schwartz MR, Miller RH. Anaplastic thyroid carcinoma. Association with differentiated thyroid cancer. Arch Otolaryngol Head Neck Surg 1988;114(1):40–44

99. Sherman SI. Thyroid carcinoma. Lancet 2003;361(9356):501–511

100. Besic N. The role of initial debulking surgery in the management of anaplastic thyroid carcinoma. Surgery 2003;133(4):453–454; author reply 454–455

101. Busnardo B, Daniele O, Pelizzo MR, et al. A multimodality therapeutic approach in anaplastic thyroid carcinoma: study on 39 patients. J Endocrinol Invest 2000;23(11):755–761

102. Kebebew E, Greenspan FS, Clark OH, et al. Anaplastic thyroid carcinoma. Treatment outcome and prognostic factors. Cancer 2005;103(7):1330–1335

103. Voutilainen PE, Multanen M, Haapiainen RK, et al. Anaplastic thyroid carcinoma survival. World J Surg 1999;23(9):975–979

104. Levendag PC, De Porre PM, van Putten WL. Anaplastic carcinoma of the thyroid gland treated by radiation therapy. Int J Radiat Oncol Biol Phys 1993;26(1):125–128

105. Mitchell G, Huddart R, Harmer C. Phase II evaluation of high dose accelerated radiotherapy for anaplastic thyroid carcinoma. Radiother Oncol 1999;50(1):33–38

106. Tennvall J, Lundell G, Wahlberg P, et al. Anaplastic thyroid carcinoma. Doxorubicin, hyperfractionated radiotherapy and surgery. Acta Oncol 1990;29(8):1025–1028

107. Sugitani I, Kasai N, Fujimoto Y, et al. Prognostic factors and therapeutic strategy for anaplastic carcinoma of the thyroid. World J Surg 2001;25(5):617–622

108. Haigh PI, Ituarte PH, Wu HS, et al. Completely resected anaplastic thyroid carcinoma combined with adjuvant chemotherapy and irradiation is associated with prolonged survival. Cancer 2001;91(12):2335–2342

109. Jereb B, Stjernsward J, Lowhagen T. Anaplastic giant-cell carcinoma of the thyroid. A study of treatment and prognosis. Cancer 1975;35(5):1293–1295

110. Buckwalter JA, Gurll NJ, Thomas GC Jr. Cancer of the thyroid in youth. World J Surg 1981;5(1):15–25

111. Goepfert H, Dichtel WJ, Samaan NA. Thyroid cancer in children and teenagers. Arch Otolaryngol 1984;110(2):72–75

112. Vassilopoulou-Sellin R, Goepfert H, Raney B, et al. Differentiated thyroid cancer in children and adolescents: clinical outcome and mortality after long-term follow-up. Head Neck 1998;20(6):549–555

113. Farahati J, Bucsky P, Parlowsky T, et al. Characteristics of differentiated thyroid carcinoma in children and adolescents with respect to age, gender, and histology. Cancer 1997;80(11):2156–2162

114. Harness JK, Thompson NW, McLeod MK, et al. Differentiated thyroid carcinoma in children and adolescents. World J Surg 1992;16(4):547–554

115. Khurana KK, Labrador E, Izquierdo R, et al. The role of fine-needle aspiration biopsy in the management of thyroid nodules in children, adolescents, and young adults: a multi-institutional study. Thyroid 1999;9(4):383–386

116. Mestman JH, Goodwin TM, Montoro MM. Thyroid disorders of pregnancy. Endocrinol Metab Clin North Am 1995;24(1):41–71

117. Moosa M, Mazzaferri EL. Outcome of differentiated thyroid cancer diagnosed in pregnant women. J Clin Endocrinol Metab 1997;82(9):2862–2866

118. Schlumberger M, Labrador E, Izquierdo R, et al. 131I therapy for elevated thyroglobulin levels. Thyroid 1997;7(2):273–276

6

Carcinoma of the Salivary Glands

Mark K. Wax, Neil D. Gross, and Peter E. Andersen

◆ Epidemiology

The etiology of carcinoma of the salivary glands is believed to be multifactorial. A combination of environmental factors as well as certain genetic abnormalities may all contribute to the development of a carcinoma in one of the salivary glands (**Table 6–1**).

Salivary gland neoplasms are rare occurring with a prevalence of 1 per 50,000 per year. Cancer of the salivary glands is rare accounting for up to 0.9% of all cancers in the United States according to the 1999 National Cancer Database Report. The incidence of malignant salivary tumors in the United States is ~1.2 per 100,000 population, with a mean age at the time of diagnosis of 60 years with no gender prevalence. The majority of tumors arise in the parotid gland: 80% of these tumors are be-

Table 6–1 Factors That May Contribute to the Development of Salivary Carcinoma

Factor
Environmental
Radiation
Ionizing
Subtherapeutic
Hazardous nuclear plant exposure
Ultraviolet light
Dietary
High intake of polyunsaturated fats
Silica dust exposure
Hormonal
Early menarche
Multiparity
Viral
Epstein-Barr virus
Genetic
Allelic loss
Structural rearrangement
Monosomy/polysomy

nign and 20% are malignant. In contrast, 80% of minor salivary gland tumors are malignant whereas only 20% are benign.[1,2]

◆ Etiology

Tumors of the salivary glands represent a diverse class of neoplasms whose biological aggressiveness ranges from indolent to aggressive. Unlike epidermoid carcinoma, the etiology of carcinoma of the salivary gland is unclear. Tobacco and alcohol have not been implicated in the development of salivary gland neoplasms; however, radiation has been implicated as a possible etiology.

As with other endocrine and solid organ tumors of the head and neck, ionizing radiation has been shown to increase the risk for the development of carcinoma in the salivary glands. Patients who are exposed to radiation have been shown to be more prone to the development of both benign and malignant salivary gland tumors. Data accumulated over time has demonstrated that patients who have received radiation therapy for head and neck cancer have a 4.5-fold incidence of developing a salivary tumor within 11 years of treatment, and mucoepidermoid carcinoma is the most predominant type.

There is some evidence to suggest that exposure to silica dust can cause an increased risk of cancer in the salivary glands. Other factors such as a history of early menarche and multiparity may also contribute to an increased risk. Several studies have examined the role of Epstein-Barr virus in the development of certain types of salivary gland tumors. Whether this is because of the high prevalence of Epstein-Barr virus in these patient populations is unknown.[3]

The salivary glandular system is composed of the major salivary glands, including the parotid, submandibular, and sublingual glands, and the minor salivary glands, which occur diffusely throughout the lining of the oral cavity (**Fig. 6–1**). The majority of benign tumors occur in the major salivary gland system, whereas the majority of malignant neoplasms occur in the minor salivary glands.

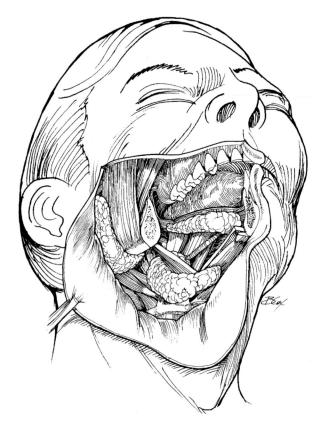

Figure 6–1 The three major paired salivary glands in the head and neck include the parotid glands, the submandibular glands, and the sublingual glands.

◆ Anatomy of the Salivary Glands

Parotid Gland

The parotid gland is the largest of the major salivary glands. The body of the gland lies over the ramus of the mandible and the masseter muscle. The inferior aspect of the gland, known as the tail of the gland, descends into the upper neck. The stylomandibular tunnel serves as a conduit connecting the deep and superficial lobes of the parotid gland. The deep lobe passes through the stylomandibular tunnel and extends into the prestyloid compartment of the parapharyngeal space. Tumors arising within the deep lobe of the parotid gland develop medial to the mandible in the parapharyngeal space and not uncommonly present with an oropharyngeal component. Although there is no fascial separation between the deep and superficial lobes of the parotid gland, the facial nerve and the retromandibular vein are used as anatomic markers between the lobes. Within the parotid gland, the facial nerve divides into two or three main trunks at pes anserinus. The lower branch is primarily composed of the marginal mandibular nerve, which supplies the muscles that allow for depression of the lower lip. The middle branch supplies the buccal, zygomatic, and lower eyelid areas, and the upper branch supplies the forehead and upper eyelid. Identification of the distal branches of the nerve as they exit the parotid gland is important when one considers reconstruction of the defect.[4]

Submandibular Gland

The submandibular gland is situated in the submandibular triangle. The marginal mandibular nerve crosses superficially to the facial vein and along the anterior aspect of the glandular capsule. The deep portion of the gland extends around the free posterior border of the mylohyoid muscle. The gland is intimately related to the lingual nerve and ganglion, which provides parasympathetic innervation to the gland. The submandibular duct (Wharton's duct) runs anterior in close association with the lingual nerve. It enters the anterior oral cavity adjacent to the frenulum. The facial artery and the facial vein course through the gland providing multiple branches to the gland.[4]

Sublingual Gland

The sublingual gland lies beneath the mucous membrane and superior to the mylohyoid muscle in the anterior floor of the mouth. It does not have a single duct that excretes into the floor of the mouth but instead has multiple ducts that may converge to form Bartholin's duct, which often joins the submandibular duct. The parasympathetic fibers that derive from the submandibular ganglion also provide innervation to the sublingual duct.

Minor Salivary Glands

The minor salivary glands are composed of between 500 and 1000 glands distributed throughout the upper aerodigestive tract. Although they can be found in the nasal cavity, larynx, and trachea, they are most prominent in the oral cavity.

◆ Development

There are currently two accepted theories on the cellular origins of salivary gland neoplasms; the multicellular theory and the bicellular theory.[5] The multicellular theory suggests that the origin of a neoplasm is derived from a distinctive cell type within the salivary gland structure. According to this theory, acinic cell tumors are thought to arise from acinar cells, whereas squamous and mucoepidermoid carcinomas are thought to arise from the excretory duct cells. An alternative theory, the bicellular theory, suggests that the basal cells of the intercalated duct cells and excretory duct cells act as reserve cells for more differentiated cells in the salivary gland unit. The basal cells give rise to the columnar and squamous cells of the excretory duct and from there it follows that the excretory duct reserve cells give rise to squamous cell carcinoma and mucoepidermoid carcinoma. The intercalated duct reserve cells give rise to the acinic cell and mixed tumor type carcinomas. The intercalated reserve duct cells are believed to be less aggressive than those tumors arising from the excretory reserve duct cells.

◆ Presentation

Salivary gland neoplasms commonly present as a firm mass within the gland. Although both benign and malignant tumors may present as a firm mass, malignancies may be fixed to the underlying soft tissue or, in advanced cases, present with a facial nerve palsy. Pain is considered an ominous sign and is usually associated with perineural invasion. Clinical presentation is often dictated by the stage and the gland afflicted with the tumor.

Parotid Gland

Tumors arising in the parotid gland often present as an asymptomatic mass. The tail of the gland is the most common site, and, depending on the physical habitus of the patient, tumors may achieve an advanced stage before being detected. As the tumor increases in size, it may begin to affect facial nerve function. This usually is associated with a high-grade malignancy such as squamous cell carcinomas, high-grade mucoepidermoid carcinomas, and/or adenoid cystic cancer. Less aggressive salivary tumors may grow extensively before causing a facial nerve palsy.[6]

Submandibular Gland

Tumors of the submandibular gland typically present as a painless mass in the submandibular triangle. The structures arising in this area such as the lingual and hypoglossal nerves are uncommonly affected unless there is extracapsular spread.

Sublingual Gland and Minor Salivary Glands

Tumors of the sublingual glands and minor salivary glands often present as a painless mass. Seldom is there ulceration; however, advanced tumors may present as an ulcerative lesion. If the lingual or hypoglossal nerves are invaded, the patient may present with dysarthria. The propensity for high-grade malignancies to metastasize to the neck is unusual and occurs in less than 20% of cases. As a result, it is rare that a salivary gland tumor presents as a neck mass distinct from the primary glandular tumor.

◆ Diagnosis and Workup

Imaging

Imaging is recommended for all salivary gland lesions because it allows for defining the size and extent of the tumor in addition to its relationship to critical structures such as the facial nerve. It is particularly helpful for minor salivary gland cancers where assessment of bone invasion or submucosal spread is critical for treatment planning. Specific indications for anatomic imaging include clinical uncertainty of tumor extent, evaluation of deep lobe or extraglandular involvement, identification of facial nerve invasion, and identification of potential cervical lymph node metastasis. Anatomic imaging is also useful for evaluating recurrent disease where differentiation between tumor and scar can be difficult. Functional imaging has limited utility for the evaluation of salivary gland malignancies except to identify rare distant metastasis.

Computed tomography (CT) and magnetic resonance imaging (MRI) can be useful in evaluating salivary gland tumors. Although each modality has inherent advantages and disadvantages, both techniques can provide valuable information. CT is capable of ruling out a salivary duct stone, which is poorly visualized using MRI. CT is also better suited for evaluating erosion of the mastoid or mandible. In contrast, bone marrow involvement is better demonstrated with MRI; however, CT is less expensive than MRI and is more widely available. Contrast-enhanced CT provides the advantage of being able to better define areas of necrosis in highly vascularized tumors but is more subject to dental artifact (**Fig. 6–2**). By comparison, MRI provides greater soft tissue detail. MRI allows for visualization of pathology in three orthogonal planes: axial, coronal, and sagittal. MRI provides better delineation of tumor architecture compared with conventional CT. MRI is particularly well-suited for differentiating deep-lobe parotid tumors, classically located in the prestyloid compartment, from other lesions of the parapharyngeal space. Perineural spread of tumor is also best visualized using MRI. For these reasons, MRI is more widely accepted as the imaging modality of choice for the evaluation of salivary gland malignancies (**Fig. 6–3**).

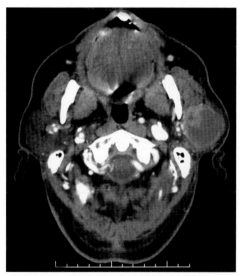

Figure 6–2 An extensive tumor of the parotid gland is visualized on this CT scan. The tumor is not well defined and demonstrates invasion of the surrounding structures.

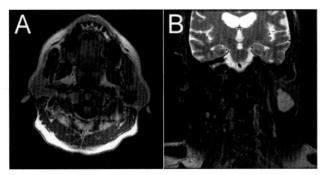

Figure 6–3 Deep-lobe left parotid tumor visualized using (**A**) axial T1-weighted (without gadolinium) and (**B**) coronal T2-weighted MRI.

The benefit of preoperative imaging for salivary gland cancer is roughly proportional to the stage of the disease. Early-stage salivary gland cancer can be managed without imaging if the clinical exam is reliable. For advanced-stage malignancies, both CT and MRI may be required to fully evaluate the extent of tumor involvement and often provide complimentary information. For example, CT may be used to assess bone destruction and to survey potential cervical metastasis. MRI can be used then to further define tumor composition and position relative to nearby soft tissue structures, as well as to assess for perineural invasion. MRI can be essential for evaluating potential intracranial extension of disease. Additional special studies may be useful for evaluating aggressive, advanced-stage salivary malignancies. Angiography and magnetic resonance angiography can be used to assess carotid invasion. Functional imaging such as positron emission tomography (PET) can be used to screen for distant metastasis.

The utility of [18F]fluoro-2-deoxy-D-glucose positron emission tomography (FDG-PET) for the routine evaluation of salivary gland malignancies has yet to be established. Both benign and malignant histology are well visualized using FDG-PET. The sensitivity of FDG-PET in the detection of salivary gland cancer is high but carries also a false-positive rate of nearly 30%.[7] Warthin's tumors and oncocytomas are most likely to be confused with salivary malignancy using FDG-PET, presumably because of the high mitochondrial content of these lesions. Although the standard uptake value (SUV) is generally higher for malignant salivary lesions compared with benign neoplasms, there is considerable overlap.[7] Given current technology, functional imaging technique cannot reliably differentiate benign from malignant salivary pathology. FDG-PET does not provide anatomic information and therefore cannot be used in place of CT or MRI in the evaluation of a salivary gland malignancy. FDG-PET can be used to screen for distant metastasis; however, the incidence of distant metastasis is low, limiting the clinical utility of FDG-PET in the routine workup of salivary cancers.

Fine-Needle Aspiration Biopsy

Fine-needle aspiration biopsy (FNAB) represents the standard of care for the workup of an unknown neck mass. The role of FNAB for salivary gland tumors, however, is less clearly

defined. This apparent discrepancy stems from the inherent difficulty of confirming the histologic diagnosis of a salivary malignancy. The majority of unknown cervical metastases are easily identified as squamous cell carcinoma; however, the variety of salivary gland histology often requires special expertise for interpretation. Further, low-grade salivary cancers are easily confused with benign neoplasms even on permanent pathologic analysis. Unlike an unknown neck mass where the histologic diagnosis profoundly impacts therapeutic strategy, the results of FNAB will seldom change the initial surgical treatment of a salivary gland tumor. For parotid tumors, the minimal uniformly accepted resection of a suspicious lesion is a superficial parotidectomy. Similarly, excisional biopsy of the submandibular gland is the core treatment of any submandibular neoplasm. Despite these logistic limitations, many clinicians rely on FNAB in the preoperative workup of patients with suspected salivary cancer.

The safety and accuracy of FNAB for salivary gland malignancies is well established. Early concerns of tumor seeding from the needle track have been dispelled. In high-volume centers with qualified personnel, FNAB is a simple, safe, and informative test. Multiple large studies from across the globe have confirmed FNAB to be exceptionally accurate and reliable when performed by an experienced cytopathologist. The distinction between benign and malignant tumors is possible in most cases. The sensitivity of FNAB for salivary gland tumors has been reported as high as 85 to 95% with a specificity approaching 100%.[8,9] FNAB is far less accurate when interpreted by less-experienced practitioners.

The results of FNAB should always be interpreted with caution. FNAB results are typically reported as benign, malignant, indeterminate, or inadequate. A "negative" FNAB has little meaning as this usually represents either an inadequate or indeterminate specimen. Inadequate sampling of the lesion is the most common diagnostic error.[10] If recognized immediately, inadequate FNAB results should prompt a second biopsy. Even when an FNAB is indeterminate, the description of histologic findings often offers clues that may help direct further workup. Therefore, it is incumbent upon the clinician to carefully analyze every detail of the written pathology report. For example, monomorphic lymphocytes noted on FNAB may be suggestive of salivary gland lymphoma prompting further investigation. Such indeterminate FNAB results, albeit helpful, are unlikely to be resolved by repeated FNAB. A more invasive approach is frequently required to pinpoint a diagnosis in these cases.

Not all patients with salivary tumors require FNAB. FNAB is best employed when the results will impact treatment or patient counseling. The results of FNAB may change the planned extent of surgical resection. Specifically, patients with confirmed malignancy on FNAB would be considered for selective cervical lymph node dissection based on the stage and grade of disease. Special attention may also be given to the preoperative planning of possible facial nerve resection and reconstruction for those patients in whom an FNAB confirms parotid malignancy. FNAB is important for differentiating tumors of salivary origin from those that are systemic or metastatic. For example, the diagnosis of lymphoma may be suggested by FNAB and, if confirmed with more tissue, could spare the patient extensive surgery. FNAB can also be helpful in counseling patients who are poor surgical candidates. An unsuitable surgical patient with the diagnosis of benign disease on FNAB can be observed. Thus, FNAB may be more important for defining those patients who will not need surgery rather than in helping to plan surgery for known operative cases.

◆ Staging

Staging of salivary gland tumors was revised in 2002 by the American Joint Committee on Cancer (AJCC). The TNM staging system is based according to the size, mobility, and in parotid tumors whether or not the facial nerve is involved. Diagnostic imaging studies may be used in staging but are not mandated. As in other sites, the TNM staging system qualifies the tumor, the node, and metastatic disease. The T stage is primarily based on the size of the tumor and whether or not extraparenchymal extension is present. The nodal staging system is the same for all tumors based in the aerodigestive tract, and the metastatic system is also the same. AJCC stage groupings follow the standard formula (**Table 6–2**).

The minor salivary glands are staged according to the site upon which they arise.[11] For example, a minor salivary gland tumor originating in the oral cavity will be staged according to the oral cavity tumor.

Table 6–2   TNM Staging System for Major Salivary Gland Cancer

Primary Tumor (T)

TX	Primary tumor cannot be assessed
T0	No evidence of primary tumor
T1	Tumor 2 cm or less in greatest dimension without extraparenchymal extension*
T2	Tumor >2 cm but not >4 cm in greatest dimension without extraparenchymal extension*
T3	Tumor >4 cm and/or tumor having extraparenchymal extension*
T4a	Tumor invades skin, mandible, ear canal, and/or facial nerve
T4b	Tumor invades skull base and/or pterygoid plates and/or encases carotid artery

Regional Lymph Nodes (N)

NX	Regional lymph nodes cannot be assessed
N0	No regional lymph node metastasis
N1	Metastasis in a single ipsilateral lymph node, 3 cm or less in greatest dimension
N2	Metastasis in a single ipsilateral lymph node, >3 cm but not >6 cm in greatest dimension, or in multiple ipsilateral lymph nodes, none >6 cm in greatest dimension, or in bilateral or contralateral lymph nodes, none >6 cm in greatest dimension
N2a	Metastasis in a single ipsilateral lymph node, >3 cm but not >6 cm in greatest dimension
N2b	Metastasis in multiple ipsilateral lymph nodes, none >6 cm in greatest dimension
N2c	Metastasis in bilateral or contralateral lymph nodes, none >6 cm in greatest dimension
N3	Metastasis in a lymph node >6 cm in greatest dimension

Distant Metastasis (M)

MX	Distant metastasis cannot be assessed
M0	No distant metastasis
M1	Distant metastasis

Stage Grouping

Stage I	T1	N0	M0
Stage II	T2	N0	M0
Stage III	T3	N0	M0
	T1	N1	M0
	T2	N1	M0
	T3	N1	M0
Stage IVA	T4a	N0	M0
	T4a	N1	M0
	T1	N2	M0
	T2	N2	M0
	T3	N2	M0
	T4a	N2	M0
Stage IVB	T4b	Any N	M0
	Any T	N3	M0
Stage IVC	Any T	Any N	M1

*Note: Extraparenchymal extension is clinical or macroscopic evidence of invasion of soft tissues. Microscopic evidence alone does not constitute extraparenchymal extension for classification purposes.

◆ Classification

Salivary gland cancers represent a diverse array of pathology, spanning the spectrum from low-grade, indolent neoplasms to highly aggressive malignancies. Therefore, the histologic classification of salivary gland cancers requires special skill. The World Health Organization (WHO) has compiled the most comprehensive classification, which was revised in 1991 to include nearly 40 distinct histologic entities of salivary origin.[12,13] The distribution of salivary gland cancers classified by the WHO is presented in **Table 6–3**.

Whereas the majority of salivary tumors are benign, nearly one third are malignant. Salivary gland cancers can be broadly divided into epithelial and nonepithelial lesions. Epithelial-derived salivary malignancies are far more common than those that are nonepithelial in origin. Among malignant tumors of the salivary glands, mucoepidermoid carcinoma is the most common accounting for nearly 15% of all salivary neoplasms. The largest single-institution experience with salivary gland tumors was reported by Spiro in 1986.[14] For this cancer-enriched cohort, mucoepidermoid carcinoma was the most common followed by adenoid cystic carcinoma, adenocarcinoma, and malignant mixed tumor.

Salivary gland malignancies demonstrate great variability with respect to natural history. The aggressiveness of a salivary cancer is often represented by the grade of the tumor. For example, mucoepidermoid carcinomas can be categorized into high-, medium-, or low-grade disease. High-grade mucoepidermoid carcinomas show a rapid and aggressive

clinical course with early cervical metastasis and a propensity for local recurrence and distant disease.[14] Conversely, low-grade mucoepidermoid carcinomas typically demonstrate a protracted, indolent course. Not surprisingly, management decisions are often made more on histologic grade than cell type. Classic high-grade salivary cancers include squamous cell carcinoma, mixed malignant tumor, and undifferentiated carcinoma. Acinic cell carcinoma and polymorphous low-grade adenocarcinoma are representative low-grade salivary malignancies.

Adenoid cystic carcinomas display a unique natural history that deserves special mention. These tumors share some features of both high- and low-grade salivary malignancies. Adenoid cystic carcinomas have a characteristic clinical course with a tendency for perineural invasion, local recurrence, and pulmonary metastasis. Yet, cervical metastases are infrequently encountered, and recurrence or spread of disease may take years to manifest. Even when distant metastases are documented, patients with adenoid cystic carcinoma can live for decades.[15] Therefore, the management and counseling of patients with adenoid cystic carcinoma is complex and cannot be extrapolated from experience with other malignancies.

◆ Treatment

In most cases, the treatment of salivary gland tumors is primarily surgical with the use of adjuvant postoperative radiation therapy based on the presence of adverse pathologic factors including high-grade histopathology; large tumors; extracapsular extension; extension into skin, temporal bone, skull base, or mandible; facial nerve involvement; or cervical lymphatic metastasis. Radiation therapy has been used in cases where the tumor is unresectable because of either technical factors or patient comorbidities. Surgical resection should be focused on complete resection with adequate margins of normal tissues, and undue morbidity should be avoided. Of particular concern is facial nerve function. When the facial nerve is not invaded or encased by tumor, every attempt should be made to preserve the nerve. If, however, the tumor cannot be completely removed without resecting all or a portion of the nerve, then the nerve should be sacrificed. On occasion, salivary gland tumors will involve the skin of the face, mandible, or temporal bone. All of these structures can be resected *en bloc* with the tumor and represent more of a reconstructive challenge than one of resection. If for technical reasons or because of patient wishes a tumor cannot be completely resected, then consideration should be given to alternative, nonoperative management as there is little evidence that partial resection benefits the patient in terms of survival and probably just results in added morbidity to the treatment.

Table 6–3 Revised World Health Organization Classification of Salivary Gland Tumors

Histology
Epithelial tumors (carcinomas)
Acinic cell carcinoma
Mucoepidermoid carcinoma
Adenoid cystic carcinoma
Polymorphous low-grade adenocarcinoma (terminal duct adenocarcinoma)
Epithelial-myoepithelial carcinoma
Basal cell carcinoma
Sebaceous carcinoma
Papillary cystadenocarcinoma
Mucinous adenocarcinoma
Oncocytic carcinoma
Salivary duct carcinoma
Adenocarcinoma
Malignant myoepithelioma (myoepithelial carcinoma)
Carcinoma in pleomorphic adenoma (malignant mixed tumor)
Squamous cell carcinoma
Small cell carcinoma
Undifferentiated carcinoma
Other carcinomas
Nonepithelial tumors
Malignant lymphomas
Secondary tumors (metastasis)

Parotid Gland

Tumors of the parotid gland that are small and located within the superficial lobe of the parotid gland can often be managed by superficial parotidectomy. Deep-lobe tumors or those that involve both the superficial and deep lobes usually require total parotidectomy (**Fig. 6–4**). The term *total parotidectomy* is a misnomer as it is technically difficult to remove all of the parotid gland due to its extensions around the external auditory canal and deep to the mandible. When extension outside of the parotid fascia occurs, surgical resection of the involved structures should be performed in an *en bloc* fashion. This may require resection of the skin overlying the parotid, the mandible, or portions of the temporal bone. When such structures require resection, various reconstructive options exist that are discussed elsewhere in this chapter.

Preservation of the facial nerve should be preserved unless there is direct invasion. When the surgeon encounters facial nerve invasion or encasement by a malignant neoplasm, the involved portion of the nerve should be resected. The nerve can be repaired primarily if a neurorrhaphy can be accomplished without tension. This is uncommon, and in most cases a nerve graft is required. Defects less than 4 cm can often be repaired with a graft obtained from the great auricular nerve if the nerve is available. When the defect is longer than 4 cm or the great auricular nerve is unavailable, then the sural nerve is a good reconstructive option.

When the tumor approaches the stylomastoid foramen or if perineural extension extends into the temporal bone, a mastoidectomy and removal of the mastoid tip can provide enhanced exposure. Mastoidectomy and intratemporal identification of the facial nerve can be particularly helpful in the case of reoperative parotid surgery as it allows identification of the nerve in a previously unoperated field.

Submandibular Gland

Neoplasms of the submandibular glands are less common than tumors of the parotid gland. Management of submandibular gland tumors in general carries less risk of damage to the facial nerve (except for its marginal mandibular branch) but there are other nerves located within proximity to the submandibular gland, specifically the lingual and hypoglossal nerves.

Surgery for tumors of the submandibular gland should be performed differently than surgery for benign inflammatory conditions of the gland. Whereas the latter can often be managed with a subcapsular enucleation of the gland, malignant tumors should be removed with a more comprehensive procedure. When the exact nature of the tumor is unclear, the procedure should be directed to adequately resect the tumor as if it were malignant. If the condition ultimately is found to represent an inflammatory condition, there are little adverse consequences to the patient.

Minor Salivary Glands

Management of the Neck

Management of the neck can be divided into two clinical scenarios: patients with clinically evident lymph node metastasis and those with a clinically N0 neck. In patients with clinical evidence of metastasis, a neck dissection is an essential aspect of management. In general, this should consist of a comprehensive neck dissection. Decisions regarding preservation of nonlymphatic structures (modified and selective neck dissections) should be based on clinical findings during the time of operation. There is little data regarding the use of selective neck dissection in the setting of neck disease, and therefore its use cannot be commented upon.

In patients with a clinically N0 neck, the risk of occult cervical metastasis depends upon multiple factors. Tumors larger than 4 cm, those with high-grade histology, extension beyond the capsule of the parotid gland, and those with preoperative facial nerve paralysis have a high rate of occult cervical lymph node metastasis. Therefore, an elective cervical lymphadenectomy is indicated. There is no consensus regarding the type of neck dissection to perform. Certainly, it seems acceptable to preserve the spinal accessory nerve in these patients. As well, the use of selective neck dissection in this setting as a staging operation seems a reasonable consideration.

◆ Prognostic Factors

Stage

The stage at presentation of a patient with a salivary gland malignancy is the most well studied prognostic factor.[16–18] With regard to adenoid cystic carcinoma, survival at 10 years posttreatment is highly correlated with stage, with 75%, 43%, and 15% of patients with stage I, stage II, and stages III or IV surviving, repectively.[16]

Surgical Margins

The adequacy of surgical resection has been found in numerous studies to be highly predictive of ultimate survival.[19] The effect is so large that in one study of patients with adenoid cystic carcinoma, those with negative surgical margins had a disease-free survival of 84% contrasted with a rate of only

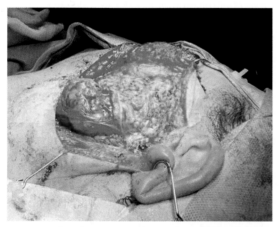

Figure 6–4 In this photo, one can see a deep-lobe tumor that splays the lower branches of the facial nerve. Meticulous dissection allows for removal with anatomic preservation of the nerve.

17% in those with residual tumor at the margin of resection.[20] There is evidence that the use of postoperative radiation in patients with positive margins can effect a substantial improvement in survival and should be considered in these patients.[21]

Grade/Histology

With the numerous different histologic types of salivary gland malignancies, much work has been done to determine whether histologic type correlates with prognosis. Most authors divide salivary gland cancers into high- or low-grade histology (**Table 6–4**). Although often considered a high grade cancer, adenoid cystic carcinoma is unusual in that it often exhibits slow, relentless growth and with late recurrences both locally and distantly.

In mucoepidermoid carcinoma, high-grade histology has been found by several authors to predict increased incidence of local and regional recurrence as well as decreased survival.[22,23]

Facial Nerve Paralysis

Preoperative facial nerve paralysis has been found by multiple authors to be an adverse prognostic factor in patients with salivary gland carcinoma. It is difficult to isolate the effect of stage in these patients because patients with facial palsy tend to have larger tumors. Nevertheless, several studies[24,25] have confirmed the relatively grim prognosis of patients with this factor.

Cervical Metastasis

As with other head and neck malignancies, the presence of cervical lymph node metastasis in patients with salivary gland cancer has been found to adversely impact survival.

◆ Treatment

Nonsurgical Treatment

Surgery is the primary therapeutic modality for malignant tumors of salivary origin. Nonsurgical management is currently restricted to the management of inoperable tumors or to palliative management.

Table 6–4 Classification of Salivary Gland Malignancies

Low Grade	High Grade
Low-grade mucoepidermoid carcinoma	Squamous carcinoma
Acinic cell carcinoma	High-grade mucoepidermoid carcinoma
Polymorphous low-grade adenocarcinoma	Adenoid cystic carcinoma
	Undifferentiated carcinoma
	Salivary duct carcinoma
	Malignant mixed tumor

Radiation Therapy

Postoperative adjuvant radiation therapy augments locoregional control of appropriately selected patients with aggressive salivary cancers.[19] There is additional evidence to suggest it may improve survival as well for this cohort.[26] Postoperative radiotherapy is typically advised for advanced-stage and or high-grade disease where the risk of locoregional failure is high. Additional indications for adjuvant postoperative radiation therapy include positive surgical margins, recurrent disease, and other unfavorable pathologic characteristics.

The role of radiotherapy for palliation of inoperable or recurrent salivary malignancy is also increasingly recognized. Fast neutron radiation therapy may offer a biologic advantage for treating inoperable salivary gland cancer, particularly adenoid cystic carcinoma. A randomized study comparing neutron therapy versus conventional photon or electron radiotherapy for unresectable salivary malignancy demonstrated improved locoregional control for the neutron therapy cohort.[27] The study, however, failed to show any difference in overall survival between groups. Increased morbidity was noted for the patients receiving neutron beam radiotherapy. For this reason, and because few facilities are capable of delivering neutron therapy, conventional photon beam radiotherapy is still recommended for the majority of patients with unresectable salivary gland cancer.

Chemotherapy

The aggressive nature and tendency for distant metastasis of high-grade salivary cancer highlights the need for systemic therapy. Unfortunately, the results of chemotherapy for treating salivary gland malignancy have been disappointing. Small, single-cohort studies have shown sporadic, unpredictable responses to cisplatin-based regimens.[28] Given the lack of evidence of efficacy observed to date, adjunctive chemotherapy is not currently advised. The use of chemotherapy for salivary gland tumors, then, remains limited to the palliative and investigational setting. Targeted molecular therapies offer the promise of improved systemic therapy for salivary cancers in the future.

Reconstruction

Reconstruction of defects after ablation for salivary gland tumors primarily deals with parotid gland defects. Minor salivary gland tumors when they are resected require some form of composite resection, which is not much different from a composite resection of the overlying oral cavity mucosa and surrounding structures. Their reconstructive paradigms follow the reconstruction for that particular anatomic subsite. The same can be said for submandibular gland tumors, which usually only require reconstructive consideration when they involve the mandible or extend up into the tongue.

Defects of the parotid gland have undergone an evolution in terms of the reconstructive aspects. Management of parotid gland tumors depends significantly on whether the facial nerve is or is not involved. If the facial nerve is involved, then sacrifice is usually mandated. Reconstruction of patients who have had their facial nerve resected is complex, and the reader is referred to a reconstructive textbook. Needless to say, management of the eye is of paramount importance at the initial setting. Gold weight placement and lateral tarsal strip have been found to be quite useful in these instances. The facial nerve usually can be reconstructed at the initial setting by using a nerve graft. There are many sites available for a nerve graft. The sural nerve is the most common, but the medial antebrachial as well as greater auricular have been used with equal success (**Fig. 6–5**). In the setting of malignancy involving the facial nerve, postoperative radiotherapy is often administered. There has been some concern that this may inhibit or affect the ultimate outcome of the facial nerve, but it has been well documented that preoperative or postoperative radiotherapy has no impact on ultimate facial nerve function.

Another issue that has arisen is the effect of perineural invasion at the margin of the resection. Several carcinomas are notorious for traveling along the nerve and leaving perineural positive margins either peripherally or centrally. A recent study has documented that this has no effect on ultimate outcome and should not influence whether or not to reconstruct the facial nerve. Most patients who have parotid malignancies, even if they do involve the facial nerve, have good 2- to 5-year survival, and reconstruction should be undertaken in all of these patients.

Ancillary measures to immediately protect those functions that the facial nerve governs such as the eye (**Fig. 6–6**) and nasal valve (**Fig. 6–7**) should be undertaken at the initial setting. It is relatively easy to perform a gold weight placement to rehabilitate the upper eye and a lateral tarsal strip to re-habilitate the lower eyelid and thus protect the cornea. The nasal valve is an area that is often overlooked because of the complexity of the patient's underlying problems. Simple stitches can be used to stent open the nasal valve and provide for an adequate airway.

Management of the lateral commissure is more problematic. Loss of the facial nerve will result in a drooping of the lateral commissure and relaxation of the elevators at the corner of the mouth. This has a significant effect not only on cosmesis but also on function (from a drooling and deglutition perspective). Patients are often quite debilitated by this. We have found that immediate reconstruction with an Allogenic sling or using suture is a technique that is quite viable and provides immediate relief of the symptomatology (**Fig. 6–8**).

The other area of major concern in total parotidectomy or in patients who have also undergone neck dissection is the cosmetic defect. The skin is the only outer envelope that is retained, and the masseter muscle as well as mandible is the next layer. This leaves quite an indentation on the lateral aspect of the facial skeleton and should be reconstructed. Free fat grafts have been used in the past, but their survival and retention of bulk is quite variable. We would suggest that a soft tissue reconstruction should be done on all of these patients. Free tissue transfer in using an anterolateral thigh flap or a de-epithelialized radial forearm flap will provide enough soft tissue to fill in the soft tissue defect. The trade-off is a cosmetic defect on the volar aspect of the forearm. The gain in a permanent predictable soft tissue augmentation in the cheek is considerable. Patients are usually pleased with their outcome and do not feel they are cosmetically deformed. True quality of life measures are absent.

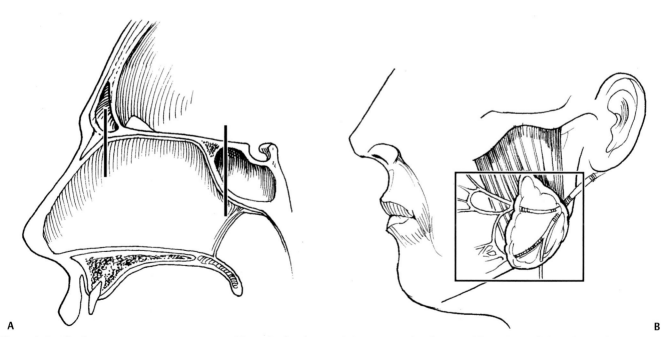

Figure 6–5 The first step in reconstruction is to address the facial nerve. (**A**) A nerve graft is harvested from the medial antebrachial nerve. (**B**) The graft is used to connect the proximal facial nerve to the distal branches.

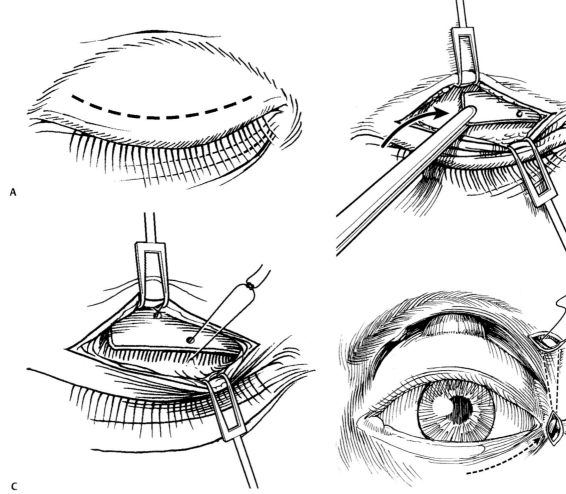

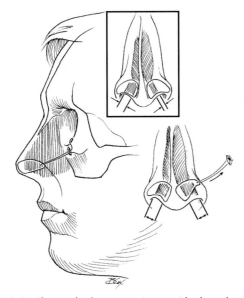

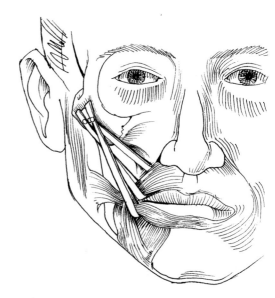

Figure 6–6 (**A**) The incision for placement of the gold weight is planned in the supratarsal crease. (**B**) The gold weight is placed deep to the skin muscle flap. (**C**) The gold weight is secured with three absorbable sutures. (**D**) The canthopexy is achieved by securing the lateral canthal tendon superior and posterior to the lateral orbital rim.

Figure 6–7 The nasal valve suspension provides lateral retraction of the nasal ala and improves the nasal airway.

Figure 6–8 The facial suspension should include three vectors of retraction to provide a natural elevation and symmetry.

Controversies

There continue to be several long-standing controversies in the management of salivary gland cancers. Debated topics include the workup, the use of intraoperative aids, and the extent of resection.

Imaging and Fine-Needle Biopsy

Historically, the greatest controversy surrounding the management of salivary gland cancers has revolved around the utility of preoperative imaging and FNAB. As discussed previously, neither anatomic imaging nor FNAB is required for every salivary malignancy. The clinical utility of FNAB for salivary cancer depends largely on the interest and expertise of the cytopathologist. Similarly, the utility of anatomic imaging depends on accurate interpretation of the study. No investigation can supplant clinical acumen. Even so, many clinicians utilize one or more of these investigations routinely. The decision to use preoperative imaging or FNAB, then, tends to rest more on personal philosophy and logistics rather than on science. Experienced head and neck surgeons selectively employ anatomic imaging and FNAB tailored to the tumor location and clinical presentation of each patient. Patients with advanced-stage tumors will frequently benefit from both investigations. Conversely, patients with small, well-circumscribed, low-grade lesions can be managed based on clinical examination alone.

Intraoperative Monitors

Controversy also exists regarding the use of special equipment to assist in intraoperative decision-making. Nerve monitoring is used routinely by neurootologists for procedures that place the facial nerve at risk. It is increasingly utilized for complex thyroid surgery as well. Facial nerve monitoring has also been advocated as a tool to help minimize nerve trauma and to help predict function after parotid surgery. Facial nerve monitoring cannot assist in the difficult decision of when facial nerve sacrifice is required. Facial nerve sacrifice is a clinical decision made at the time of surgery based on gross nerve invasion. Frozen-section biopsy is also argued to be a useful intraoperative tool in the management of suspected salivary gland cancer. Like FNAB, the utility of frozen-section analysis of salivary lesions is highly dependent on the experience of the pathologist. Some head and neck surgeons insist on frozen-section confirmation of malignancy before sacrificing a preoperatively functional facial nerve involved by tumor. Opponents of frozen section contend that all important intraoperative decisions should be made based on clinical judgment rather than on pathologic examination.

Resection and Dissection

There is no consensus regarding the extent of primary tumor resection and or neck dissection required for salivary gland malignancies. Although most head and neck surgeons re-commend at least superficial parotidectomy for any parotid neoplasm, the extent of facial nerve dissection is debatable. Tumors isolated to the tail of the parotid, for example, can be resected via a modified superficial parotidectomy where only the inferior division of the facial nerve is dissected. Similarly, some surgeons will resect deep-lobe parotid lesions without identifying the full extent of the facial nerve. The most explicit example of controversy related to extent of dissection involves the appropriateness of sentinel lymph node biopsy (SLNB) involving the parotid gland without identification of the facial nerve. This form of lymph node "plucking," previously rebuked, has now gained increasing enthusiasm. SLNB involving the parotid gland has been reported to be safe.[29] Yet, many surgeons remain reluctant to embrace the concept of blind intraparotid dissection. The extent of and need for neck dissection in the setting of a clinically N0 neck is also debated. Although most authors reserve neck dissection in this setting for large or high-grade tumors, there is no consensus about which cervical levels require dissection. This is particularly true for minor salivary gland tumors where the location of disease can be quite variable, and the incidence of cervical metastasis is low.

◆ Clinical Cases

Case 1 Management of long-standing parotid mass.

Presentation An 83-year-old woman presented with a slow-growing mass in the left parotid region. The mass was ~5 cm in size and had been present for the past 20 years. When she originally consulted a physician 20 years ago, she was scheduled to have the mass removed but suffered a stroke and in the recovery phase neglected to have the parotid mass followed.

Physical Examination Physical examination revealed an immobile mass located in the tail of the parotid. Facial nerve function, cranial facial exam, and head and neck exam were negative. The patient was wheelchair bound, slightly aphasic, and had a history of cardiac myopathy with tenuous status due to her congestive heart failure.

Diagnosis and Workup CT and MRI scans demonstrated a cystic-appearing mass with distinct borders. FNAB confirmed a Warthin's tumor.

Treatment of the Primary Tumor The pathology and radiographic findings combined with a 20-year history of slow growth confirm that this is a benign lesion. Given this woman's tenuous medical status and the lack of concern for cosmesis, a decision is made to continue to follow the tumor.

Over the next 2 to 3 years, the mass slowly increases in size to ~6 cm. No active intervention was undertaken, and the woman passed away one evening in her sleep.

Summary of Treatment This case demonstrates how watchful waiting and observation is appropriate in a certain patient population with well-defined histopathology.

Case 2 Management of the subacute parotid mass.

Presentation A 24-year-old man presented with a 1.5-cm nodule anterior to the tragus. This mass was first noticed ~2 to 3 months prior to presentation. It had slowly increased in size but was otherwise asymptomatic. The patient had no complaints concerning the ear, nose, and throat. He had no infectious etiology or exposure.

Physical Examination His physical exam was unremarkable with the exception of a mobile 2.5-cm mass anterior and inferior to the tragus.

Diagnosis and Workup In view of the gentleman's recent exposure to a cat, an FNAB was performed. Pathologic features consistent with a pleomorphic adenoma were identified on cytology. A CT scan confirmed the presence of a superficial lobe parotid tumor with well-defined borders.

Treatment of the Primary Tumor Through a standard parotidectomy incision, the lesion was removed after identification of the facial nerve. The mass was found to lie between the buccal and the ramus mandibularis branch of the facial nerve. These nerves were preserved, and a sternocleidomastoid flap was positioned into the defect to preserve cosmesis. Final pathology revealed a pleomorphic adenoma, and the patient healed well with no sequelae.

Summary of Treatment This case demonstrates how a careful history is required to rule out etiologies other than benign neoplasms. Cat scratch fever, though a rare cause of a lymphadenopathy in the parotid gland, should always be considered. FNAB was performed for that reason in this case, and imaging was believed to not contribute to either the diagnosis or management so was not done. Although a large number of surgeons do not reconstruct the parotid defect, given this gentleman's young age and concern over cosmesis, a small myogenous rotational flap was used to obliterate the dead space and improve the postoperative cosmetic appearance.

Case 3 Management of a low-grade malignant parotid lesion.

Presentation A 56-year-old man presented with a 3-month history of a facial mass located at the angle of the mandible. It was noticed while he was shaving and has not bothered him. He thinks that it may have increased in size over the past month or so but has not been associated with other symptoms.

Physical Examination Physical examination revealed a firm indistinct mass in the angle of the mandible. It was ~3 cm and mobile. Cranial facial exam demonstrated that the facial nerve and the head and neck exam were normal.

Diagnosis and Workup An FNAB was performed and revealed a mixed population of cells suggestive of a malignancy; however, a definitive diagnosis could not be made. An MRI scan was performed because of the indistinctness of the mass, and it revealed a bilobed tumor that extends into the parapharyngeal space. The borders were indistinct suggesting a malignant etiology.

Treatment of the Primary Tumor The patient was counseled and taken to the operating room. A standard parotid-

ectomy was performed through a standard approach, and the facial nerve was identified. Intraoperative examination revealed a tumor that was deep to the ramus mandibularis nerve extended into the parapharyngeal space. Through a standard approach, the mass was resected, and pathology revealed a low-grade mucoepidermoid carcinoma. Because the tumor was "low grade," no adjuvant therapy was recommended.

Summary of Treatment This case demonstrated how a mass that is indistinct in the parotid on examination requires radiographic investigation to determine the anatomic boundaries. Fine-needle aspiration was essential in helping counsel the patient regarding possible facial nerve resection. The grading of mucoepidermoid carcinoma is based on the cystic component of the tumor, neural invasion, necrosis, mitoses, and anaplasia. In general, the more squamoid and less mucinous features associated with the histology, the more high-grade the tumor. Whereas high-grade mucoepidermoid carcinoma is commonly treated with postoperative radiation therapy after surgery, low-grade tumors can be managed with surgery followed by close observation. Intermediate-grade cancers represent a controversial subgroup. The decision to observe or radiate is usually based on the margin status.

Case 4 Management of a parotid lesion with facial nerve involvement.

Presentation The patient is a 56-year-old man who presents with a 3-month history of a gradually expanding mass in the right parotid region. His history was interesting in that approximately 7 years ago, he had a large squamous cell carcinoma removed from his temple. Margins were negative at that time. The parotid mass has been slowly increasing in size, and he finds that he is unable to elevate his brow as well as he has in the past. At the end of the day he will have trouble reading, as the brow "hangs" over the eye. He is otherwise well and asymptomatic.

Physical Examination His physical examination confirms that the upper branch of his facial nerve is not functioning well. There was a weakness of the closure apparatus of his eye. He is able to close the eye, but when the examiner attempts to open the eye, it is relatively easy to do compared with the contralateral side. Furthermore, the eyebrow is seen to hang down over the eye producing a hooding effect. He can lift the eyebrow but movement is sluggish. The rest of his facial nerve and craniofacial examination was normal. He has a 4-cm, firm, hard mass in the right parotid gland that appears fixed to the underlying tissues. There is no other lymphadenopathy present. A CT scan and MRI scan reveal a single 4-cm inhomogeneous mass in the right parotid gland. It appears fixed to the inferior portion of the zygomatic process. There is no other lymphadenopathy present.

Diagnosis and Workup An FNAB confirmed squamous cell carcinoma. The patient is presented at tumor board, and the parotid tumor is believed to be a metastatic squamous cell carcinoma from a primary on his temple. It is believed that combined modality treatment with surgery followed by postoperative radiotherapy would be his best management.

Treatment of the Primary Tumor He proceeded to the operating room where a total parotidectomy and level II to IV neck dissection are performed. In conjunction with this, the facial nerve is sacrificed.

At the time of his initial ablative procedure, a de-epithelialized radial forearm fascial cutaneous free flap is placed in the wound bed. This allows for rehabilitation and reconstruction of the soft tissue defect. A nerve graft of the medial antebrachial nerve is harvested and connected from the facial nerve stump to the peripheral branches. At the same time, the upper eye is rehabilitated with the placement of a 1.2-mg gold weight, and a lateral canthal strip procedure is performed. A stitch to expand and stabilize the nasal valve is placed, and an AlloDerm sling is used to suspend the lower lip.

Summary of Treatment This case demonstrates that large ablative procedures involving the facial nerve and the soft tissues of the face are best rehabilitated by reconstructing the facial nerve with a graft for long-term rehabilitation and then by various facial plastic procedures to rehabilitate the eye, both its upper and lower lid components as well as the mid-face and lower face. The contour secondary to the soft tissue loss is reconstructed with a free tissue flap.

References

1. Spitz MR, Batsakis JG. Major salivary gland carcinoma. Descriptive epidemiology and survival of 498 patients. Arch Otolaryngol 1984;110(1):45–49

2. Pinkston JA, Cole P. Incidence rates of salivary gland tumors: results from a population-based study. Otolaryngol Head Neck Surg 1999;120(6):834–840

3. Zheng W, Shu XO, Ji BT, Gao YT. Diet and other risk factors for cancer of the salivary glands: a population-based case-control study. Int J Cancer 1996;67(2):194–198

4. Carlson GW. The salivary glands. Embryology, anatomy, and surgical applications. Surg Clin North Am 2000;80(1):261–273, xii.

5. Kirkbride P, Liu FF, O'Sullivan B. Outcome of curative management of malignant tumours of the parotid gland. J Otolaryngol 2001;30(5):271–279

6. Pohar S, Gay H, Rosenbaum P, et al. Malignant parotid tumors: presentation, clinical/pathologic prognostic factors, and treatment outcomes. Int J Radiat Oncol Biol Phys 2005;61(1):112–118

7. Uchida Y, Minoshima S, Kawata T, et al. Diagnostic value of FDG PET and salivary gland scintigraphy for parotid tumors. Clin Nucl Med 2005;30(3):170–176

8. Orell SR. Diagnostic difficulties in the interpretation of fine needle aspirates of salivary gland lesions: the problem revisited. Cytopathology 1995;6(5):285–300

9. Stewart CJ, MacKenzie K, McGarry GW, et al. Fine-needle aspiration cytology of salivary gland: a review of 341 cases. Diagn Cytopathol 2000;22(3):139–146

10. MacLeod CB, Frable WJ. Fine-needle aspiration biopsy of the salivary gland: problem cases. Diagn Cytopathol 1993;9(2):216–224; discussion 224–225

11. Numata T, Muto H, Shiba K, et al. Evaluation of the validity of the 1997 International Union Against Cancer TNM classification of major salivary gland carcinoma. Cancer 2000;89(8):1664–1669

12. Seifert G, Sobin LH. The World Health Organization's Histological Classification of Salivary Gland Tumors. A commentary on the second edition. Cancer 1992;70(2):379–385

13. Simpson RH. Classification of salivary gland tumours–a brief histopathological review. Histol Histopathol 1995;10(3):737–746

14. Spiro RH. Salivary neoplasms: overview of a 35-year experience with 2,807 patients. Head Neck Surg 1986;8(3):177–184

15. Spiro RH, Huvos AG, Berk R, et al. Mucoepidermoid carcinoma of salivary gland origin. A clinicopathologic study of 367 cases. Am J Surg 1978;136(4):461–468

16. Spiro RH, Huvos AG. Stage means more than grade in adenoid cystic carcinoma. Am J Surg 1992;164(6):623–628

17. Hocwald E, Korkmaz H, Yoo GH, et al. Prognostic factors in major salivary gland cancer. Laryngoscope 2001;111(8):1434–1439

18. Tullio A, Marchetti C, Sesenna E, et al. Treatment of carcinoma of the parotid gland: the results of a multicenter study. J Oral Maxillofac Surg 2001;59(3):263–270

19. Theriault C, Fitzpatrick PJ. Malignant parotid tumors. Prognostic factors and optimum treatment. Am J Clin Oncol 1986;9(6):510–516

20. Perzin KH, Gullane P, Clairmont AC. Adenoid cystic carcinomas arising in salivary glands: a correlation of histologic features and clinical course. Cancer 1978;42(1):265–282

21. Garden AS, Weber RS, Morrison WH, et al. The influence of positive margins and nerve invasion in adenoid cystic carcinoma of the head and neck treated with surgery and radiation. Int J Radiat Oncol Biol Phys 1995;32(3):619–626

22. Auclair PL, Goode RK, Ellis GL. Mucoepidermoid carcinoma of intraoral salivary glands. Evaluation and application of grading criteria in 143 cases. Cancer 1992;69(8):2021–2030

23. Hicks MJ, el-Naggar AK, Flaitz CM, et al. Histocytologic grading of mucoepidermoid carcinoma of major salivary glands in prognosis and survival: a clinicopathologic and flow cytometric investigation. Head Neck 1995;17(2):89–95

24. Eneroth CM. Facial nerve paralysis. A criterion of malignancy in parotid tumors. Arch Otolaryngol 1972;95(4):300–304

25. Spiro RH, Huvos AG, Strong EW. Cancer of the parotid gland. A clinicopathologic study of 288 primary cases. Am J Surg 1975;130(4):452–459

26. Armstrong JG, Harrison LB, Spiro RH, et al. Malignant tumors of major salivary gland origin. A matched-pair analysis of the role of combined surgery and postoperative radiotherapy. Arch Otolaryngol Head Neck Surg 1990;116(3):290–293

27. Laramore GE, Krall JM, Griffin TW, et al. Neutron versus photon irradiation for unresectable salivary gland tumors: final report of an RTOG-MRC randomized clinical trial. Radiation Therapy Oncology Group. Medical Research Council. Int J Radiat Oncol Biol Phys 1993;27(2):235–240

28. Creagan ET, Woods JE, Rubin J, et al. Cisplatin-based chemotherapy for neoplasms arising from salivary glands and contiguous structures in the head and neck. Cancer 1988;62(11):2313–2319

29. Schmalbach CE, Nussenbaum B, Rees RS, et al. Reliability of sentinel lymph node mapping with biopsy for head and neck cutaneous melanoma. Arch Otolaryngol Head Neck Surg 2003;129(1):61–65

7

Carcinoma of the Nasal Cavity and Paranasal Sinus

Houtan Chaboki, Georges B. Wanna, Richard Westreich, Johnny Kao, Stuart H. Packer, and William Lawson

◆ Epidemiology

Tumors of the nasal cavity and paranasal sinuses are uncommon. The estimated annual incidence of these tumors in the United States is less than 1 per 100,000 persons. This represents ~3 to 5% of cancers of the upper aerodigestive tract and 0.2% of all cancers.[1-4] The reported incidence of sinonasal tumors varies widely likely because of the multifocal nature of this tumor type and the different classification schemes.[4] The majority of carcinomas arise within the maxillary sinus (70 to 80%), followed by the ethmoid sinus (10 to 20%) and finally the sphenoid and frontal sinuses (<5%).[4] The nasal cavity is involved in 35% of the cases primarily by extension from the paranasal sinuses or nasopharynx; however, advanced lesions often preclude identification of the origin.[2]

Cancers of the paranasal sinuses arise most often during the fifth and sixth decades of life with a male to female ratio of ~2:1. Given the rarity of these neoplasms, differences in histology, and the variety of sites within this region, there is a paucity of prospective studies examining management and outcomes. Consequently, management is controversial, and the reported results are based commonly on experience with inhomogeneous groups of patients.

◆ Anatomy and Lymphatic Drainage

The paranasal sinuses and nasal cavity are in proximity to many vital structures that can easily be involved through contiguous spread of a tumor. Extension to these areas through preformed pathways and intervening thin lamellae of bone influences the extent of surgical resection and risk of local recurrence. In addition, the paranasal sinuses have lymphatic and venous drainage pathways, which provide additional routes of tumor spread intracranially.

Historically, the maxillary sinus was originally divided by a line drawn from the medial canthus to the angle of the mandible. This line, often referred to as Ohngren's line (**Fig. 7–1**),

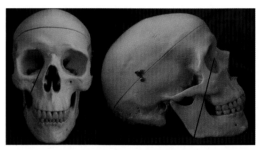

Figure 7–1 Ohngren's line: a line drawn from the medial canthus to the angle of the mandible separating the maxillary suprastructure from the maxillary infrastructure.

separates the maxillary suprastructure from infrastructure. Lesions occurring superior or posterior to this imaginary line are associated with a poor prognosis because of the proximity of the orbit and the pterygopalatine and intratemporal fossae. The pterygopalatine and intratemporal fossae possess a confluence of vascular and lymphatic channels connecting the mid-face with the cranial vault. When these areas are invaded, tumors gain access to the middle cranial fossa, orbit, nose, nasopharynx, and palate.

Despite extensive local growth, these tumors have a low propensity for lymphatic and hematogenous spread at the time of diagnosis. Nasal and maxillary sinus mucosa have distinct superficial and deep longitudinal lymphatic capillary networks, directed toward the maxillary sinus natural ostium.[5] The capillary networks connect directly to nasal vessels transmurally through natural bony gaps of the uncinate process. The primary lymphatic drainage basin of the nasal cavity and paranasal sinuses is to lateral and retropharyngeal nodes; however, tumors of the paranasal sinuses that do not manifest regional disease in levels I to IV rarely harbor retropharyngeal disease.

Superiorly, the fovea ethmoidalis and cribriform plate are thin and perforate providing a tenuous barrier to tumor spread from the nasal cavity and ethmoid sinuses. Laterally, the thin medial plate of the ethmoid bone, the lamina papyracea, also provides little resistance to orbital invasion (**Fig. 7–2**).

Malignancies of the sphenoid sinus are usually unresectable. The optic nerve, carotid artery, and cavernous sinus are intimately involved with the sphenoid sinus. The close relationship of the carotid artery with the sphenoid sinus makes it vulnerable to invasion and injury. Cadaveric dissection revealed that 71% of cavernous carotid arteries project into the lateral sphenoid sinus, with 66% having a bony covering of less than 1 mm and 4% totally dehiscent.[6] Therefore, tumors originating in the sphenoid can easily gain access to the carotid artery and cavernous sinus.

The anatomy of this region explains why nasal cavity and paranasal sinus tumors often present in an advanced stage involving several critical structures. Understanding this anatomy is essential in understanding the behavior of paranasal sinus carcinoma and the common routes of spread. The American Joint Committee on Cancer (AJCC) staging system functions to classify tumors based on location and extent (**Table 7–1**).

◆ Etiology

Several environmental factors have been implicated in the development of tumors of the sinonasal region. Specifically, woodworkers, shoe workers, and furniture makers have been demonstrated to have an occupational risk of developing adenocarcinoma as a result of inhaled mutagens. The specific mutagens involved are unknown, but combinations of one or more toxic substances from the wood itself, preservatives, stains, and paints have been implicated in the carcinogenic process. Wood-dust particles have been shown to reduce mucociliary clearance resulting in prolonged exposure of the sinonasal mucosa to toxins.[7] Exposure of epithelial cells and seromucous glands to wood dust has been shown to lead to overexpression of p53 protein, which may be linked to p53 gene mutations and subsequent malignant transformation.[8]

The pathologic process leading to adenocarcinoma may follow a pathway of distinct morphologic stages wherein metaplasia and dysplasia precede invasive carcinoma.[9,10] It is thus possible that the same pathologic process could occur within the nasal cavity and paranasal sinuses after exposure to wood dust. Other mutagens such as formaldehyde have been shown to increase the risk of both sinonasal adenocarcinoma and squamous cell carcinoma.[11] In addition, exposure to asbestos may increase the risk of squamous cell carcinoma.[11] A recent epidemiologic review of sinonasal carcinoma demonstrated that tobacco is associated with an average relative risk of 1.5 to 2.5 for the development of sinonasal cancer, and most studies demonstrate a dose-response relationship.[12] Additionally, cessation of tobacco results in a significant decrease in risk of cancer with increasing number of years since cessation. When histologic types were analyzed separately, the relative risk is increased for squamous cell carcinomas but not for adenocarcinoma.

Human papilloma virus (HPV) has also been associated with the development of squamous cell carcinoma. Although the specific molecular mechanism remains unknown, patients with HPV type 16 and 18 harbor a risk of developing carcinoma transformation from inverted papilloma in ~10% of cases. Other risk factors include radiation exposure.

Sarcomas are the most common radiation-related tumors of the sinonasal cavity; however, for any tumor to be considered "radiation induced," (1) the tumor must arise in a

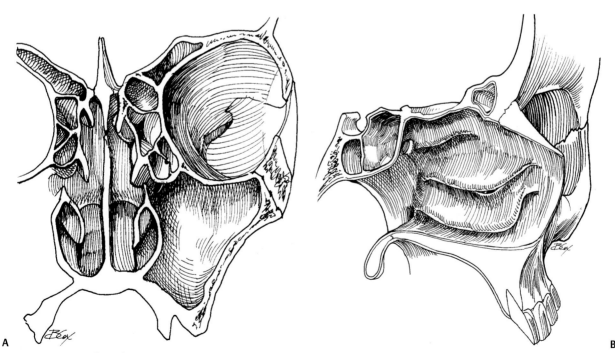

Figure 7–2 Anatomy of nasal cavity and paranasal sinuses. **(A)** Note the thin layer of bone (lamina papyracea) separating the ethmoid sinuses from the orbital contents. **(B)** Note the superior, middle, and inferior turbinates.

Table 7–1 TNM Staging of Nasal Cavity and Paranasal Sinus Cancers According to the AJCC *Cancer Staging Manual*, 6th Edition

Maxillary Sinus	Criteria
T1	Tumor limited to maxillary sinus mucosa with no erosion or destruction of bone
T2	Tumor causing bone erosion or destruction including extension into hard palate and/or middle nasal meatus, except extension to posterior wall of maxillary sinus and pterygoid plates
T3	Tumor invades any of the following: bone of posterior wall of maxillary sinus, subcutaneous tissue, floor or medial wall of orbit, pterygoid fossa, ethmoid sinuses
T4a	Tumor invades anterior orbital contents, skin of cheek, pterygoid plates, infratemporal fossa, cribriform plate, sphenoid or frontal sinuses
T4b	Tumor invades any of the following: orbital apex, dura, brain, middle cranial fossa, cranial nerves other than maxillary division of trigeminal nerve (V2), nasopharynx, or clivus

Nasal Cavity and Ethmoid Sinus	
T1	Tumor restricted to any one subsite, with or without bone invasion
T2	Tumor invading two subsites in a single region or extending to involve an adjacent region within the nasoethmoidal complex, with or without bony invasion
T3	Tumor extends to invade the medial wall or floor of the orbit, maxillary sinus, palate, or cribriform plate
T4a	Tumor invades any of the following: anterior orbital contents, skin of nose or cheek, minimal extension to anterior cranial fossa, pterygoid plates, sphenoid or frontal sinuses
T4b	Tumor invades any of the following: orbital apex, dura, brain, middle cranial fossa, cranial nerves other than maxillary division of trigeminal nerve (V2), nasopharynx, or clivus

Regional Lymph Nodes	
NX	Regional lymph nodes cannot be assessed
N0	No regional lymph node metastasis
N1	Metastasis in a single ipsilateral lymph node, 3 cm or less in greatest dimension
N2a	Metastasis in single ipsilateral lymph node, more than 3 cm but not more than 6 cm in greatest dimension
N2b	Metastasis in multiple ipsilateral lymph nodes, none more than 6 cm in greatest dimension
N2c	Metastasis in bilateral or contralateral lymph nodes, none more than 6 cm in greatest dimension
N3	Metastasis in a lymph node, more than 6 cm in greatest dimension

Distant Metastasis	
MX	Distant metastasis cannot be assessed
M0	No distant metastasis
M1	Distant metastasis

Source: Adapted from Greene FL, Page DL, Fleming ID, et al. AJCC Cancer Staging Manual, 6th ed. New York: Springer; 2002.
Note: Nonepithelial tumors such as those of lymphoid tissue, soft tissue, bone, and cartilage are not included.

previously irradiated field; (2) the new tumor must be histologically different from the original tumor; (3) there must have been no evidence of the new tumor prior to the time of radiation therapy; and (4) a latency period of 20 years must exist between irradiation and the development of the new tumor.[13,14] Radiation-induced malignancy has an estimated incidence of less than 1.0% and has an estimated 5-year survival of 10 to 30%.[14]

◆ Presentation

Thorough inspection of the nasal cavity requires training and equipment that is not available to most general practitioners, and the sinuses themselves can only be visualized using radiographic studies. Because of these limitations and the subtle signs and symptoms associated with tumors of the paranasal sinuses, neoplasms are often diagnosed at a late stage. Typically, the clinical symptoms are nonspecific and subtle and they are often indistinguishable from benign sinonasal

diseases, such as chronic sinusitis or nasal allergy. Common presenting symptoms include nasal obstruction, anosmia, nasal and cheek pain, rhinorrhea, epistaxis, and headache; however, the index of suspicion increases greatly if proptosis, facial swelling, loose teeth, epiphora, trismus, unilateral signs and symptoms of diplopia or blurred vision, and cranial nerve paralysis are present. Extensive tumor invasion is usually underestimated based on clinical evaluation alone. In evaluating sinonasal tumors, the orbit, intracranial fossa, pterygomaxillary fissure, pterygopalatine fossa, and the infratemporal space require special attention.

◆ Diagnosis and Workup

The diagnostic workup mandates an endoscopic examination of the nasal cavity. Irregularities in the mucosa of the nasal septum, lateral nasal wall, and the turbinates should be noted in addition to bowing of the lateral nasal wall. Whereas carcinoma of the nasal mucosa may present with mucosal irregularity or ulceration, intrasinus tumors may result in a subtle bowing or deformity of the lateral nasal wall or ethmoid sinus mucosa. Because both benign and malignant disease may present with a polypoid mass, a biopsy is essential. The risk of a vascular tumor, encephalocele, or meningoencephalocele warrants imaging prior to proceeding with a biopsy.

Both computed tomography (CT) and magnetic resonance imaging (MRI) are essential tools for diagnosis, staging, and operative planning. The combination of CT and MRI is highly sensitive for identifying bone destruction, soft tissue invasion, and evaluation of the adjacent structures. In studying soft tissue structures, MRI is more accurate than the CT scan. MRI provides excellent delineation of tumor from the surrounding inflamed soft tissue and retained secretions. The latter generally have sufficient water content to produce signal hyperintensity on T2-weighted images. Most sinonasal tumors are highly cellular with little free water and therefore display low to intermediate signal intensities on both T1- and T2-weighted images. Focal, well-defined areas of intermediate to high signal intensities on T1- and T2-weighted images may represent subacute or chronic hemorrhage. Areas of low to intermediate signal intensities may be present in T1-weighted images, and areas of high intensity on T2-weighted images usually represent fluid-filled sites of necrosis. Gadolinium enhances the mucosa more than the tumor and helps differentiate an obstructed sinus and inflammation from tumor. Finally, MRI is the standard imaging modality for postoperative surveillance.

For evaluation of the fine bony structures, high-resolution CT is an excellent tool. High-resolution CT provides an unmatched view of the bony anatomy that is essential is evaluating sinus carcinoma. The combination of CT and MRI yields a sensitivity and specificity for identification of extrasinus extension of nearly 98% with the exception of identifying invasion of periorbital and dural invasion, which are best identified intraoperatively.[15] Positron emission tomography (PET) scanning plays a limited role in the evaluation of local and regional disease; however, it has become more commonly used for assessment of distant disease in the initial metastatic workup. In addition, PET may play a role in post-therapy surveillance, yet future studies in this area are necessary. Early reports indicate that both [^{18}F]fluoro-2-deoxy-D-glucose (FDG) and ^{11}C-choline could distinguish squamous cell carcinoma from benign lesions of the nasal cavity and paranasal sinuses.[16] Generally, FDG uptake in malignant tumors may be variable and inconsistent whereas ^{11}C-choline uptake is uniform. In the future, PET with ^{11}C-choline may supplement FDG-PET in cases of low uptake of FDG.

◆ Treatment

Surgical Treatment

Sinonasal malignancy is optimally managed with *en bloc* surgical resection. The addition of postoperative chemotherapy and radiation is predicated on the presence of bone erosion, positive or close margins, and poor prognostic features such as advanced disease, regional disease, and perineural or vascular invasion. The proximity of the paranasal sinuses to vital structures often presents a limitation to achieving tumor-free margins. In some cases, the tumor may not be resectable. Sisson detailed four specific criteria for unresectability: (1) extension of tumor to the frontal lobes (superior extension), (2) invasion of the prevertebral fascia (posterior extension), (3) bilateral optic nerve involvement, and (4) cavernous sinus extension (lateral extension).[17] Dural or carotid artery invasion are relative contraindications to surgery, yet both findings are associated with a poor prognosis.[18] However, there is evidence that neoadjuvant radiation therapy for stage II and III tumors followed by surgery may aid in achieving tumor-free margins at the time of surgical resection.[18–21]

Surgery alone is an acceptable method of treatment for early disease (stages I and II disease). Small nasal septal lesions can be treated by wide local excision. Early-stage maxillary tumors can be removed via a sublabial approach and medial or infrastructure maxillectomy.[22] Larger tumors, however, require partial or total maxillectomy via mid-facial degloving or a Weber-Fergusson incision. Orbital exenteration is less frequently used in the management of early sinonasal carcinoma largely because it has been demonstrated that there is no survival benefit unless the orbital contents are grossly involved.[23] The periorbita must be critically evaluated intraoperatively. Although invasion through the periorbita is not a strict indication to perform an orbital exenteration, when there is demonstrable invasion of the periorbital fat or extraocular muscles, an orbital exenteration is indicated. When there is lateral extension of maxillary tumors into the infratemporal fossa, a combined anterolateral approach should be considered. This approach allows for a careful evaluation of the area and a critical evaluation of the anterior and middle cranial fossae.

Early ethmoid tumors may be resected endoscopically. The surgeon must be proficient at endoscopic techniques and confident that all margins are carefully assessed during the course of surgery. In cases where access is limited or critical structures are involved, the lateral rhinotomy approach provides ample access to the ethmoid sinus providing exposure for an *en bloc* medial maxillectomy. The degloving approach can also be utilized for limited tumors; however, larger tumors with intracranial extension require an anterior craniofacial resection.

Primary lesions of the sphenoid are very rare. The majority of these tumors are secondary to tumor extension from adjacent sites. Sphenoid tumors may be approached endoscopically or from an external approach if necessary. Similarly, early frontal sinus tumors can often be removed through an endoscopic approach; however, as these tumors become more extensive, a bicoronal incision and open frontal sinus approach is recommended. This approach may be combined with a frontal craniotomy to obtain adequate margins.

Surgical Approaches

Medial Maxillectomy Medial maxillectomy is indicated for tumors that are limited to the medial wall of the maxillary sinus and the ethmoid sinuses (**Fig. 7–3**). When performed in conjunction with a lateral rhinotomy, it is possible to achieve *en bloc* excision of the lateral nasal wall from the nasal floor to the junction of the roof and medial wall of the orbit. This procedure usually includes removal of the middle and inferior turbinates, lamina papyracea, and ethmoid labyrinth, with preservation of the globe, alveolar ridge, and nasal-facial contours. A medial maxillectomy can also be performed through an endonasal and/or sublabial approach; however, these approaches are generally used for benign lesions, and removal is often in piecemeal fashion.

Infrastructure Maxillectomy   Infrastructure maxillectomy is indicated for tumors of the floor of the maxillary sinus, palate, and alveolus with limited invasion of the nasal cavity and ethmoid. It entails removal of the medial and lateral walls of the maxilla, hard palate, and dental alveolus. The operation can be performed through either the Weber-Fergusson or mid-face degloving approach. The mid-face degloving approach has the advantage of avoiding facial incision; however, extension posteriorly to the pterygoid plates may require a lip-splitting incision for added access in some cases.

Total Maxillectomy with Orbital Preservation   Total or radical maxillectomy involves the complete removal of all walls of the maxillary sinus (**Fig. 7–4**). Preservation of the orbital contents in advanced paranasal sinus carcinoma remains a controversial issue. The two main points of contention are the oncologic safety of orbital preservation and the functional outcome of the preserved globes. A variety of indications

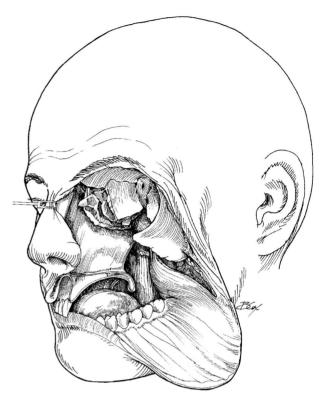

Figure 7–4   Total maxillectomy. A total maxillectomy involves resection of the maxillary sinus with or without exenteration of the orbit.

for exenteration have been proposed based on involvement of bone, periorbita, orbital fat, extraocular muscles, orbital apex, or the eyelids.[24] Sisson et al demonstrated in a series of 60 patients that orbital preservation in patients with tumor invasion limited to the bony orbit did not compromise local control or survival compared with patients undergoing orbital exenteration for tumors demonstrating soft tissue orbital invasion.[17] Similarly, Weymuller et al could not demonstrate an improved local control rate or survival advantage when the orbital contents were included in maxillectomy procedures.[25] In a series of 43 patients, Larson et al showed no difference in survival when comparing patients with orbital exenteration to patients with orbital preservation.[26] This finding was confirmed in other studies.[24] Assessment of the orbit should begin at the floor of the orbit. This area should be explored first by careful elevation of the periosteum. If the periorbita has not been penetrated, and there is no gross evidence of disease in the orbit, the globe can be preserved. A total maxillectomy is performed through the Weber-Fergusson approach. Utilizing lateral rhinotomy, lip splitting, and infraorbital incisions to create a cheek flap, the orbital contents are spared and the periorbita is elevated from the floor of the orbit to determine whether exenteration should be performed. The nasolacrimal duct is sharply divided and canalized with Silastic tubes, or marsupialized, to maintain patency. The extent of the resection, hence the placement of the osteotomies, is determined by the extent of the tumor.

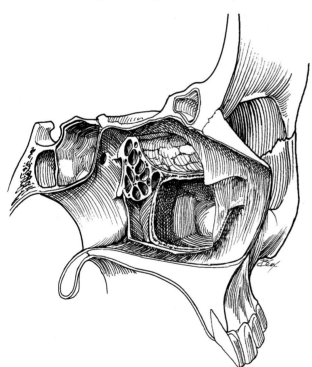

Figure 7–3   Medial maxillectomy. The medial maxillectomy involves resection of the medial wall of the nasal cavity with preservation of the remaining maxilla.

The superior extent of dissection depends on the extent of ethmoidal involvement and may be carried up to the frontoethmoidal suture line to encompass the ethmoid labyrinth, middle turbinate, and inferior turbinate. Osteotomies are made superiorly, along the medial orbital wall, along the orbital floor, and across the lateral orbital wall; anteriorly, along the frontonasal process through the piriform aperture; and inferiorly through the alveolus and hard palate at the midline. The soft palate is detached from the bony palate. Laterally, the maxilla is separated from the zygoma through the inferior orbital fissure. With tumor extension into the zygomatic recess of the antrum, the zygoma is included in the specimen by osteotomies through the middle of the lateral orbital wall and across the zygomatic-temporal suture. Posterior extension to the pterygomaxillary space, or pterygoid fossa, will require an osteotomy at the base of the pterygoid plates. Otherwise, the maxillary tuberosity may be separated from the pterygoid plates. The remaining soft tissue attachments are divided. Delivery of the specimen is performed after dividing the attachment of the pterygoid muscle and plates. Branches of the internal maxillary artery and vein are controlled with electrocautery or vascular clips. The cavity is packed with antibiotic-impregnated gauze. Before the incisions are closed, the internal aspect of the cheek flap is covered by a split-thickness skin graft to prevent mid-face contracture. The orbital floor must be reconstructed to prevent orbital dystopia, enophthalmos, diplopia, and ectropion. This can be accomplished with a soft (Prolene mesh) or rigid (titanium) implant material anchored to the cut ends of the orbital floor. The oral cavity must also be separated from the sinonasal tract by the insertion of an appliance fabricated by a prosthodontist to permit immediate swallowing and articulation.

Total Maxillectomy with Orbital Exenteration Total maxillectomy with orbital exenteration is employed for carcinoma of the maxilla invading the orbital contents. The lateral rhinotomy incision is made with extensions around the ciliary borders of the eyelids, which join beyond the lateral canthus. The skin is divided through the orbicularis oculi down to the periosteum of the orbit. The periorbita is elevated back to the optic canal. When approached medially, the optic nerve is 5 to 10 mm posterior to the posterior ethmoid artery. The optic nerve is sectioned midway between the globe and optic foramen. The dissection then proceeds in the subperiosteal plane to the superior orbital fissure. The contents of the fissure are divided, and the ophthalmic blood vessels are ligated. At this point, the eye is pedicled on the floor of the orbit. The maxillectomy then proceeds as described earlier. The tumor is delivered with the orbital contents attached to the roof of the maxillary sinus.

Craniofacial Resection Craniofacial resection (CFR) entails complete resection of tumors involving the anterior skull base, including the cribriform plate, medial orbital wall, ethmoid labyrinth, superior nasal septum, and posterior wall of the frontal sinus (**Fig. 7–5**). Any malignant tumor with involvement of these sites requires CFR for *en bloc* resection. The most common tumors requiring CFR are squamous cell carcinoma, olfactory neuroblastoma, and

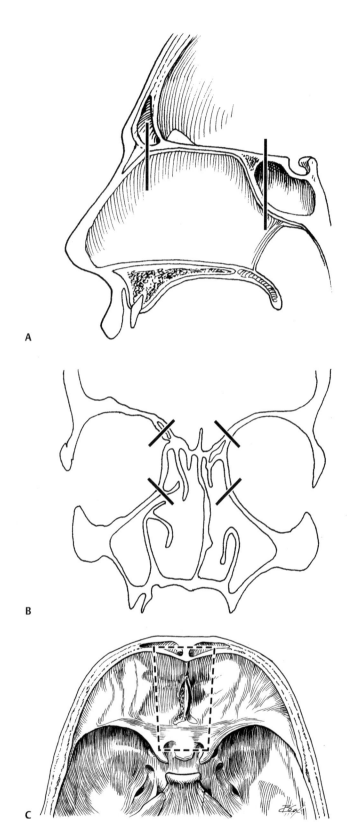

Figure 7–5 (**A**) Craniofacial resection, sagittal view. Resection of the anterior skull base extending from the posterior wall of the frontal sinus to the sphenoid sinus. (**B**) Craniofacial resection, coronal view. Bone cuts through the medial orbital wall. (**C**) Craniofacial resection, axial view. Bone cuts through the anterior cranial fossa.

adenocarcinoma. This operation requires a multidisciplinary approach involving teamwork between the head and neck surgeon and the neurosurgeon. Resection is accomplished by using a combination of superior and inferior approaches to the tumor.

Contraindications to CFR are controversial. Gross intracranial extension into the frontal lobes is a contraindication to surgery; however, isolated dural involvement is not. CFR is performed with a bicoronal incision combined with a Weber-Fergusson, lateral rhinotomy, or mid-face degloving, depending on the tumor location and extension. The bicoronal flap starts 2 to 3 cm posterior to the hairline and extends from the preauricular crease of one ear to the contralateral side. Careful subgaleal dissection is performed to preserve the supraorbital and supratrochlear neurovascular bundles.

The pericranial flap, based on the supraorbital arteries, is essential for reconstruction. It is important to maintain the periosteal layer during elevation of the scalp flap in the subgaleal plane. Once a wide and long pericranial flap has been developed, a frontal craniotomy can be performed by the neurosurgical team. Once the frontal bone flap is removed, the dura can be dissected and inspected for invasion, and the frontal lobes are retracted. Dura and brain are resected as necessary. Next, intracranial bone cuts are made to allow *en bloc* resection and tumor delivery into the nose. Lateral bone cuts are through the medial portion of the orbital roof bilaterally. The posterior bone cut is just posterior to the anterior wall of the sphenoid sinus. The anterior bone cut is through the floor of the frontal sinus and includes the posterior wall of the frontal sinus in the resection specimen. Numerous variations exist on these basic resection limits.

The inferior, transfacial portion is performed once the superior, intracranial portion is completed. A total ethmoidectomy is performed via Weber-Fergusson, lateral rhinotomy, or mid-face degloving incision. Orbital dissection is accomplished by preserving the periorbita. The anterior and posterior ethmoidal arteries are controlled. The orbital bone cuts are then completed and connected to the intracranial bone cuts. Intranasal cuts are made with scissors, and the tumor is delivered *en bloc* through the nasal cavity. Tumor removal results in a defect with a direct communication between the anterior cranial fossa and the sinonasal cavity. Dural repair is performed with a combination of free fascia and muscle grafts, and the pericranial flap. Large defects require free vascularized flaps, such as rectus abdominus or latissimus dorsi flap, to separate the brain from the sinonasal cavity.

Management of the Neck

The incidence of neck metastasis ranges between 8% and 50%.[27] Positive cervical lymph nodes have the most impact on outcome and portend a poor prognosis.[2] Neck dissection improves regional control and is required for patients with clinical or radiographic evidence of neck disease.[28,29] PET scan, multidetector CT scan, and high-resolution MRI have improved detection of neck disease and have had a significant impact on surveillance.

Management of the clinically negative neck in sinonasal carcinoma remains controversial. The risk of nodal neck relapse in untreated N0 necks ranges from 12 to 38%, respectively.[30,31] For maxillary tumors, some recommend administering elective nodal radiotherapy routinely to patients with T2 or greater squamous or undifferentiated carcinoma,[31] whereas other groups consider that neck irradiation should only be used in patients with more advanced tumors.[30]

Reconstruction

Reconstruction is a crucial consideration for patients undergoing maxillectomy. The goal of reconstruction is to preserve form and function. Mid-face reconstruction can be achieved with either a palatal prosthesis, local flap, or free tissue transfer. The method of reconstruction requires a dialogue between the surgeon and the patient prior to surgery. If the patient elects to proceed with a palatal prosthesis, a preoperative consultation with the prosthodontist is essential to perform impressions and create a temporary obturator after surgery. A variety of factors should guide the patient and the surgeon in determining the optimal approach to oral dental rehabilitation. Traditionally, defects of the palate and maxilla have been rehabilitated with palatomaxillary obturators. An obturator provides several advantages including an immediate reconstruction that does not require further surgery. There are, however, several disadvantages to an obturator. Whereas they provide excellent stability for smaller defects, larger defects loose stability and retention. This can result in difficulty with both mastication and speech. Additionally, obturators require extensive maintenance and hygiene. The goal of contemporary palatomaxillary reconstruction should be to provide patients with a permanent separation of the oral nasal cavities and stable dentition without the use of an obturator. Preliminary work has suggested that patients who undergo palatomaxillary reconstruction enjoy a superior function and quality of life when compared with patients rehabilitated with an obturator.

The three-dimensional infrastructure of the maxillary skeleton provides support for the upper dentition, buttresses for mastication, and support for the globe and the nasal airway. Additionally, the maxilla provides an aesthetic scaffold that lends form to the nose, cheek, and upper lip. The complex structure of the mid-face and the relationship between function and aesthetics make reconstruction of the mid-face a formidable task for the reconstructive surgeon. Prosthetic obturation, free bone grafts, pedicled flaps, and free tissue transfer have all played a role in the evolution of palatomaxillary restoration. Choosing the best reconstructive approach requires a comprehensive evaluation of the soft tissue defect, the bone defect, and the quality and position of the remaining dentition.

◆ Pathology

The variable histology and embryologic development of the nose and paranasal sinuses are responsible for the wide vari-

Table 7–2 Malignant Tumors of the Nasal Cavity and Sinuses

Squamous Cell Carcinoma (SCC)
Lymphoreticular
• Lymphoma
• Extramedullary plasmacytoma
Glandular
• Adenoid cystic carcinoma (ACC)
• Adenocarcinoma (AC)
Sarcomas
• Rhabdosarcoma
• Fibrosarcoma
• Hemangiopericytoma
• Chondrosarcoma
• Osteosarcoma
Miscellaneous tumors
• Olfactory neuroblastoma
• Sinonasal undifferentiated carcinoma (SNUC)
• Sinonasal neuroendocrine carcinoma (SNEC)
• Malignant melanoma
Metastatic carcinoma
• Kidney
• Lung
• Breast

ety of tumors that occur in the paranasal sinuses (**Table 7–2**). Epithelium, glandular tissue, including salivary and goblet cells, cartilage, bone, neuroendocrine, and neurovascular structures can degenerate into an array of tumors. Diagnosis is dependent upon adequate biopsy material and immunohistochemical analysis.

In most series, squamous cell carcinoma (SCC) is cited as the most common malignancy, having an incidence of roughly 80%. Adenoid cystic carcinoma (ACC) and adenocarcinoma (AC) are next in frequency at ~10%. Small numbers of a variety of other tumors complete the list.[3] Except for nonepithelial neoplasms, malignant nasal tumors are diseases of adults.[3] Metastasis to this region from distant sites is extremely rare. Renal cell carcinoma is the most frequent type, followed distantly by lung and breast cancer.

Squamous Cell Carcinoma

SCC represents greater than 70% of the soft tissue tumors found at this location. More than 95% of patients are greater than 45 years old, with a 2:1 male predominance. The maxillary sinus is the primary focus, accounting for ~70% of the cases. Intranasal primaries account for 20% of the cases, with the turbinates the most frequently affected site. The remaining 10% of the tumors are found in the ethmoid, sphenoid, and frontal sinuses in decreasing frequency. In most cases, tumor extension through at least one sinus wall has occurred at the time of diagnosis, resulting in the majority of lesions being T2 stage or greater.[32]

On rhinoscopy, SCC often appears polypoid and gray and bleeds easily with manipulation. Office biopsy should be performed only after complete radiographic evaluation to rule out intracranial origin and further delineate the lesion's location. Anterior lesions are amenable to office biopsy be-

cause they are easily accessible and control of bleeding may be easily achieved. Lesions with minimal nasal extension should be performed in an operating room setting under general anesthesia.

A metastatic workup should also be completed because distant metastases occur in ~18% of patients. Locoregional spread can be identified in 17 to 30% of patients.[32] Maxillary sinus lesions have a tendency to metastasize more frequently than tumors arising on the nasal septum or turbinates. This discrepancy may be related to earlier detection of nasal cavity tumors due to prominent symptoms of nasal obstruction and epistaxis. This is reflected in a 5-year survival rate almost double that of maxillary sinus carcinomas (**Table 7–3**).

Surgical excision is the primary treatment modality. The surgical approach is dictated by the extent of involvement and may require partial or radical maxillectomy and craniofacial resection. Postoperative radiotherapy is recommended for advanced lesions, those with close pathologic margins, and for retropharyngeal lymph node involvement. Ongoing studies using adjuvant cisplatin, 5-fluorouracil (5-FU), and hydroxyurea have demonstrated promising results for local control.[33]

Lymphoreticular

Lymphoma

Lymphoma of the sinonasal cavity is most often non-Hodgkin's type.[34] Patients are usually elderly males, except in Asian populations where young males are more commonly affected.[34] Both T- and B-cell types occur, which are more prominent in Asian and Western populations, respectively. Most lesions present at an advanced stage, with 50% classified as T4 at the time of diagnosis. A diagnostic biopsy may be attempted in the office; however, a sufficient volume of tissue is needed for immunohistochemical analysis and flow cytometry. Chemoradiotherapy or radiotherapy alone are the primary treatment modalities for sinonasal lymphoma. Surgical intervention is limited to diagnostic biopsy alone.

Extramedullary Plasmacytoma

Patients with extramedullary plasmacytoma have involvement of the nose, nasopharynx, or paranasal sinuses in 60% of cases.[34] Lesions appear polypoid, or sessile, reddish in color, and may be localized or part of a systemic disorder (i.e., multiple myeloma). In addition to CT scan and biopsy, additional studies should be performed to rule out systemic involvement (**Table 7–4**). Wide local excision with or without chemoradiotherapy is the treatment modality of choice. Five-year control rates of 78% for T1 to T3 lesions and 38% for T4 lesions have been reported.[34]

Table 7–3 Five-Year Survival Rates for Maxillary Sinus Squamous Cell Carcinoma

T1	67%
T2	40%
T3	30%
T4	18%

Table 7–4 Supplemental Diagnostic Studies for Lymphoid Tumors

Additional Laboratory and Radiology Studies
Urine protein electrophoresis
Serum protein electrophoresis
Quantitative immunoglobulins
Urine Bence-Jones protein
Bone marrow biopsy (possible)
Skeletal x-ray survey

Glandular

Glandular tumors represent ~10% of the lesions in the sinonasal cavity.[35] Similar to SCC, the maxillary sinus is the most common location, followed by the nasal cavity and the ethmoid sinuses. Lesions arise from minor salivary glands found throughout the region.[35] ACC and AC are the most frequent types encountered, followed distantly by pleomorphic adenoma, mucoepidermoid carcinoma, and undifferentiated subtypes.

Adenoid Cystic Carcinoma

ACC is the most common salivary gland tumor of the nose and paranasal sinuses. Like other locations in the head and neck, it displays neurotrophic behavior and has a propensity for spread along the infraorbital neurovascular bundle. The histology is also similar to lesions at other sites and includes cribriform, solid, and tubular patterns. The most common appearance is the cribriform type, which has been described as having a "Swiss cheese" appearance. Radiographically, there is generally a heterogeneous signal with cystic components often present. The gross appearance typically is that of a well-defined but nonencapsulated mass that can be seen infiltrating the surrounding normal tissue. Tumor grade correlates with the rate of metastasis and overall prognosis.

Surgery is the primary modality of treatment. Because of neurotrophic spread, adjuvant radiotherapy is often included and may improve locoregional control; however, adjuvant radiation has failed to demonstrate a significant improvement in long-term survival.[36] Radiotherapy may also be used for palliation or pain control in unresectable cases. Distant pulmonary metastasis may develop in one third of the patients; however, liver and bone metastasis may also occur. Wiseman reported a 5-year overall survival of 65% and a 10-year survival of 55% in patients treated with combination chemoradiation demonstrating reasonable long-term control with combined-modality therapy.[36]

Adenocarcinoma

AC is the second most common salivary gland tumor found in the sinonasal tract. Clinically, it may appear as a papillary or sessile mass within the nose and has a variable histology, which may mimic mucoepidermoid carcinoma or adenocarcinoma of the colon. The histologic grade (low vs. high) affects prognosis and the rates of locoregional metastatic disease. Involvement limited to the nose has been seen in 25 to 30% of cases, more commonly with high-grade lesions. Distant metastatic spread may be seen in 15 to 20% of cases.

Sarcoma

Sinonasal sarcomas are rare lesions, representing less than 1% of all head and neck sarcomas. Previous radiotherapy is the main risk factor. Surgery, with the exception of rhabdomyosarcoma, is the main treatment modality.

Rhabdomyosarcoma

Rhabdomyosarcoma is the most common soft tissue tumor found in patients less than 15 years of age. It is often misdiagnosed as adenoidal hypertrophy by presenting with nasal obstruction. When compared with other head and neck sites, sinonasal disease carries a poorer prognosis due to intracranial extension, which has been reported in up to 90% of patients in some series. A variety of histologic patterns occur, with the embryonal and alveolar forms predominating. The current treatment recommendation is chemoradiotherapy followed by surgical salvage.

Fibrosarcoma

Fibrosarcomas represent less than 5% of all soft tissue sarcomas. They often appear as a polypoid mass in the nasal cavity. Unlike other areas of the body, histologic grade is not predictive of overall survival and recurrence. Metastatic disease is rare but may develop up to 10 years later. Primary treatment is by surgical excision.

Hemangiopericytoma

Hemangiopericytomas have a predilection for the head and neck, accounting for 25% of the cases. These lesions are of capillary origin, arising from the pericytes of Zimmerman. On immunohistochemistry, they display factor 13a positivity. Clinically, they appear gray and rubbery and may grow rapidly. Unlike other tumors of the sinonasal cavity, the maxillary sinus is not often involved. The distribution of lesions is 60% in the nasal cavity, 30% in the sphenoethmoid complex, and 5% in both the maxilla and nasopharynx. Despite aggressive surgery and adjuvant radiation, recurrence is common. Some series have shown a 57% recurrence rate, with 50% occurring later than 5 years after definitive therapy. Long-term postoperative monitoring and evaluation is necessary.[37]

Chondrosarcoma

Chondrosarcoma is a rare lesion in the sinonasal complex. Distinguishing between a benign chondroma and chondrosarcoma is suggested by the radiologic findings of tumor size; generally, chondromas are less than 3 cm in diameter, whereas chondrosarcomas are greater than 3 cm. Calcification is often seen in both benign and malignant lesions. Histologic grading of chondrosarcomas can be used to separate these lesions into well differentiated (grade I), moderately differentiated (grade II), and poorly differentiated (grade III) lesions. The presence of a high chondroid to myxoid ratio, absent mitosis, and near-normal nuclear appearance separates the well-differentiated lesions from the other grades.

Most chondrosarcomas are well-differentiated grade I lesions. Grade II and III lesions are associated with a poorer prognosis and may histologically resemble other mesenchymal tumors, such as fibrosarcoma. Diagnosis depends on the identification of the lower-grade component that produces chondroid. Chondrosarcomas arising in the nasopharynx and sinonasal tract are associated with a poorer prognosis compared with other sites due to skull base involvement. Wide surgical resection is the primary treatment of choice, although up to 85% may recur.[38] Because of its indolent course and slow growth, vital structures are often spared in surgical planning.

Olfactory Neuroblastoma

Olfactory neuroblastoma, formerly known as esthesioneuroblastoma, is a rare lesion that arises from the olfactory epithelium of the cribriform plate, septum, or superior turbinate. It was first described by Berger and Luc in 1924.[39] The mean age of onset is between 20 and 50 years of age. A bimodal distribution is present, with two thirds of patients presenting between 10 and 34 years of age and one third presenting in older populations.[39] The lesion often appears gray-red and fleshy. Office biopsy may be performed; however, brisk bleeding may occur because of the tumor's vascularity. Additionally, differentiation from other small blue-cell tumors (**Table 7–5**) often requires immunohistochemical analysis and larger tissue blocks. S-100 staining is universally present. Similarities to sinonasal undifferentiated carcinoma (SNUC) and sinonasal neuroendocrine carcinoma (SNEC) have prompted some clinicians to consider these lesions related to one another; however, distinct differences in their clinical behavior exist.

CT and MRI are both employed, as intracranial and dural involvement will determine the surgical approach. Locoregional metastatic disease at the time of diagnosis is present in 10 to 30% of patients.[40]

Staging is usually performed using the Kadish system, although other systems exist (**Table 7–6**).[41] Short-term (less than 5 years) disease-free survival has been reported in 38 to 82% of patients; however, recurrent disease may occur 10 years after the initial presentation.

Surgical approach varies with the extent of the tumor. Commonly, the cribriform plate and/or dura are involved. In these instances, craniofacial resection is the treatment of choice. Other procedures include medial maxillectomy, external frontoethmoidectomy, and endoscopic removal. Radiation is em-

Table 7–5 Small Blue-Cell Tumors

Melanoma
Esthesioneuroblastoma
Rhabdomyosarcoma
Lymphoma
Ewing's sarcoma
SNUC/SNEC
Plasmacytoma

ployed either pre- or postoperatively, sometimes in conjunction with chemotherapy.

Sinonasal Undifferentiated Carcinoma

SNUC is an aggressive lesion that fortunately is rare. It was first described in 1986 by Frierson et al.[42] Multimodal treatment including surgery, chemotherapy, and radiotherapy is generally employed. Diagnosis is based on biopsy and immunohistochemical analysis demonstrating cytokeratin positivity and neuron-specific enolase while lacking S-100 and vimentin reactivity.

Many patients present with locally advanced disease and intracranial extension. Almost 50% will have orbital symptoms at the time of diagnosis. The average survival is approximately 1 year.[43] Although reports have suggested that certain chemoradiotherapy protocols can increase 2-year survival to ~50%,[44] statistically significant data are not yet available.

Sinonasal Neuroendocrine Carcinoma

SNEC is another related lesion that can only be distinguished from SNUC based on immunohistochemical analysis; however, the clinical behavior is much more indolent. Common sites of involvement include the nasal cavity, ethmoid sinuses, and maxillary sinuses. As with other high-grade sinonasal lesions, they are often diagnosed at a late stage. Locoregional metastatic disease develops in 40% of patients, and 10% will have distant lesions at the time of diagnosis.[45] Recurrence is common, but 5-year survival rates of 74 to 100% have been reported.[46,47] Combined surgery with chemoradiotherapy is the current standard of treatment.

Melanoma

Mucosal melanoma is a rare and extremely aggressive tumor in the sinonasal tract that carries an overall prognosis worse

Table 7–6 Staging System for Esthesioneuroblastoma

	Kadish		Biller
Stage		**Stage**	
A	Nasal cavity	T1	In nasal cavity and paranasal sinus without bone involvement Sphenoid free
B	Nasal cavity + paranasal sinuses	T2	Into orbit or anterior cranial fossa
C	Outside sinonasal cavity	T3	Intracranial
D	Regional or distal metastatic disease		

than its cutaneous types.[48] It constitutes less than 2% of all Western melanomas but represents one quarter to one third of all melanomas in Japanese patients.[48] There is no sex predilection, and patients are usually more than 60 years of age. It has a predilection for the anterior nasal septum and turbinates, and satellite lesions are common. Patients usually present with intractable epistaxis that leads to its diagnosis. The function of sinonasal melanocytes, presumably the source of malignant sinonasal melanoma, is unknown. These melanocytes were first observed in the lamina propria and around sinonasal salivary glands.[49] In addition, they appear to be acquired, as they are only seen in adults and not in children.[48]

Treatment is surgical resection of the primary site with wide margins. The average survival for sinonasal melanoma is ~9 to 12 months. Adjunctive therapy with radiation, chemotherapy, and immunotherapy has been applied with limited success. Recurrences are common, and the risk does not decrease with time. Local and regional recurrences are best managed by surgery, as this may prolong survival.[48]

Osteosarcoma

Osteosarcoma is the most common primary neoplasm of bone with an incidence of 1:100,000. Although uncommonly found in the head and neck compared with other body sites, the mandible, maxilla, and paranasal sinuses may be affected. The mean age of onset is between 20 and 40 years

of age with males being slightly more affected than females. Osteosarcoma is associated with prior radiation treatment, as well as other disease processes including Paget disease, fibrous dysplasia, Li-Fraumeni syndrome, and chronic osteomyelitis. Radiologically, these tumors display both osteolytic and osteosclerotic features, with a "sunburst" appearance generally considered diagnostic. Osteoid within a fibrous stroma is typically seen on histology, although special stains such as osteocalcin and osteonectin may be required.

Treatment is primarily surgical, with radiotherapy reserved for unresectable and medically unstable patients. The approach is determined by the extent of involvement, and very wide margins are recommended because of tumor extension through cancellous bone. Because of the limited feasibility of obtaining these margins when skull base involvement is present, 5-year survival rates for maxillary sinus and sinonasal osteosarcomas are less than 10% in most reported series.

Radiation Therapy

As with other head and neck subsites, the radiation oncologist must consider whether the primary tumor and/or neck require treatment. Because of the rarity of sinonasal malignancies, treatment recommendations are largely based on single-institutional retrospective data. Outcomes from relatively large site-specific series are summarized in **Table 7–7**. Tumors of the ethmoid and maxillary sinuses are generally

Table 7–7 Sinonasal Cancer: Outcome Data from Selected Single-Institution Experiences

Institution Reference	Site/Patients	Treatment	5-year OS (%)	Local Control (%)
University of Florida[60]	Nasal vestibule N = 39	EBRT, BT, or both	Stage I–II: 77 Stage III–IV: 73	T1–T2: 94 T3–T4: 71
Princess Margaret Hospital[71]	Nasal vestibule N = 56	EBRT	64	<2 cm: 97 >2 cm: 57
University of Florida[53]	Nasal cavity and paranasal sinuses N = 78	RT ± S ± CT	50	Stage I: 86 Stage II: 65 Stage III: 34
UCSF/Stanford[54]	Maxillary sinus N = 97	RT ± S	Stage II: 75 Stage III: 37 Stage IV: 28	43
Princess Margaret Hospital[55]	Maxillary sinus N = 110	RT ± S	30	RT alone: 36 S + RT: 57
M.D. Anderson[62]	Nasal cavity N = 45	RT ± S	75	Nasal septum: 86 Lateral wall or floor: 68
M.D. Anderson[50]	Ethmoid sinus N = 34	RT ± S ± CT	55	S + RT: 74 RT: 64
Ghent University[58]	Paranasal sinuses or nasal cavity N = 39	S + RT (IMRT)	59 (4 year)	68
University of Michigan[72]	Paranasal sinuses N = 39	RT (3D-conformal) ± S	RT alone: 32 (4 year) S + RT: 60	RT: 32 S + RT: 65
University of Chicago[33]	Paranasal sinuses N = 19	RT + CT ± S	73	76
Mayo Clinic[64]	Esthesioneuroblastoma N = 49	S ± RT	69	S + RT: 86 S: 73

Abbreviations: BT, brachytherapy; CT, chemotherapy; EBRT, external beam radiotherapy; IMRT, intensity modulated radiotherapy; RT, radiotherapy; S, surgery.

treated with primary surgery when possible; however, local control has historically been poor with surgery alone. Therefore, save for T1 N0 patients with negative margins and no perineural invasion, postoperative radiation is indicated for all patients.[34,50] As with other sites, a dose of 54 to 60 Gy is recommended to the tumor bed if margins are negative. If margins are microscopically positive or close (<2 mm), a dose of 66 Gy is recommended. If margins are grossly positive or have unresectable disease, a dose of 70 to 72 Gy is needed. The initial target volume includes not only the tumor volume with 2- to 3-cm margin but also the ipsilateral maxillary antrum, nasal cavity, ethmoid sinus, medial orbit, nasopharynx, base of skull, and pterygopalatine fossa. The boost targets only the tumor bed with 1- to 2-cm margin. Important dose-limiting normal structures include optic nerves, optic chiasm, retina, lacrimal glands, brain, brain stem, and spinal cord.[51,52] The tolerance levels for these structures are shown in **Table 7–8**.

When conventional radiation is used to treat paranasal sinus cancer, ~80% of the dose is delivered through an anterior portal that encompasses the ipsilateral optic apparatus, optic chiasm, and brain stem. These structures are blocked in the lateral portals that deliver the remaining 20%. Unfortunately, with this technique, the anterior tumor extension is often blocked on the lateral fields to protect the eyes. With surgery followed by conventional radiotherapy (RT), local control is ~70 to 80% for T1 to T2 and 35 to 55% for T3 to T4.[30,50,53] Local control is ~20 to 40% for unresectable lesions treated with conventional RT.[54–56] The incidence of unilateral blindness secondary to retinopathy or optic neuropathy is ~30% with conventional RT, and the incidence of bilateral blindness is 5%.[30,53]

Intensity-modulated radiation therapy (IMRT) allows for the high-dose region to conform to the shape of the target volume. In this technique, the target volumes and avoidance structures, often based on MRI fusion, are contoured on axial CT slices obtained at the time of simulation. Computer-controlled optimization of beam intensity allows for optimal dose distributions. Therefore, the tumor volume will receive the prescription dose while keeping the critical normal structures within their tolerance doses.[57] Examples of dose distributions that can be achieved with this technique are shown in **Fig. 7–6**. IMRT offers the possibility of radiation dose escalation. Although, not proven to improve outcome, this strategy holds great promise. IMRT results in perhaps the most significant improvement in dose distribution of any head and neck subsite. A preliminary report of

Table 7–8 Recommended Maximum Doses

Structure	Dose (Gy)	Complication
Lens	12	Cataract
Lacrimal glands	30	Dry-eye syndrome
Retina	50	Blindness
Optic nerve	54	Blindness
Optic nerve adjacent to tumor	60	Blindness
Optic chiasm	54	Bilateral blindness
Brain stem	54	Cranial nerve deficits
Spinal cord	50	Myelitis

39 patients with sinonasal malignancy treated with surgery and adjuvant IMRT yielded a 4-year local control rate of 68% in a cohort of patients with mostly T3 to T4 disease with no radiation-induced blindness.[58] IMRT is also effective at reducing the incidence of dry-eye syndrome.[59]

Elective radiation of the clinically N0 neck is indicated for T3 to T4 disease and high-grade histologies including squamous and undifferentiated carcinoma.[30,31] Unlike other head and neck primary sites, only levels I, II, and retropharyngeal nodes need to be covered. For patients with a clinically N+ neck, neck dissection and comprehensive nodal irradiation are indicated.

Radiation for Uncommon Sinonasal Malignancies

Radiation alone is the preferred treatment for SCC of the nasal vestibule cancer for all cases except superficial lesions. Radiation consisting of external beam radiation with or without interstitial brachytherapy results in ~90 to 95% local control for T1 to T2 lesions and 70% local control for T3 to T4 lesions.[60,61] Complications including necrosis, nasal stenosis, and epistaxis occur in less than 5% of patients.[60] Because of the difficulty of resection and reconstruction for nasal vestibule cancers, the cosmesis after radiation is superior to primary surgery. For bulky, infiltrative lesions, multimodality therapy consisting of surgery followed by radiation or chemoradiation is indicated.

Localized squamous cell lesions of the nasal septum may be treated with an iridium-192 interstitial implant to a dose of 65 Gy over 6 to 7 days. Local control with this approach is ~85%.[62] Tumors of the lateral wall or floor of the nasal cavity and bulky nasal septum lesions require surgery followed by postoperative radiation. Local control with this approach is ~70%.[62]

For Kadish stage A olfactory neuroblastoma, surgery followed by radiation results in good locoregional control (85%), although surgery alone (50% local control) can be considered for patients with widely negative margins.[63] For stage B to C olfactory neuroblastoma, the most promising results have been achieved with both combined surgery and radiation with local control ranging from 70 to 80%.[63,64] Chemotherapy is considered for stage C disease.[65] When radiation is used for gross disease, a dose of 60 to 66 Gy is required. A dose of 54 Gy is recommended when combined with surgery with negative margins.

Natural killer cell–like CD56+/CD3+ T-cell sinonasal lymphoma, formerly known as lethal midline granuloma, is an EBV latent membrane protein positive malignancy that is more common in Asia. Most patients are treated with both radiation and chemotherapy, although the efficacy of anthracycline-based chemotherapy regimens typically used for B-cell lymphomas is poor. A dose of at least 45 to 50 Gy results in improved local control compared with chemotherapy alone or lower-dose radiation.[66] Despite multimodality therapy, the prognosis is poor with a 30% disease-free survival.[66] Localized (Ann Arbor stage I to II) intermediate grade B cell sinonasal lymphomas have a more favorable prognosis and should be treated with chemotherapy (cyclophosphamide, doxorubicin, vincristine, prednisone, and rituximab) followed by radiation.[34]

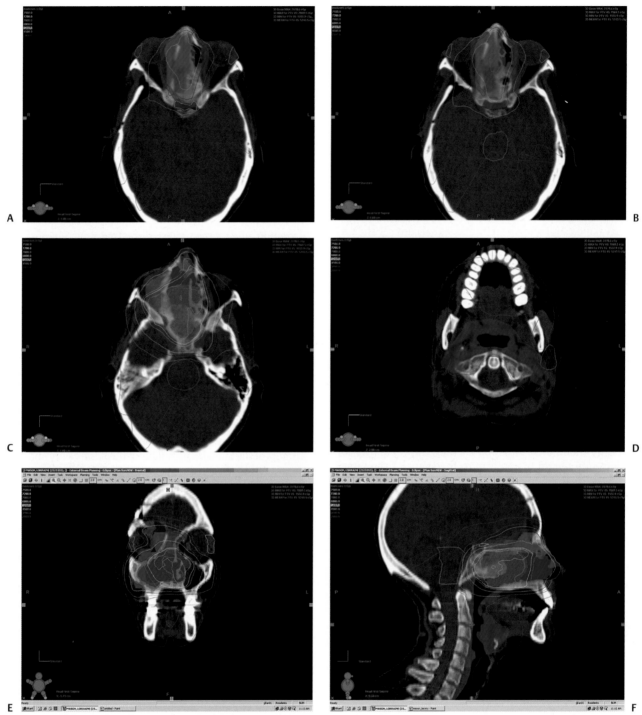

Figure 7–6 (**A**) Recurrent ethmoid sinus carcinoma treated with chemoradiation to 72 Gy conformal radiation of ethmoid sinuses with sparing of the bilateral optic nerves, lacrimal glands, and optic chiasm. The right optic nerve receives less than 60 Gy and the optic chiasm and left optic nerve receives less than 54 Gy. (**B**) Coverage of the ethmoid sinuses with sparing of the bilateral optic nerves and lacrimal glands. (**C**) High-dose radiation of the recurrent tumor, sparing of the brain stem. (**D**) The retropharyngeal and level II nodes are covered while sparing the parotid glands and oral cavity. (**E**) Coronal view of the dose distribution demonstrating sparing of the orbits, lacrimal glands, brain, and oral cavity. (**F**) Sagittal view demonstrates sparing of the brain, brain stem, spinal cord, and oral cavity while covering the tumor bed and regional nodes.

Sinonasal plasmacytoma should be treated with radiation to the primary site. Elective nodal irradiation is only needed if the lesion arises in Waldeyer's ring. Local control is ~80 to 85% with 15% of patients progressing to multiple myeloma.[67] A dose of 50 Gy is recommended for optimal local control.

Sinonasal rhabdomyosarcoma is considered a parameningeal site. Current guidelines are as per the International Rhabdomyosarcoma Study Group V.[68] Guidelines are extremely complex, but indications for radiation after surgery include microscopic positive margins (36 Gy) or positive nodes (41.4 Gy). Patients with gross residual disease after biopsy only or incomplete resection require definitive chemoradiation. Most patients will start with induction chemotherapy followed by reassessment at week 12. If the patient had no clinical or radiographic evidence of skull base involvement prior to chemotherapy and achieves a biopsy-proven complete response after chemotherapy, the radiation dose is 41.4 Gy. All other patients receive 50.4 Gy. Patients with intracranial extension should receive chemotherapy and radiation (50.4 Gy) starting on day 0. With appropriate multidisciplinary care, patients with parameningeal rhabdomyosarcoma now have a 5-year overall survival approaching 75%.[69]

Chemotherapy

There are no randomized trials specifically addressing the role of chemoradiation in this subsite of head and neck malignancies. Therefore, standard treatment paradigms of head and neck cancers are used as the basis for treatment recommendations for squamous cell cancers of the nasal cavity and paranasal sinus. For patients with locoregionally advanced unresectable disease, concurrent chemoradiotherapy has become the standard of treatment.[70] As in other head and neck cancers, the integration of chemotherapy into the multimodality treatment of nasal cavity and paranasal sinus cancers has shown encouraging results. In some instances, induction therapy with chemotherapy and/or radiotherapy has allowed subsequent surgical resection.

In an early study, 12 patients with locally advanced paranasal sinuses and nasal fossa cancers were treated with cisplatin and infusional 5-FU followed by radiation therapy and subsequent surgery. There was a 70% response rate, and local control was achieved in 11 of 12 patients. Ten patients were alive and free of disease at 27 months. Rosen et al reported 12 patients with locally advanced paranasal sinus carcinoma treated with induction cisplatin and infusional 5-FU followed by surgical resection and adjuvant radiotherapy. Eleven were alive and free of disease at a median follow-up of 55 months. These same authors reported on a cohort of 19 patients with stage III to IV paranasal sinus carcinoma treated in phase II trials with concurrent chemoradiation (most commonly induction cisplatin and 5-FU followed by surgery and adjuvant chemoradiation consisting of 60 Gy and 5-FU and hydroxyurea): the 5-year local control was 76% and 5-year overall survival was 73%.[33] In a subgroup of 11 patients with unresectable T4 sinonasal carcinoma treated in a phase II trial with 70 Gy and concomitant cisplatin, the 3-year local control was 78%.[68] Based on these promising results, chemo-radiation should be strongly considered in historically poor prognosis patients with squamous cell histology, including T3 to T4, N+, or unresectable disease.

Postoperatively, patients with adverse prognostic features such as extranodal extension have improved local control and in some series improved overall survival with concurrent chemoradiotherapy compared with radiation alone. In light of the frequent presentation of advanced disease in these patients, postoperative adjuvant therapy is often indicated.

Chemotherapy for Uncommon Sinonasal Malignancies

There are several relatively uncommon neoplasms in the nasal cavity and paranasal sinuses that are chemotherapy sensitive. Olfactory neuroblastoma (ONB) is a rare tumor of neuroectodermal origin that often presents with advanced disease. Craniofacial resection followed by radiation therapy has been the standard of care. Some series advocate concurrent chemoradiotherapy in an attempt to improve local control. Induction chemoradiotherapy prior to craniofacial resection has also been evaluated. In one series of 34 patients, 66% had significant reduction in tumor burden with induction therapy. Five-year and 10-year disease-free survival rates were 81% and 55%, respectively.

Sinonasal undifferentiated carcinoma is a rare and extremely malignant tumor of the paranasal sinuses. Chemotherapy is an important aspect of the multimodality treatment of these neoplasms, although its exact sequence with radiation and surgery is uncertain. Most patients are treated with craniofacial resection followed by postoperative chemoradiotherapy. Unresectable patients are treated with induction chemoradiotherapy followed by surgical resection if possible. Some investigators advocate that all patients be treated with induction chemoradiotherapy prior to resection.

◆ Clinical Cases

Case 1   T4a N3c M1 adenocarcinoma ethmoid sinus.

Clinical Presentation   A 68-year-old woman presented with a history of sudden onset of diplopia after more than a year of nonspecific nasal symptoms, including nasal obstruction, sneezing, and rhinorrhea. Past medical history was significant for diabetes mellitus and hypertension. Exam revealed a mass in the left nasal cavity and facial paresthesia over V2 distribution. She had left medial rectus palsy, but no proptosis or chemosis.

Diagnosis and Workup   A CT scan revealed an expansile and destructive lesion of the left sinonasal complex, involving the maxillary, ethmoid, and sphenoid sinuses, with extension into the left orbit (**Fig. 7–7A,B**). MRI showed a heterogeneous signal within this multisinus expansile mass (**Fig. 7–7C**). Biopsy revealed poorly differentiated adenocarcinoma. Metastatic workup revealed bilateral cervical and mediastinal disease, as well as multiple bone lesions.

Options for Treatment   Given the metastatic nature of this advanced tumor, palliative chemoradiotherapy was recommended.

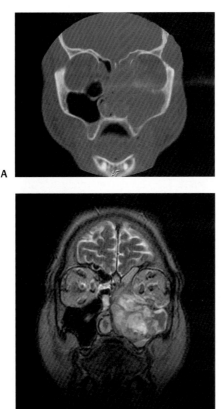

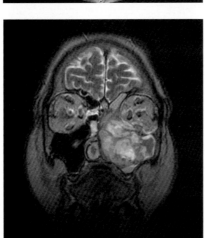

Figure 7-7 (**A**) Adenocarcinoma, CT scan, coronal view. This scan demonstrates an expansile lesion involving the maxillary sinus with erosion of the ethmoid labyrinth. (**B**) Adenocarcinoma, CT scan, axial view. This scan demonstrates the invasion into the sphenoid sinus. (**C**) Adenocarcinoma, MRI, coronal view. This scan is essential in identifying orbital invasion and separating tumor from sinus secretions. This scan demonstrated an intact orbit without obvious invasion.

Treatment of the Primary Tumor The patient underwent radiation therapy with IMRT with eye-sparing protocol to a dose of 250 cGy in 15 fractions. She also received concomitant chemotherapy with Taxotere (Aventis Pharmaceuticals, Inc., New Jersey; docetaxel and carboplatin).

Treatment of the Neck She received radiation to the bilateral cervical lymph nodes.

Treatment of Distant Sites The systemic chemotherapy was the treatment for the distant sites.

Reconstruction No reconstruction was necessary, given the nonoperative therapy.

Summary of Management Adenocarcinoma is primarily treated with *en bloc* resection followed by combined chemoradiation therapy in resectable cases. This tumor was unresectable because of middle cranial fossa involvement and distant metastatic disease. The orbital involvement was not a contraindication to surgery.

Case 2 Olfactory neuroblastoma, Kadish stage B.

Clinical Presentation A 44-year-old man presented with chronic right nasal obstruction and headaches. He denied any visual changes or rhinorrhea. Past medical history was significant for hepatitis C for which he had been on immunosuppressive therapy. Exam revealed a gray-red and fleshy mass filling the right nasal cavity. Ophthalmologic exam was unremarkable.

Diagnosis and Workup A CT scan of the paranasal sinuses revealed a heterogeneous mass filling the nasal cavity and thinning the right medial orbital wall (**Fig. 7-8A**). MRI demonstrated a right nasal cavity mass extending to the medial orbital wall and superiorly to the olfactory groove, but no gross involvement of the dura or periorbita (**Fig. 7-8B**). Metastatic workup was negative. Biopsy was consistent with olfactory neuroblastoma.

Options for Treatment Olfactory neuroblastoma is generally treated by surgery with postoperative radiation therapy to the primary site for resectable cases. This particular tumor involved the bone of the medial orbital wall and cribriform plate, and required a craniofacial resection for complete tumor removal.

Treatment of the Primary Tumor The patient underwent a craniofacial resection (**Fig. 7-8C,D**). The tumor perforated

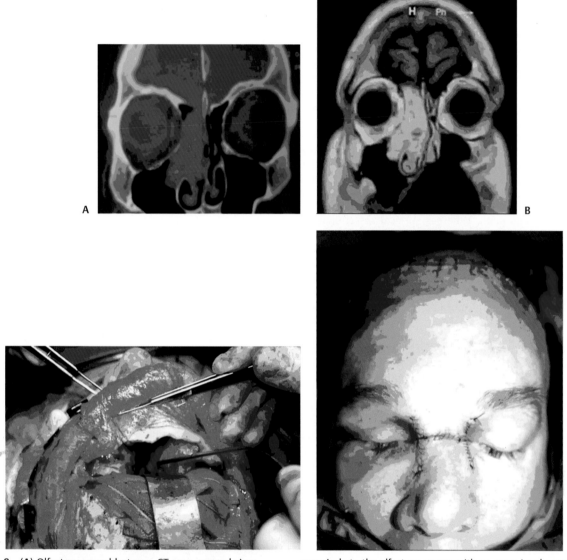

Figure 7–8 (**A**) Olfactory neuroblastoma, CT scan, coronal view. The scan demonstrates a heterogeneous mass filling the nasal cavity and thinning the right medial orbital wall. (**B**) Olfactory neuroblastoma, MRI, coronal view. The MRI demonstrated a right nasal cavity mass extending to the medial orbital wall and superiorly to the olfactory groove with no gross involvement of the dura or periorbita. (**C**) Olfactory neuroblastoma. Craniofacial resection viewed from cranially through the craniotomy. (**D**) Olfactory neuroblastoma. Craniofacial resection after closure.

the lamina papyracea and a small portion of the periorbita, which was included with the specimen. The tumor extended to the dura but did not violate it. The adjacent dura was resected and the dural defect repaired with a pericranial flap. The specimen was removed *en bloc* without gross evidence of residual disease. The final pathologic margins were negative. The patient received postoperative radiation with IMRT to a dose of 6000 cGy in 30 treatments. The patient did not receive chemotherapy.

Treatment of the Neck As the incidence of occult regional metastasis is low, the neck was observed.

Treatment of Distant Sites Although the risk of occult distant metastatic disease is low, annual evaluation with PET scanning is indicated.

Reconstruction The anterior skull base defect was reconstructed with a pericranial flap.

Summary of Treatment Olfactory neuroblastoma is a rare lesion that arises from the olfactory epithelium of the superior nasal cavity. Differentiating it from other small blue-cell tumors requires immunohistochemical analysis. Locoregional and distant metastatic disease is uncommon. The surgical approach for resectable cases is craniofacial resection given the superior origin of this tumor at the cribriform plate.

Case 3 T3 N0 M0 mucosal melanoma left ethmoid sinus.

Clinical Presentation An 81-year-old woman presented with left-sided intractable epistaxis and nasal obstruction. Past medical history was noncontributory. Exam revealed

133

a large mass filling the left nasal cavity and no orbital changes or facial paresthesia.

Diagnosis and Workup   A CT scan of the paranasal sinuses revealed left-sided pan-sinus opacification with maxillary expansion and thinning of the left medial orbital wall and cribriform plate (**Fig. 7–9A**). MRI demonstrated a left nasal cavity mass with involvement of the lamina papyracea and cribriform plate, with obstructed secretions in the maxillary, sphenoid, and frontal sinuses (**Fig. 7–9B**). Biopsy of the mass revealed malignant melanoma, with immunohistochemical studies positive for S-100, human melanoma black (HMB)-45, vimentin, and cytokeratin, but negative for leukocyte common antigen (LCA). Metastatic workup with a whole-body bone scan and CT scan were negative.

Options for Treatment   Whereas surgical resection may not impact overall survival, it will improve local control and quality of life. Given the location of the tumor, an *en bloc* surgical resection with postoperative radiation therapy offers the patient local control. Other options include primary radiation therapy or no therapy. Because of the possibility of satellite lesions, a wide resection margin is required.

Treatment of the Primary Tumor   The patient underwent medial maxillectomy and lateral rhinotomy. Intraoperatively, the lacrimal fossa was filled with tumor and the medial orbital wall was eroded. The tumor was bluntly dissected off the periorbita, which was not violated. The specimen was removed *en bloc* without gross evidence of residual disease, but on final pathology the intranasal mucosal margin was positive and satellite lesions were present. The patient received postoperative radiation with IMRT dosing of 6000 cGy in 30 treatments. The patient did not receive chemotherapy.

Treatment of the Neck   The neck was observed.

Treatment of Distant Sites   The risk of occult distant metastatic disease is low.

Reconstruction   No reconstruction is required after medial maxillectomy.

Summary of Treatment   Mucosal melanoma is a rare and aggressive tumor with a poor prognosis. The tumor often arises from the anterior nasal septum and turbinates. Surgical resection followed by radiation, chemotherapy, and immunotherapy has been applied with limited success but may provide acceptable local control.

Case 4   A T1 N0 M0 squamous cell carcinoma within an inverting papilloma.

Clinical Presentation   The patient is a 57-year-old man with no significant past medical history who presented with right-sided unilateral nasal obstruction.

Diagnosis and Workup   On examination, a right-sided unilateral polypoid lesion was found. A CT scan was obtained and demonstrated a lesion involving the lateral nasal wall and medial wall of the maxillary sinus. A biopsy performed in the office demonstrated an inverting papilloma. The patient was taken to the operating room where an endoscopic resection of the medial maxilla was performed. The intraoperative margins were free of tumor, and the patient was discharged on postoperative day 2. The final pathology demonstrated a 1-cm focus of moderately differentiated SCC within the specimen.

Options for Treatment   Endoscopic management of sinonasal tumors has become progressively more popular because it obviates the need for a facial incisions and patients recover quickly with less pain; however, there is a great deal of controversy regarding this technique for the management of high-grade benign and malignant lesions. Because a piecemeal resection is performed, monitoring margins and control of tumor spill are exceptional concerns. This case

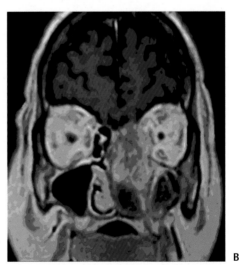

A   B

Figure 7–9 (**A**) Melanoma, CT scan, coronal view. This scan demonstrates a left-sided pan-sinus opacification with maxillary expansion and thinning of the left medial orbital wall and cribriform plate. (**B**) Melanoma, MRI, coronal view. The MRI demonstrates a left nasal cavity mass with involvement of the lamina papyracea and cribriform plate, with obstructed secretions in the maxillary, sphenoid, and frontal sinuses.

highlights the potential shortcomings of the endoscopic approach and the necessity for intraoperative frozen-section analysis. The options for management include observation, external beam radiation, or re-resection.

Treatment of the Primary Tumor Because an endoscopic resection was performed for an inverted papilloma, and the margins of resection were assessed and considered clear of disease at the time of surgery, re-resection is probably not necessary. Because this is considered a T1 carcinoma, surgical resection is considered adequate therapy and observation is appropriate.

Treatment of the Neck Management of the neck is not warranted.

Treatment of Distant Sites Not applicable.

Reconstruction Not required.

Summary of Treatment Management of this case highlights the potential problems with endoscopic surgery of malignant disease. Because this case was performed for the management of an inverted papilloma and the margins were assessed throughout the surgery, the surgical resection is considered adequate for a T1 cancer of the maxillary sinus. In the event that the original surgery was performed for a nasal polyp or another pathology where margins were not assessed, a re-resection would be recommended.

References

1. Grant RN. Cancer Statistics. New York, NY: American Cancer Society; 1970:8, 14
2. Myers LL, Nussenbaum B, Bradford CR, et al. Paranasal sinus malignancies: an 18-year single institution experience. Laryngoscope 2002;112(11):1964–1969
3. Shao W. Malignant tumors of the nasal cavity. Emedicine.com. 2002
4. Waldron J, Witterick I. Paranasal sinus cancer: caveats and controversies. World J Surg 2003;27(7):849–855
5. Hosemann W, Kühnel TH, Burchard AK, et al. Histochemical detection of lymphatic drainage pathways in the middle nasal meatus. Rhinology 1998;36(2):50–54
6. Renn WH, Rhoton AL Jr. Microsurgical anatomy of the sellar region. J Neurosurg 1975;43(3):288–298
7. Ahman M, Holmström M, Cynkier I, et al. Work related impairment of nasal function in Swedish woodwork teachers. Occup Environ Med 1996;53(2):112–117
8. Valente G, Ferrari L, Kerim S, et al. Evidence of p53 immunohistochemical overexpression in ethmoidal mucosa of woodworkers. Cancer Detect Prev 2004;28(2):99–106
9. Wilhelmsson B, Hellquist H, Olofsson J, et al. Nasal cuboidal metaplasia with dysplasia. Precursor to adenocarcinoma in wood-dust-exposed workers? Acta Otolaryngol 1985;99(5–6):641–648
10. Boysen M, Voss R, Solberg LA. The nasal mucosa in softwood exposed furniture workers. Acta Otolaryngol 1986;101(5–6):501–508
11. Luce D, Leclerc A, Bégin D, et al. Sinonasal cancer and occupational exposures: a pooled analysis of 12 case-control studies. Cancer Causes Control 2002;13(2):147–157
12. Sasco AJ, Secretan MB, Straif K. Tobacco smoking and cancer: a brief review of recent epidemiological evidence. Lung Cancer 2004;45(Suppl 2):S3–S9
13. Murray EM, Werner D, Greeff EA, et al. Postradiation sarcomas: 20 cases and a literature review. Int J Radiat Oncol Biol Phys 1999;45(4):951–961
14. Sale KA, Wallace DI, Girod DA, et al. Radiation-induced malignancy of the head and neck. Otolaryngol Head Neck Surg 2004;131(5):643–645
15. Lloyd G, Lund VJ, Howard D, et al. Optimum imaging for sinonasal malignancy. J Laryngol Otol 2000;114(7):557–562
16. Ninomiya H, Oriuchi N, Kahn N, et al. Diagnosis of tumor in the nasal cavity and paranasal sinuses with [^{11}C]choline PET: comparative study with 2-[^{18}F]fluoro-2-deoxy-D-glucose (FDG) PET. Ann Nucl Med 2004;18(1):29–34
17. Sisson GA Sr, Toriumi DM, Atiyah RA. Paranasal sinus malignancy: a comprehensive update. Laryngoscope 1989;99(2):143–150
18. Galati L. Malignant tumors of the sinuses. Emedicine.com. 2005
19. Laramore G. Radiation Therapy of Head and Neck Cancer. Berlin, Germany: Springer-Verlag; 1989
20. Thawley SE. Comprehensive Management of Head and Neck Tumors. New York, NY: W.B. Saunders; 1986
21. Schantz S. Tumors of the nasal cavity and paranasal sinuses, nasopharynx, oral cavity, and oropharynx. In: Cancer: Principles and Practice of Oncology. Philadelphia, PA: Lippincott-Raven; 1997:741–801
22. Fowler JF, Lindstrom MJ. Loss of local control with prolongation in radiotherapy. Int J Radiat Oncol Biol Phys 1992;23(2):457–467
23. Carrau RL, Segas J, Nuss DW, et al. Squamous cell carcinoma of the sinonasal tract invading the orbit. Laryngoscope 1999;109(2 Pt 1):230–235
24. Imola MJ, Schramm VL Jr. Orbital preservation in surgical management of sinonasal malignancy. Laryngoscope 2002;112(8 Pt 1):1357–1365
25. Weymuller EA Jr, Reardon EJ, Nash D. A comparison of treatment modalities in carcinoma of the maxillary antrum. Arch Otolaryngol 1980;106(10):625–629
26. Larson DL, Christ JE, Jesse RH. Preservation of the orbital contents in cancer of the maxillary sinus. Arch Otolaryngol 1982;108(6):370–372
27. Day TA, Beas RA, Schlosser RJ, et al. Management of paranasal sinus malignancy. Curr Treat Options Oncol 2005;6(1):3–18
28. Robbins KT, Clayman G, Levine PA, et al. Neck dissection classification update: revisions proposed by the American Head and Neck Society and the American Academy of Otolaryngology-Head and Neck Surgery. Arch Otolaryngol Head Neck Surg 2002;128(7):751–758
29. McHam SA, Adelstein DJ, Rybicki LA, et al. Who merits a neck dissection after definitive chemoradiotherapy for N2–N3 squamous cell head and neck cancer? Head Neck 2003;25(10):791–798
30. Jiang GL, Ang KK, Peters LJ, et al. Maxillary sinus carcinomas: natural history and results of postoperative radiotherapy. Radiother Oncol 1991;21(3):193–200
31. Le QT, Fu KK, Kaplan MJ, et al. Lymph node metastasis in maxillary sinus carcinoma. Int J Radiat Oncol Biol Phys 2000;46(3):541–549
32. Stern SJ, Goepfert H, Clayman G, et al. Squamous cell carcinoma of the maxillary sinus. Arch Otolaryngol Head Neck Surg 1993;119(9):964–969
33. Lee MM, Vokes EE, Rosen A, et al. Multimodality therapy in advanced paranasal sinus carcinoma: superior long-term results. Cancer J Sci Am 1999;5(4):219–223
34. Logsdon MD, Ha CS, Kavadi VS, et al. Lymphoma of the nasal cavity and paranasal sinuses: improved outcome and altered prognostic factors with combined modality therapy. Cancer 1997;80(3):477–488
35. Reino AJ. Factors in the pathogenesis of tumors of the sphenoid and maxillary sinuses: a comparative study. Laryngoscope 2000;110(10 Pt 2 Suppl 96):1–38
36. Wiseman SM, Popat SR, Rigaul NR, et al. Adenoid cystic carcinoma of the paranasal sinuses or nasal cavity: a 40-year review of 35 cases. Ear Nose Throat J 2002;81(8):510–517
37. Batsakis JG. Tumors of the Head and Neck. Baltimore, MD: The Williams & Wilkins Company; 1979
38. Harwood AR, Krajbich JI, Fornasier VL. Radiotherapy of chondrosarcoma of bone. Cancer 1980;45(11):2769–2777
39. Broich G, Pagliari A, Ottaviani F. Esthesioneuroblastoma: a general review of the cases published since the discovery of the tumour in 1924. Anticancer Res 1997;17(4A):2683–2706
40. Resto VA, Deschler DG. Sinonasal malignancies. Otolaryngol Clin North Am 2004;37(2):473–487
41. Kadish S, Goodman M, Wang CC. Olfactory neuroblastoma. A clinical analysis of 17 cases. Cancer 1976;37(3):1571–1576
42. Frierson HF Jr, Mills SE, Fechner RE, et al. Sinonasal undifferentiated carcinoma. An aggressive neoplasm derived from schneiderian epithelium and distinct from olfactory neuroblastoma. Am J Surg Pathol 1986;10(11):771–779
43. Gorelick J, Ross D, Marentette L, et al. Sinonasal undifferentiated carcinoma: case series and review of the literature. Neurosurgery 2000;47(3):750–755
44. Musy PY, Reibel JF, Levine PA. Sinonasal undifferentiated carcinoma: the search for a better outcome. Laryngoscope 2002;112(8 Pt 1):1450–1455

45. Smith SR, Som P, Fahmy A, et al. A clinicopathological study of sinonasal neuroendocrine carcinoma and sinonasal undifferentiated carcinoma. Laryngoscope 2000;110(10 Pt 1):1617–1622

46. Fitzek MM, Thornton AF, Varvares M, et al. Neuroendocrine tumors of the sinonasal tract. Results of a prospective study incorporating chemotherapy, surgery, and combined proton-photon radiotherapy. Cancer 2002;94(10):2623–2634

47. Perez-Ordonez B, Caruana SM, Huvos AG, et al. Small cell neuroendocrine carcinoma of the nasal cavity and paranasal sinuses. Hum Pathol 1998;29(8):826–832

48. Brandwein MS, Rothstein A, Lawson W, et al. Sinonasal melanoma. A clinicopathologic study of 25 cases and literature meta-analysis. Arch Otolaryngol Head Neck Surg 1997;123(3):290–296

49. Zak FG, Lawson W. The presence of melanocytes in the nasal cavity. Ann Otol Rhinol Laryngol 1974;83(4):515–519

50. Jiang GL, Morrison WH, Garden AS, et al. Ethmoid sinus carcinomas: natural history and treatment results. Radiother Oncol 1998;49(1):21–27

51. Parsons JT, Bova FJ, Fitzgerald CR, et al. Radiation optic neuropathy after megavoltage external-beam irradiation: analysis of time-dose factors. Int J Radiat Oncol Biol Phys 1994;30(4):755–763

52. Parsons JT, Bova FJ, Fitzgerald CR, et al. Severe dry-eye syndrome following external beam irradiation. Int J Radiat Oncol Biol Phys 1994;30(4):775–780

53. Katz TS, Mendenhall WM, Morris CG, et al. Malignant tumors of the nasal cavity and paranasal sinuses. Head Neck 2002;24(9):821–829

54. Le QT, Fu KK, Kaplan M, et al. Treatment of maxillary sinus carcinoma: a comparison of the 1997 and 1977 American Joint Committee on cancer staging systems. Cancer 1999;86(9):1700–1711

55. Waldron JN, O'Sullivan B, Warde P, et al. Ethmoid sinus cancer: twenty-nine cases managed with primary radiation therapy. Int J Radiat Oncol Biol Phys 1998;41(2):361–369

56. Jansen EP, Keus RB, Hilgers FJ, et al. Does the combination of radiotherapy and debulking surgery favor survival in paranasal sinus carcinoma? Int J Radiat Oncol Biol Phys 2000;48(1):27–35

57. Huang D, Xia P, Akazawa P, et al. Comparison of treatment plans using intensity-modulated radiotherapy and three-dimensional conformal radiotherapy for paranasal sinus carcinoma. Int J Radiat Oncol Biol Phys 2003;56(1):158–168

58. Duthoy W, Boterberg T, Claus F, et al. Postoperative intensity-modulated radiotherapy in sinonasal carcinoma: clinical results in 39 patients. Cancer 2005;104(1):71–82

59. Claus F, Boterberg T, Ost P, et al. Short term toxicity profile for 32 sinonasal cancer patients treated with IMRT. Can we avoid dry eye syndrome? Radiother Oncol 2002;64(2):205–208

60. McCollough WM, Mendenhall NP, Parsons JT, et al. Radiotherapy alone for squamous cell carcinoma of the nasal vestibule: management of the primary site and regional lymphatics. Int J Radiat Oncol Biol Phys 1993;26(1):73–79

61. Langendijk JA, Poorter R, Leemans CR, et al. Radiotherapy of squamous cell carcinoma of the nasal vestibule. Int J Radiat Oncol Biol Phys 2004;59(5):1319–1325

62. Ang KK, Jiang GL, Frankenthaler RA, et al. Carcinomas of the nasal cavity. Radiother Oncol 1992;24(3):163–168

63. Chao KS, Kaplan C, Simpson JR, et al. Esthesioneuroblastoma: the impact of treatment modality. Head Neck 2001;23(9):749–757

64. Foote RL, Morita A, Ebersold MJ, et al. Esthesioneuroblastoma: the role of adjuvant radiation therapy. Int J Radiat Oncol Biol Phys 1993;27(4):835–842

65. Eden BV, Debo RF, Larner JM, et al. Esthesioneuroblastoma. Long-term outcome and patterns of failure—the University of Virginia experience. Cancer 1994;73(10):2556–2562

66. Cheung MM, Chan JK, Lau WH, et al. Early stage nasal NK/T-cell lymphoma: clinical outcome, prognostic factors, and the effect of treatment modality. Int J Radiat Oncol Biol Phys 2002;54(1):182–190

67. Tsang RW, Gospodarowicz MK, Pintilie M, et al. Solitary plasmacytoma treated with radiotherapy: impact of tumor size on outcome. Int J Radiat Oncol Biol Phys 2001;50(1):113–120

68. Raney RB, Anderson JR, Barr FG, et al. Rhabdomyosarcoma and undifferentiated sarcoma in the first two decades of life: a selective review of intergroup rhabdomyosarcoma study group experience and rationale for Intergroup Rhabdomyosarcoma Study V. J Pediatr Hematol Oncol 2001;23(4):215–220

69. Raney RB, Meza J, Anderson JR, et al. Treatment of children and adolescents with localized parameningeal sarcoma: experience of the Intergroup Rhabdomyosarcoma Study Group protocols IRS-II through -IV, 1978–1997. Med Pediatr Oncol 2002;38(1):22–32

70. Harrison LB, Raben A, Pfister DG, et al. A prospective phase II trial of concomitant chemotherapy and radiotherapy with delayed accelerated fractionation in unresectable tumors of the head and neck. Head Neck 1998;20(6):497–503

71. Wong CS, Cummings BJ, Elkhaim T, et al. External irradiation for squamous cell carcinoma of the nasal vestibule. Int J Radiat Oncol Biol Phys 1986;12(11):1943–1946

72. Roa WH, Hazuka MB, Sandler HM, et al. Results of primary and adjuvant CT-based 3-dimensional radiotherapy for malignant tumors of the paranasal sinuses. Int J Radiat Oncol Biol Phys 1994;28(4):857–865

8

Carcinoma of the Nasopharynx

William I. Wei and Jonathan S. T. Sham

◆ Anatomy of the Nasopharynx

The nasopharynx is the region located behind the nasal cavities and above the soft palate. The undersurface of the body of the sphenoid bone forms the slanting roof that merges inferiorly with the posterior wall, which is formed by the arch of the atlas and the upper part of the body of the axis vertebra. The floor of the nasopharynx opens downward into the oropharynx at the level of the soft palate. The lateral wall is formed by the superior constrictor muscle with the opening of the eustachian tube situated in the upper part. The cartilage that surrounds the orifice of this auditory tube is an incomplete ring, deficient in the inferolateral portion. The medial portion of the cartilage elevates the mucosa to form the medial crura. The slit-like space situated medial to this crura is the fossa of Rosenmüller; its size and depth varies between individuals, and nasopharyngeal carcinoma is commonly found in this recess.

The posterior wall of the nasopharynx is lined with stratified squamous cell, and pseudostratified ciliated epithelium is found in the region of the nasopharynx near the choana. The epithelium lies on a well-defined basement membrane and then the lamina propria, which contains abundant lymphoid tissue. The superior constrictor forms the muscular layer of the nasopharynx, and investing this muscle on the outside is the pharyngobasilar fascia. This fascia joins its counterpart from the opposite side to form the median raphe, which extends from the skull base to the posterior pharyngeal wall. The pharyngobasilar fascia together with the prevertebral fascia encloses the retropharyngeal space, which harbors the node of Rouviere. This retropharyngeal space is part of the retrostyloid space of the paranasopharyngeal space (**Fig. 8–1**). The last four cranial nerves, the carotid sheath, and the sympathetic trunk are located in this retrostyloid space, and they can be affected by direct tumor extension or lymphatic permeation. Important structures located in the prestyloid space are the maxillary artery and nerves.

The lymphatic supply of the nasopharynx is found mainly in the submucosal region, which drains into the retropharyn-

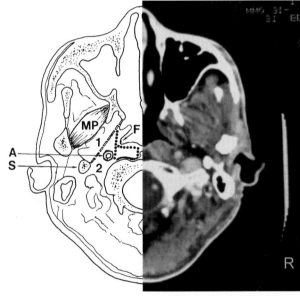

Figure 8–1 Axial view of the nasopharynx showing its relationship with the surrounding structures. A, internal carotid artery; F, fossa of Rosenmüller; MP, medial pterygoid muscle; S, styloid process. The semisolid line is the imaginary line joining the medial pterygoid plate to the styloid process. (*1*) The space in front of the dashed line is the prestyloid space; (*2*) behind the dashed line is the poststyloid space. The dotted line is the pharyngobasilar fascia, which joins with the fascia of the opposite side to form the median raphe. This fascia together with the prevertebral fascia (*solid line*) encloses the retropharyngeal space.

geal lymph nodes. Efferents from these nodes together with some lymphatics that come directly from the nasopharynx drain to the deep cervical lymph nodes. The lymphatic drainage then goes in an orderly fashion, from the high neck nodes to the lower ones, and this is also the pattern of metastasis of nasopharyngeal carcinoma in the cervical lymph nodes.[1]

◆ Epidemiology

Nasopharyngeal carcinoma (NPC) is a squamous cell carcinoma with a varying degree of differentiation, arising from any part of the epithelial lining of the nasopharynx, most frequently from the fossa of Rosenmüller, the recess located medial to the medial crura of the eustachian tube. The malignant squamous cells of NPC are large polygonal cells with a syncytial character. These cells are frequently intermingled with lymphoid cells in the nasopharynx, giving rise to the term *lymphoepithelioma*.[2] Electron microscopy studies have however confirmed the squamous origin of these malignant cells.

The histologic classification of NPC proposed by the World Health Organization (WHO)[3] in 1978 categorized the tumors into three groups:

1. Type I are those typical keratinizing squamous cell carcinomas.
2. Type II includes nonkeratinizing epidermoid carcinomas.
3. Type III includes undifferentiated carcinomas or poorly differentiated carcinoma. These cells have indistinct cell margins with hyperchromatic nuclei and respond favorably to radiation treatment.

In North America, around 25% of NPC patients have type I histology, 12% type II, and 63% type III. The respective histologic distribution in Chinese patients is 3%, 2%, and 95%, respectively.[4]

◆ Etiology

NPC is frequently seen in the inhabitants of southern China, northern Africa, and Alaska. The recent reported incidence of NPC among men and women in Hong Kong, which is geographically adjacent to Guangdong Province in southern China, was 30 per 100,000 and 20 per 100,000, respectively.[5] This malignancy is however uncommon in other countries; the age-adjusted incidence for both sexes is less than 1 per 100,000.[5]

The incidence of NPC still remains high among Chinese who have immigrated to Southeast Asia or North America but is lower among those Chinese born in North America when compared with those born in southern China.[6,7] Thus genetic, ethnic, and environmental factors may all play a role in the etiology of the disease.

One commonly suggested etiologic factor is the consumption of salted fish. Dimethylnitrosamine, a carcinogenic compound, has been detected in the salted fish,[8] and this might lead to the development of NPC. Subsequent case-control study, however, showed that only frequent consumption of salted fish before 10 years of age was associated with increased risk of developing NPC.[9]

The Epstein-Barr virus (EBV) has also been considered to play an oncogenic role in the development of this tumor, as the EBV genome is frequently detected in the biopsy specimens of this tumor.[10] As EBV is present in many races of the human population, it is unlikely that EBV is the only causative agent of NPC. The first-degree relatives of NPC patients have a 6-times greater chance of developing NPC than controls,[11] and comparative genomic hybridization studies have demonstrated alterations in multiple chromosomes such as the deletion of regions at 14q, 16p, 1p and amplification of 12q and 4q.[12,13] Tumor suppressive genes have also been recently located in chromosome 14q.[14] This suggests that genetic factors have an important etiologic role in NPC.

◆ Presentation

The incidence of NPC in general is 3 times more in men than in women; the median age is 50 years. Symptoms are related to the location of the primary tumor, their infiltration of structures in the vicinity of the nasopharynx, or metastasis to the cervical lymph nodes. The symptoms of epistaxis, nasal obstruction, and discharge are related to the presence of tumor mass in the nasopharynx; deafness and tinnitus are likely the result of dysfunction of the eustachian tube, following the posterolateral extension of the tumor to the paranasopharyngeal space. Serous otitis media was noted in 41% of 237 newly diagnosed NPC patients. Thus, when a Chinese adult patient presents with serous otitis media, the possibility of NPC should be considered.[15] A headache or multiple cranial nerve neuropathies including cranial nerves III, IV, V, and/or VI may be a result of superior extension of the tumor into the skull base. Neck masses, usually appearing first in the upper neck due to metastasis to the cervical lymph nodes (**Fig. 8–2**). As the nasopharynx is located in the midline, it is not uncommon to see patients presenting with bilateral cervical lymph nodes.

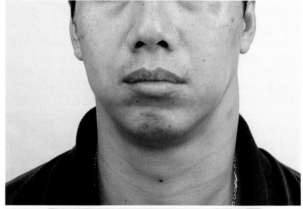
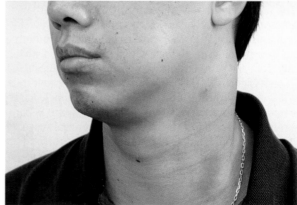

Figure 8–2 Clinical photograph of a patient showing enlarged left upper cervical lymph node.

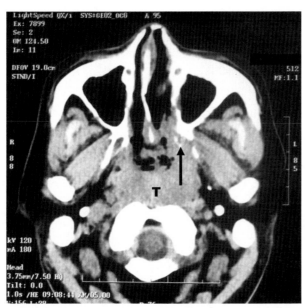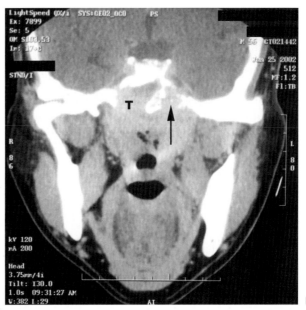

Figure 8–3 (**A**) CT scan (axial view) showing tumor (*T*) in the nasopharynx that has eroded the pterygoid plate (*arrow*). (**B**) CT scan (direct coronal view) showing tumor (*T*) in the nasopharynx that has eroded the skull base (*arrow*).

Many of these symptoms are inconspicuous and non-specific; the painless, enlarged lymph nodes are frequently under the cover of the sternomastoid muscle and remained unnoticed until they reach a significant size. Thus, many patients suffering from NPC only seek medical advice when the disease is in the advanced stage. A retrospective study of 4768 patients reported that the symptoms at presentation were neck mass in 76%, nasal symptoms in 73%, aural symptoms in 62%, and cranial nerve palsy in 20% of patients.[16]

◆ Diagnosis and Workup

Where patients present with symptoms suggestive of NPC, they should be clinically evaluated for physical signs of the disease including the regional lymph nodes and whether there were distant metastasis. Indirect examination of the postnasal space with a mirror should be performed together with an x-ray of the chest. Complete blood count and renal and liver function tests should also be done. Cross-sectional imaging by computed tomography (CT) or magnetic resonance imaging (MRI) may show abnormal structural alterations in the nasopharynx and its vicinity (**Figs. 8–3** and **8–4**). The neck should also be included in the imaging studies for the detection of occult metastasis to the neck. Serology test showing elevated EBV antititer will give further grounds for suspicion and would justify an endoscopic examination and a biopsy of the nasopharynx. A definitive diagnosis of NPC requires a positive biopsy taken from the tumor in the nasopharynx. When there are palpable cervical lymph nodes, fine-needle aspiration cytology should be performed. Even when there is no clinically evident neck lymph nodes, ultrasound examination of the neck should be performed, and any suspicious nodes should have fine-needle aspiration cytology examination under ultrasound guidance. This will give additional information as to the extent of disease at the time of presentation.

Serology

In patients suffering from NPC, the antibody immunoglobulin A (IgA) responds to the early antigen (EA), and the viral capsid antigen (VCA) of EBV has been shown to be of diagnostic value.[17]

The IgA anti-VCA is more sensitive but less specific than the IgA anti-EA. In population screening studies of more than thousands of apparently healthy individuals, for those with elevated titers of these antibodies, their incidence of harboring subclinical NPC ranged from 3[18] to 5%.[19] The value of EBV serology in the

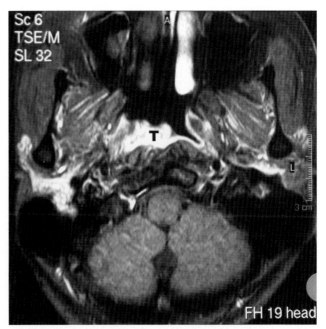

Figure 8–4 MRI scan (axial view) showing tumor in the nasopharynx, extending to the paranasopharyngeal space (*T*).

diagnosis of NPC was confirmed by a recent report. In this study, the initial EBV serologies of 9699 subjects were cross-checked against the cancer registry and death registry in the ensuing 15-year period. It was found that the longer the duration of follow-up, the greater the difference in the cumulative incidence of NPC between seropositive and seronegative subjects.[20] The level of IgA anti-VCA has also been shown to be related to the stage of the disease, and the level may decrease after therapy.[21]

Recently, cell-free DNA of the EBV has been detected in NPC patients, and it has been evaluated as a tumor marker.[22] However, it has a moderate sensitivity for the detection of recurrent tumor after radiotherapy, especially when the primary tumor is small.[23]

Imaging Studies

Cross-sectional imaging studies provide information on the deep extension of the tumor including skull base erosion and intracranial spread. These investigations are essential nowadays to document the extent of the disease in the nasopharynx and in the planning of delivery of radiation.[24] This is particularly applicable when intensity-modulated radiation therapy (IMRT) is the treatment modality. IMRT delivers targeted radiation more accurately to the tumor while at the same time sparing adjacent normal tissues. MRI in the delineation of the extent of tumor involvement and volume is essential for the IMRT form of radiotherapy.[25]

CT demonstrates the soft tissue extent of the tumor in the nasopharynx and into the paranasopharyngeal space.[26] It is sensitive in detecting bone erosion especially that of the skull base. Tumor extension intracranially through the foramen ovale with the perineural spread can also be detected and provides evidence of cavernous sinus involvement without skull base erosion.[27] CT is capable of showing bone regeneration after therapy, and this indicates complete eradication of tumor.[28]

MRI provides multiplanar imaging abilities and is better than CT in the differentiation of tumor from inflammation of soft tissues. MRI is also more sensitive at evaluating retropharyngeal and deep cervical nodal metastases (**Fig. 8–5**).[29]

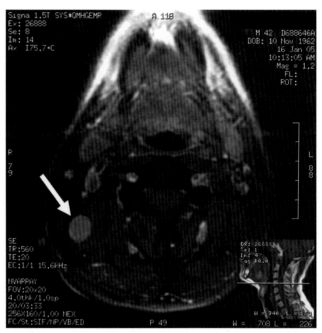

Figure 8–5 MRI scan showing metastatic cervical lymph node (*arrow*).

MRI is able to detect bone marrow infiltration by tumors, whereas CT cannot detect this kind of infiltration unless there is associated bony erosion. It is important to detect this marrow infiltration as it is associated with an increased risk of distant metastases.[30] MRI, however, is unable to evaluate details of bone erosion, and CT should be performed when the status of the base of the skull needs to be evaluated.

Recurrent NPC after radiotherapy may exhibit a range of signal intensities, and these can be difficult to interpret.[31] Both CT and MRI, however, have relatively low sensitivity in detection of tumor recurrence.[32] Positron emission tomography (PET) has been reported to be more sensitive than cross-sectional imaging studies in detecting persistent and recurrent NPC,[33] both at the primary site and in the neck (**Fig. 8–6**).

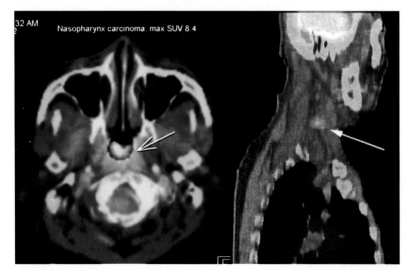

Figure 8–6 PET scan. **Left**: Tumor in nasopharynx (*arrow*). **Right**: Tumor in the cervical lymph node (*arrow*).

Endoscopic Examination

The nasopharynx can be adequately examined under topical anesthesia with either the rigid or flexible endoscope (**Fig. 8–7**). The rigid Hopkin endoscope is 4 mm in diameter, and both the 0-degree and 30-degree scopes give an excellent view of the nasopharynx and tumor on the side of insertion (**Fig. 8–8**). A 70-degree endoscope inserted behind the soft palate allows visualization of the roof of the nasopharynx and both eustachian tube openings and provides a good view of extension of the tumor across the midline (**Fig. 8–9**). These telescopes, however, do not have a suction channel, and the biopsy forceps has to be inserted by the side of the endoscope for a biopsy.

The fiberoptic flexible endoscope on the other hand allows thorough examination of the entire nasopharynx even when it is inserted through one nasal cavity. It has a suction channel for the removal of nasal secretions during examination, and a biopsy forceps can be inserted through this channel to take a biopsy of the tumor under direct vision. It can also be manipulated upward behind the soft palate to examine the nasopharynx from the inferior aspect. In view of the size of the endoscope and its flexibility, it is well tolerated by most patients. Despite all these advantages, the visual image gathered with the flexible endoscope is inferior to that of the rigid endoscope and the cup size of the biopsy forceps is also small, thus the amount of tissue obtained for histologic examination may be suboptimal. Thus, multiple biopsies might have to be taken to increase the yield. Occasionally, the NPC may be located in the submucosal region, thus the mucosal surface has to be broken with the forceps to enable deeper tissue to be obtained.[34]

◆ Staging

There are several staging systems that have been used for NPC. The Ho system is often used in Asia,[35] whereas the American Joint Committee on Cancer/Union Internationale Contre le Cancer (AJCC/UICC) systems are more frequently used in Europe and the United States.[36] The nodal classifica-

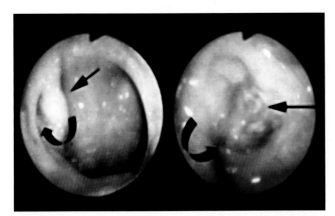

Figure 8–7 Fiberoptic flexible endoscopic views. **Left**: Normal nasopharnyx of right side. Eustachian tube opening (*curved arrow*) and fossa of Rosenmüller (*straight arrows*). **Right**: Tumor arising from the fossa of right side. Eustachian tube opening (*curved arrow*) and tumor (*straight arrow*).

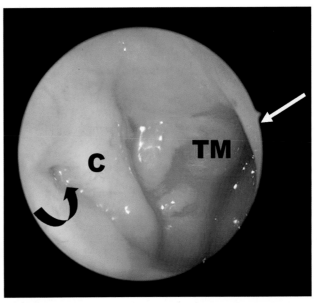

Figure 8–8 Rigid endoscopic view of the right nasopharynx showing tumor in the central posterior wall. (*TM*). The opening of the right eustachian tube (*curved arrow*) and medial crura (*C*) can be seen. The *straight arrow* identifies the posterior edge of the nasal septum.

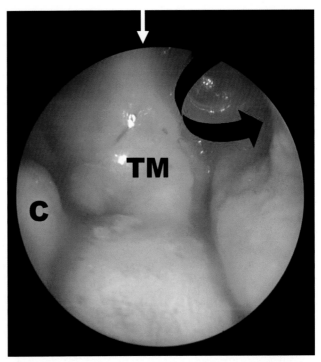

Figure 8–9 Rigid endoscope (70 degree) inserted through the oral cavity, inspecting the nasopharynx from below. Posterior edge of the nasal septum (*straight arrow*), left eustachian tube orifice (*curved arrow*), medial crura of the right eustachian tube orifice (*C*), and nasopharyngeal tumor can be seen extending from the posterior wall onto the roof of the nasopharynx (*TM*).

tion in Ho's staging system has been shown to reflect prognostic evaluation, but its stratification of the T stages into five levels differs from most staging systems for cancer.

With the recent identification of some factors that have prognostic significance such as skull base erosion, involvement of cranial nerves,[37] primary tumor extension to paranasopharyngeal space,[38] and the level and size of the cervical nodes,[39] there is a need for the proposal of a revised staging system, taking all these factors into consideration.

A revised AJCC/UICC staging system was published in 1997[40] (**Table 8–1**). In this new staging system, the T stage has included local tumor extension such as involvement of the nasal fossa, oropharynx, or paranasopharyngeal space. The erosion of skull base, the involvement of infratemporal fossa, orbit, hypopharynx, and cranium or the cranial nerves were all incorporated. The nodal staging has also been revised, and the new staging system has been shown to reflect more precisely patient survival.[41,42]

Table 8–1 American Joint Committee on Cancer Staging System of Tumor in the Nasopharynx

Tumor in Nasopharynx (T)

T1	Tumor confined to the nasopharynx
T2	Tumor extends to soft tissues of oropharynx and/or nasal fossa
T2a	Without parapharyngeal extension
T2b	With parapharyngeal extension
T3	Tumor invades bony structures and/or paranasal sinuses
T4	Tumor with intracranial extension and/or involvement of cranial nerves, infratemporal fossa, hypopharynx, or orbit

Regional Lymph Nodes (N)

The distribution and the prognostic impact of regional lymph node spread from nasopharynx cancer, particularly of the undifferentiated type, is different than that of other head and neck mucosal cancers and justifies use of a different N classification scheme.

NX	Regional lymph nodes cannot be assessed
N0	No regional lymph node metastasis
N1	Unilateral metastasis in lymph node(s), 6 cm or less in greatest dimension, above the supraclavicular fossa
N2	Bilateral metastasis in lymph node(s), 6 cm or less in greatest dimension, above the supraclavicular fossa
N3	Metastasis in a lymph node(s)
N3a	Greater than 6 cm in dimension
N3b	Extension to the supraclavicular fossa

Distant Metastasis (M)

MX	Distant metastasis cannot be assessed
M0	No distant metastasis
M1	Distant metastasis

Stage Grouping

Stage 0	T1s	N0	M0	
Stage I	T1	N0	M0	
Stage IIA	T2a	N0	M0	
Stage IIB	T1	N1	M0	
	T2	N1	M0	
T2a	N1	M0		
	T2b	N0	M0	
T2b	N1	M0		
Stage III	T1	N2	M0	
	T2a	N2	M0	
	T2b	N2	M0	
T3	N0	M0		
T3	N1	M0		
T3	N2	M0		
Stage IVA	T4	N0	M0	
T4	N1	M0		
T4	N2	M0		
Stage IVB	Any T	N3	M0	
Stage IVC	Any T	Any N	M1	

◆ Treatment

As NPC is radiosensitive, radiotherapy alone has been employed as the primary treatment modality for decades both for early and advanced stages of the disease. In recent years, it has been shown that adding chemotherapy is also beneficial and thus the alternative initial treatment is concomitant chemoradiation especially in advanced-stage disease.

Radiotherapy

Radiotherapy is the standard treatment for NPC. Radical radiotherapy should be attempted even with the most advanced locoregional disease, as long as there is no evidence of distant metastases; cure is still a realistic goal. The target volume of radiotherapy includes the primary tumor in the nasopharynx and the involved neck nodes. Because of the high incidence of occult metastases to the cervical lymphatics, prophylactic neck irradiation is a standard for the N0 cases.[43] Good locoregional control should be the prime objective of treatment, as locoregional relapses represent a significant risk factor for the development of distant metastases.[44]

Radiotherapy treatment is usually divided into two phases; with phase I, the radiation field covers the nasopharynx and the upper-neck lymphatics, including the spinal accessory group of lymph nodes, in one target volume using large lateral opposing faciocervical fields, with matching lower anterior cervical field for lower-neck lymphatics. When the spinal cord dose reaches its tolerance dose of 40 to 45 Gy, there are two common options for phase II treatment. Treatment can be continued either using the lateral opposing faciocervical fields but with shrinkage of fields to avoid the spinal cord or by treating the superior-posterior neck lymphatic using matching electron fields. Alternatively, treatment can be changed to lateral opposing facial fields, with matching anterior cervical field for the neck lymphatics.[45,46] During the phase II treatment, an additional anterior facial field is usually added to cover the primary tumor to cut down the radiation dose to the temporomandibular joints.

The major shortcoming of treating the primary tumor and the neck lymphatics in two separate volumes including both of the phase II treatment techniques is the potential for underdosing target volumes for the treatment of the paranasopharyngeal extension of the tumor and the upper-neck nodes at the junction between the primary tumor and neck lymphatics.

The radiotherapy dose of 65 to 75 Gy is normally given to the primary tumor and 65 to 70 Gy to the involved neck nodes, whereas the dose for prophylactic treatment for a node-negative neck is 50 to 60 Gy. This treatment has successfully controlled T1 and T2 tumors in 75 to 90% of cases and T3 and T4 tumors in 50 to 75% of cases.[47–49] Nodal control is achieved in 90% for N0 and N1 cases, but the control rate drops to 70% for N2 and N3 cases.[47]

For T1 and T2 tumors, a booster dose using intracavitary brachytherapy has been shown to improve tumor control by 16%,[50] and for more advanced stage diseases, adjuvant use of chemotherapy is often considered.

Acute Side Effects

During radiotherapy, patients often experience the sensation of dry mouth starting at the end of the first week, and the degree of dryness will progress toward the end of radiotherapy. For most patients, the dryness of mouth becomes permanent if the conventional two-dimensional (2-D) planning of radiotherapy treatment was used. Mucositis involving the posterior part of the oral cavity and the upper part of the oropharynx usually appear toward the end of the fourth week of radiotherapy, and this will progress toward the end of radiotherapy. The mucositis, however, will improve within a few weeks after completion of radiotherapy. Treatment of mucositis is mainly supportive such as the use of gargle and analgesic. For a small percentage of patients, when the mucositis affects adequate oral feeding, nasogastric tube feeding may be required.

Late Sequelae of Therapy

Unfortunately, because of the location of the nasopharynx, it is in close proximity to several radiosensitive, dose-limiting organs. These are the brain stem, temporal lobes, pituitary-hypothalamic axis, middle and inner ears, spinal cord, eyes, and parotid glands. Radical radiotherapy when including these organs may produce undesirable complications. The radiation field sometimes has to include these organs in view of the infiltrative behavior of NPC and the proximity of tumor extension to these organs especially when disease is advanced. It is difficult to protect these structures without reducing the radiation delivered to treat the primary tumor.

These sequelae of radiotherapy for NPC include auditory[51] and neuroendocrine[52] complications, dry mouth, poor oral and dental hygiene,[53,54] radiation-induced soft tissue fibrosis,[55] and carotid artery stenosis.[56] The most debilitating sequelae are the neurologic complications. These may include serious disorders such as temporal lobe necrosis,[57] cranial nerve palsies,[58] and dysphagia,[59] and less obvious effects such as memory,[60] cognitive,[61] and neuropsychological dysfunctions.[62] The use of chemotherapy in more advanced cases further augments the side effects, which include ototoxicity associated with cisplatin.[63]

Reducing the late complications of treatment is one of the main objectives of many current clinical trials. It has been demonstrated that shielding of the pituitary-hypothalamic axis in 2-D planning and treatment can significantly reduce neuroendocrine complications.[64]

The major limitations of 2-D planning for NPC can now be overcome with three-dimensional (3-D) conformal radiotherapy (3-D CRT) and IMRT.[65,66] For extensive tumors, and when the tumor extension was close to the dose-limiting organs, IMRT is distinctly preferable to 3-D CRT because it further improves the dose differential between the tumor and the dose-limiting organs.[67,68] As IMRT allows the primary tumor and the upper-neck nodes to be treated in one volume throughout, the problem of dose uncertainty at the junction between the primary tumor and neck lymphatic target volumes in 2-D planning and treatment is also resolved.

Although IMRT theoretically allows very good dose differential between the tumor and the sensitive adjacent normal tissue structures, the optimal safety margin required between gross tumor and adjacent tissues has not yet been determined. Randomized prospective trials would help to define the optimal safety margin and clinical target volume.

IMRT has achieved excellent locoregional control of NPC,[69] and the degree of short-term control is encouraging.[70] An IMRT study that evaluated prospectively salivary functions confirmed the gradual recovery of parotid function within 2 years after completion of IMRT.[71]

Adjuvant Chemotherapy to Radical Radiotherapy

For the stage III and IV cases, treatment results using radical radiotherapy alone were not satisfactory, and the role of adding chemotherapy has been explored. The Intergroup 1997 study was the first study to demonstrate that the use of *concurrent chemoradiotherapy* (i.e., three courses of adjuvant chemotherapy in addition to initial chemoradiotherapy) improved overall survival when compared with radiotherapy alone.[72] A subsequent report from Taiwan[73] confirmed the benefit of this approach. Despite the use of *concomitant chemoradiotherapy*, distant metastases remain the major cause of failure,[74] and the prognosis for stage IV patients remains grim.[75] Several studies had been launched in different parts of Asia where NPC is endemic to confirm the efficacy of concomitant use of chemotherapy during radical radiotherapy. Because of the poor tolerance of patients to further adjuvant chemotherapy after concomitant chemoradiotherapy, the use of induction chemotherapy to be followed by concurrent chemoradiotherapy has also been studied. The 2004 meta-analysis using updated and pooled patient data from the Sun Yat-sen University, Guangzhou 2001, and Asian Oceanian Clinical Oncology Association 1998 studies noted improvements in relapse-free survival and disease-specific survival.[76] However, overall survival showed no improvement. This is because of the increased intercurrent patient mortality in the treatment group.

Chemotherapy for Metastatic and Advanced Recurrent Nasopharyngeal Carcinoma

Cisplatin-based combination chemotherapy is the most effective treatment for metastatic NPC. Cisplatin and infusional 5-fluorouracil (5-FU) has become the standard treatment, achieving a 66 to 76% response rate.[77]

Several phase II studies on the newer agents have been reported; these included capecitabine, gemcitabine, ifosfamide, paclitaxel, and irinotecan.[78–82] More intensive combinations give a higher response rate, though such intensive chemotherapy is usually associated with increased toxicities.[83–85] Despite the promising results reported for these other chemotherapy combinations, none of them had been compared with the combination of cisplatin and infusional 5-FU in a prospective randomized study.

It is generally agreed that treatment of metastatic NPC using chemotherapy is essentially palliative, though long-term disease-free survivors have been reported.[86] For selected patients with limited metastases, more aggressive additional local treatment can be considered. Resection of lung metastases may result in prolonged control for patients where the spread of the carcinoma to the lung has been limited.[87] When there is limited spread to the mediastinal nodes, the addition of radiotherapy to chemotherapy may also result in more prolonged tumor control.[88]

Treatment of Recurrence

Despite the fact that concomitant chemoradiation has improved the outcome of patients suffering from NPC, there are some patients who still develop local or regional recurrence after the initial radical chemoradiation management. These failures could present either as persistent or recurrent tumor. When the tumor did not regress completely after therapy or reappeared within 3 months after treatment, it was recognized as persistent tumor. For recurrent disease, the tumor showed complete regression after treatment and reappeared only 3 months after completion of treatment.

To successfully manage these persistent or recurrent diseases in the nasopharynx, early detection is essential. The PET is superior both to CT[89] and MRI[33] under these circumstances, and an endoscopic examination with biopsy should be performed to confirm the presence of malignancy in the nasopharynx. Persistent or recurrent tumor in the neck node after chemoradiotherapy, however, is notoriously difficult to confirm, as in some lymph nodes only clusters of tumor cells are present.[90] Thus, fine-needle aspiration cytology aiming to confirm the presence of malignant cells in the nodes is frequently not helpful. The clinical course of the neck node and the findings of PET scan guide the clinician toward further management of these patients.

Locally or regionally persistent or recurrent NPC should be treated whenever possible, because although survival after salvage treatment for extensive disease remains poor, the outcomes of these patients were still superior to those of patients who were given supportive treatment only. Even for those NPC patients with synchronous locoregional failures, aggressive treatment should also be considered for selected patients.[91]

Persistent or Recurrent Tumor in Neck Lymph Nodes

After combined chemoradiation for NPC, the incidence of isolated failure in the neck node was less than 5%.[92] For patients with neck nodes harboring the malignant cells when managed with a second course of external radiotherapy, the reported overall 5-year survival rate was only 19.7%.[93] Radical neck dissection as a form of surgical salvage has been reported to achieve a 5-year local tumor control rate of 66% in the neck and a 5-year actuarial survival of 38%.[94] Frequently, the persistent or recurrent disease in the neck after radiotherapy presents with only one clinically palpable lymph node, and simple excision of the lymph node might be considered sufficient for tumor eradication. Pathology studies of the serial sectioning of the neck dissection specimens obtained from these patients, however, have shown that for those with persistent or recurrent cervical lymph nodes in the neck, the extent of tumor involving local tissue was extensive (**Fig. 8–10**). There were 3 times more pathologic lymph nodes in the neck than what could be detected at clinical examination. There was a 70% incidence of extracapsular spread among the malignant nodes. The affected nodes were closely associated with the sternomastoid muscle, spinal accessory nerve, and the internal jugular vein. Thus, in ensuring the removal of all the tumor-bearing nodes in the neck, a radical neck dissection was considered essential for salvage. Under this clinical situation, the radical neck dissection should be performed to achieve the best outcome.[90]

When tumor in the neck node extends beyond the confines of the lymph node, then radical neck dissection may still fail to remove all malignant tissue. To achieve a similar tumor control rate as when radical neck dissection was performed for less extensive neck disease, further therapy to the tumor bed is essential. This includes further external radiotherapy or brachytherapy. After-loading brachytherapy has been used and has achieved acceptable results.[95] Hollow nylon tubes were placed accurately on the surgical bed at the completion of the radical neck resection, and single-source, high-dose-rate iridium wires were inserted after the neck wound had healed as the after-loading brachytherapy radiation source. As the neck skin was included in the initial radiation field and could not stand further radiation, the skin overlying the planned brachytherapy area should be removed and replaced. The reconstruction of the neck skin is achieved with either a deltopectoral flap or a pectoralis major myocutaneous flap. The former provides full-thickness skin coverage and requires a second-stage operation 3 weeks later to return the deltopectoral flap to the anterior chest wall. The latter is a one-stage procedure, but the chest

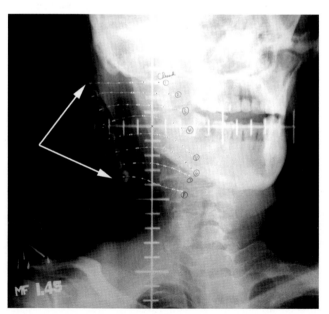

Figure 8–10 Postoperative cheek film of the neck showing the eight nylon tubes with dummy radiation source (*arrows*).

wall would be disturbed. With this new cutaneous coverage, full-dose brachytherapy can be administered for salvage.[95] After the completion of the brachytherapy, the hollow nylon tubes can be removed and the patient returned to general wound healing.

Persistent or Recurrent Tumor in the Nasopharynx

A second course of radiation has been shown to be effective in the treatment of the persistent or recurrent tumor in the nasopharynx after the initial radical radiation. The radiation dose has to be greater than the first treatment, and a salvage rate of 32% has been reported together with a treatment mortality of 1.8%.[96] The sequelae developed after the second course of external radiotherapy are not negligible and affect significantly the quality of life of these patients. Thus, alternative salvage treatment options have been introduced for small persistent or recurrent tumor localized in the nasopharynx. The aim is to eradicate the disease without producing the undesirable side effects. These include stereotactic radiotherapy, brachytherapy, and surgical resection.

Stereotactic Radiotherapy

A small number of patients have been treated with this modality of treatment.[97] For small localized persistent or recurrent tumor treated with stereotactic radiotherapy, a local tumor control rate of 86% at 3 years has been reported.[98] The long-term follow-up results on local tumor control rate, disease-free survival rate, and incidence of complication, however, were not documented.

Brachytherapy

When brachytherapy is employed for the management of persistent or recurrent NPC in the nasopharynx, the radiation source is placed close to or inserted directly into the tumor, delivering high radiation dose at the brachytherapy source, and the radiation dose then declines with increasing distance from the tumor. Thus, the persistent or recurrent tumor in the nasopharynx receives the highest therapeutic radiation while the surrounding tissue was irradiated with a much smaller dose. Intracavitary brachytherapy has been used traditionally for NPCs both as a boost of the primary treatment and as salvage treatment for persistent or recurrent disease.[99] The radiation source such as iridium-192 (^{192}Ir) can be placed in a mold, and this is then inserted into the nasopharynx, delivering 40 Gy for persistent disease and 50 to 60 Gy for recurrent disease. Good local tumor control rates and survival rates have been reported.[100] To circumvent the problem of irregular contour of the primary tumor within the nasopharynx, radioactive interstitial implants were used as a brachytherapy source, and these radiation sources were inserted directly into the tumor. Thus, high-dose radiation is delivered to each region of the localized persistent or recurrent tumor in the nasopharynx.[101]

A frequently employed brachytherapy source is radioactive gold grains (^{198}Au). Gold grains can be implanted either transnasally or using the split-palate approach.[102] The transnasal route is simple but has technical problems. The bleeding encountered during the insertion of the initial gold grains will obscure the viewing of the tumor making subsequent insertions difficult. The split-palate approach was done under general anesthesia. The soft palate was incised in the midline and lifted with the mucoperiosteum of the hard palate. After the retraction of the palatal flaps, the tumor in the nasopharynx was exposed, and accurate implantation of the desired number of gold grains could be performed under direct vision. Thus, an ideal dosimetry for the radiation of the persistent or recurrent tumor could be achieved. The surgical procedure is simple, and the morbidity related to surgery is low.[103] With interstitial gold grain implants in the treatment of persistent and recurrent NPC after radiotherapy, the morbidity related to the second course of radiation is minimal. The 5-year local tumor control rates were 87% and 63%, respectively, and the corresponding 5-year disease-free survival rates were 68% and 60%, respectively.[104]

Surgical Treatment

Nasopharyngectomy

The persistent or recurrent tumor in the nasopharynx on presentation might be bulky or exhibit extensive involvement thus making the application of brachytherapy not satisfactory. Brachytherapy is also not applicable when the tumor extends either directly to the paranasopharyngeal space or affects the lymph nodes in this space. Salvage surgery in the form of nasopharyngectomy with resection of lymph nodes in the paranasopharyngeal space has been shown to be effective to eradicate localized tumor in selected patients.[105]

The nasopharynx is situated in the central part of the head. Tumor located in the region and its vicinity is difficult to be exposed adequately to allow an oncologic resection. Few approaches have been reported to be useful in the exposure of the nasopharynx to allow salvage nasopharyngectomy. Superior and posterior approaches are not practical, as the brain and the vertebral column limit the movement of tissue to get good exposure. The transantral and mid-facial degloving procedures allow the approach of the nasopharynx from the front but do not provide adequate exposure of the whole nasopharynx, including the superior and lateral walls. These anterior approaches, even with controlled fracture of the hard palate followed by its downward displacement, only expose the posterior wall of the nasopharynx and not its lateral walls and its vicinity where most tumors are located.

The nasopharynx can be approached from the inferior aspect employing the transpalatal, transmaxillary, and transcervical approach.[106,107] This approach is useful for tumors located in the central and lower posterior wall of the nasopharynx. For more extensive tumors, especially those situated on the roof and on the lateral wall, the dissection of the paranasopharyngeal space is difficult with this inferior approach. As the lateral extension of the persistent or recurrent NPC frequently extends to tissue planes lying close to the internal carotid artery, this vessel has to be protected during the resection of tumor with this inferior approach.

To approach the nasopharynx from the lateral aspect, approach through the infratemporal fossa to remove pathologic tissue in the region has been described.[108] With this route, a radical mastoidectomy has to be performed and some important structures have to be mobilized; these include the internal carotid artery, the fifth cranial nerve, and the floor of the middle cranial fossa. The resultant morbidities after this approach are not negligible, and considerable surgical expertise is required to carry out this procedure. This approach exposes directly the lateral wall of the nasopharynx including the internal carotid artery on the side of the surgery, thus it is useful for laterally located disease. It however does not provide access to the lateral wall of the nasopharynx on the opposite side.

The nasopharynx can also be approached from the anterolateral route following the lateral swinging hard palate and the maxillary antrum (**Fig. 8–11**). This maxillary swing approach exposes the nasopharynx and its vicinity adequately to allow salvage nasopharyngectomy. The facial incision employed is similar to that of maxillectomy except that there is no incision along the upper alveolar ridge as the anterior cheek flap is not to be separated from the anterior wall of the maxilla. A total of three osteotomies are required to detach the maxilla. The first horizontal osteotomy on the anterior wall of the maxilla is placed below the inferior rim of the orbit, thus the orbital floor is not disturbed. The oscillating saw then goes through the maxillary antrum to separate the posterior wall of the maxilla from its superior attachments. The second osteotomy divides the hard palate in the midline, and the third osteotomy is to separate the maxillary tuberosity from the pterygoid plates with a curved osteotome. After the osteotomies, the maxilla with half of the hard palate attached to the anterior cheek flap can be swung laterally as one osteocutaneous flap (**Fig. 8–12**).[109] The operative procedure involved is similar to that of a maxillectomy, only that here the maxilla is left attached to the anterior cheek flap and is returned to its original position after the nasopharyngectomy. A dental plate is usually made before the operation as this ensures the correct repositioning of the maxilla after removal of tumor. For similar reasons, the holes for the titanium plates that would be used to fix the maxilla to the rest

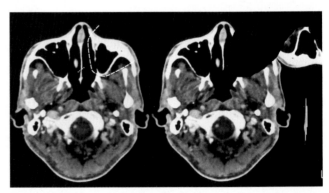

Figure 8–11 Schematic CT image. **Left:** Planned osteotomies of the maxilla and the posterior part of the nasal septum. **Right:** The maxilla is swung laterally while still attached to the cheek flap.

of the facial skeleton were drilled before the osteotomies. After the maxilla is swung laterally, pterygoid plates are removed and the attached pterygoid muscles are retracted, then the entire nasopharynx and the paranasopharyngeal space are exposed to allow an oncologic surgical procedure to be performed. The posterior part of the nasal septum is removed to improve exposure of the opposite nasopharynx. The cartilaginous portion of the eustachian tube together with the lateral wall of the nasopharynx including the fossa of Rosenmüller on the side of the swing is removed with the tumor *en bloc*. The prevertebral muscle could be removed together with the tumor to improve the resection margin, and for similar reason, the anterior wall of the sphenoid sinus is removed. The sphenoid sinus is opened and its mucosa is not disturbed.

The wide exposure achieved after the maxilla is swung laterally allows the dissection of the paranasopharyngeal space under direct vision. Thus, lymph nodes or the tumor that has extended to the paranasopharyngeal space can be removed. The internal carotid artery lying outside the pharyngobasilar fascia can be identified by palpation during the dissection of the paranasopharyngeal space and thus safeguarded (**Fig. 8–13**).

The mortality associated with this salvage surgical procedure is low and acceptable. With the modification of the palatal incision, the complication of postoperative pala-

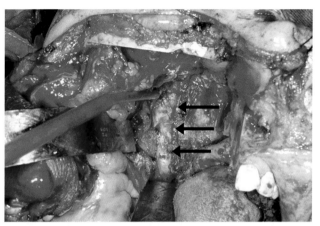

Figure 8–13 After removing the tumor in the nasopharynx and the lymph node in the paranasopharyngeal space, the internal carotid artery can be seen (*arrows*).

tal fistula has been eliminated.[110] Many patients developed some degree of trismus after operation. This is related to the previous radical radiotherapy and the development of additional fibrosis after the dissection around the pterygoid muscle region. The trismus frequently improves with passive stretching.

When the persistent or recurrent tumor can be resected with a clear margin, the long-term results have been satisfactory. The 5-year actuarial control of tumors in the nasopharynx after salvage nasopharyngectomy has been reported to be around 65%, and the 5-year disease-free survival rate is around 54%.[111,112]

◆ Clinical Cases

Case 1 T4 N0 M0 squamous cell carcinoma of the nasopharynx.

Clinical Presentation A 53-year-old Chinese woman presented with right facial pain and tinnitus for 3 months. The patient had no other symptoms, and there was no recent change in appetite and body weight. The patient had no prior history of tobacco, and she is a social drinker.

Examination Clinical examination confirmed palsy of the mandibular division of the right fifth cranial nerve. Otoscopy examination showed right serous otitis media, and tuning fork test confirmed conductive deafness in the right ear. There was no palpable cervical lymph node. Examination of the nasopharynx revealed an exophytic mass in the right fossa of Rosenmüller extending to the right roof. Biopsy of the mass confirmed the presence of undifferentiated carcinoma.

Diagnosis and Workup Complete blood count and renal and liver function tests were normal, and an antibody against VCA of EBV was elevated at 1:40 dilution. MRI of the nasopharynx confirmed erosion of the clivus and tumor extension through the foramen ovale to the right middle cranial fossa and cavernous sinus. There was no

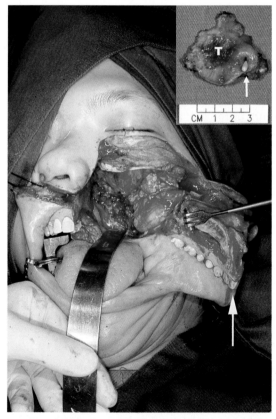

Figure 8–12 The left maxilla is swung laterally to expose the nasopharynx with recurrent tumor. The hard palate and the left central incisor tooth (*arrow*) are shown. **Inset**: Nasopharyngectomy specimen showing tumor (*T*). The eustachian tube opening is marked with a tube (*arrow*)

evidence of neck node involvement. The patient also had a PET scan performed, which confirmed the extent of tumor in the nasopharynx, and there was no evidence of distant metastases.

The patient had a pure tone audiogram performed, which showed air-bone gap confirming conductive deafness. Dental examination showed early carious teeth formation in several teeth, and extraction was performed for the two most badly involved teeth, and dental preventive measures were also performed.

Management After discussion with the patient and her relatives, in view of the presence of skull base erosion and cranial nerve involvement, which are poor risk factors for tumor control, the patient agreed to adjuvant chemotherapy in addition to standard radiotherapy. IMRT was employed for her. A total tumor dose of 68 Gy in 34 fractions over 7 weeks was given, concomitant intravenous chemotherapy (carboplatin) was given on days 1, 22, and 43, and this was followed by three courses of adjuvant intravenous chemotherapy using cisplatin and infusional 5-FU.

Assessment of response of tumor at 8 weeks after completion of radiotherapy using endoscope examination showed complete remission of tumor in the nasopharynx, and this was confirmed by biopsy taken from the initial site of tumor. MRI of the nasopharynx performed at 3 months after completion of radiotherapy also confirmed complete remission.

The patient was regularly followed up with clinical examination and endoscope once every 2 months in the first year and every 3 months in the second and third years. MRI of the nasopharynx and neck was repeated every 6 months in the first 3 years, and the patient remained in remission.

Case 2 T1 N1 M0 squamous cell carcinoma of the nasopharynx.

Clinical Presentation A 35-year-old Chinese woman noted a left upper cervical lymph node with no other symptoms.

Examination Clinical examination demonstrated a 2-cm-diameter, firm lymph node in the left upper neck under the cover of the sternomastoid muscle. The node had a smooth surface and was mobile. There were no other palpable lymph nodes, and there were no other masses or lesions in the head and neck region.

Diagnosis and Workup Fine-needle aspiration cytology showed the presence of metastatic undifferentiated carcinoma, and flexible endoscopic examination of the upper aerodigestive tract revealed an exophytic growth 0.5 cm in diameter in the nasopharynx obscuring the left fossa of Rosenmüller. Biopsy of the lesion in the nasopharynx showed undifferentiated carcinoma.

Management The patient was managed with radical radiation to the nasopharynx and also to both necks. The total radiation dose to the nasopharynx was 68 Gy and to the neck 64 Gy; these were delivered with daily fractions of 200 cGy over 6 weeks. Complete regression of the tumor in the nasopharynx and the cervical lymph nodes was seen at the fourth week after completion of radiation.

The patient remained asymptomatic for 2 years and then she noticed a progressively enlarging left neck swelling. Clinical examination showed a 2-cm-diameter hard mass under the cover of the upper part of the left sternomastoid muscle. The mass was indurated, nontender, and had an ill-defined border. The mass was also attached to underlying structure and thus immobile. The overlying skin however was mobile, and there was no other lymph node detected. There was no hoarseness, no swallowing problem, and also no nasal symptom. Endoscopic examination of the nasopharynx revealed normal findings, and both vocal cords were mobile. There was no serous otitis media. CT showed the presence of a 2-cm-diameter, enlarged lymph node in the upper neck under the cover of the sternomastoid muscle; the border was not clearly defined. EBV titers were not elevated.

Fine-needle aspiration cytology was performed twice and only revealed suspicious cells. Chest x-ray and metastatic workup showed no distant metastasis. In view of the progressively enlarging neck mass and the likelihood of recurrent tumor in the neck lymph node, salvage surgery was planned.

At the time of surgery, excision biopsy of the neck node was performed first, and frozen section of the specimen confirmed the presence of recurrent tumor in the cervical lymph node. The deep surface of the lymph node was also found to be infiltrating the muscular floor of the upper neck, posterior to the carotid sheath. Radical neck dissection was performed removing the sternomastoid muscle, internal jugular vein, and the accessory nerve. Part of the muscle on the floor of the posterior triangle where the node was attached was also removed together with the skin overlying the area. There was no macroscopic tumor left in the operative field. In view of the extensive infiltrative nature of the tumor harboring lymph node, six parallel hollow nylon tubes separated from each other by 1 cm were placed on the tumor bed. The overlying skin defect was reconstructed with a left deltopectoral flap from the left side. Split-thickness skin graft was used to cover the donor site.

Starting from the eighth postoperative day, six iridium wires were inserted into the hollow nylon tubes to deliver a daily dose of 12 Gy to the tumor bed in the neck to a total of 40 Gy. The nylon tubes were removed on the 15th day after the neck dissection, and the deltopectoral flap pedicle was divided and returned to the chest wall on the 28th day after the initial operation. The patient was last seen at 3 years after the radical neck dissection together with the after-loading brachytherapy; there was no evidence of disease.

Case 3 T1 N0 M0 squamous cell carcinoma of the nasopharynx.

Clinical Presentation A 50-year-old Chinese man presented with partial nasal obstruction together with intermittent epistaxis for 1 month.

Examination Flexible endoscopic examination demonstrated a mass in the nasopharynx.

Diagnosis and Workup A biopsy of the mass demonstrated poorly differentiated carcinoma. Clinically, there were no palpable cervical lymph nodes, and subsequent investigation showed no distant metastasis.

Management The patient was treated with radical external radiotherapy delivering 70 Gy to the nasopharynx and 52 Gy to the neck bilaterally. This was completed in July 1997.

The patient recovered from the radiotherapy and remained well for 8 months. He then noticed increased postnasal drip associated with altered blood, especially in the morning. Flexible endoscopic examination of the nasopharynx showed a 1-cm-diameter mucosal irregularity in the right posterior wall of the nasopharynx; the fossa of Rosenmüller was not involved. MRI showed that the recurrent tumor was superficially localized in the nasopharynx, not infiltrating the prevertebral muscle. Multiple biopsies were performed around the edge of the tumor under direct vision of the flexible endoscope. This was to confirm the extent of the recurrent tumor. In view of the small tumor localized in the nasopharynx, brachytherapy using radioactive gold grains (^{198}Au) was chosen. This was performed under general anesthesia with the split-palate approach. Oral endotracheal tube was used during anesthesia. A total of seven gold grains were inserted under direct vision into the tumor achieving good dosimetry. After insertion of the gold grains, to reduce the radiation hazards to the theater personnel, lead shields were used to separate the patient from personnel working in the operating room. The palate wound was closed under direct vision in three layers. The patient recovered from the operation and the palatal wound healed primarily despite the two courses of radiation.

The patient remained well for 15 months and then he noticed repeated episodes of epistaxis, and endoscopic examination revealed an exophytic growth arising from the right fossa of Rosenmüller. Biopsy of the mass confirmed recurrence of the NPC, and subsequent investigations showed no evidence of regional or distant metastasis. MRI showed that the tumor was localized in the nasopharynx and there was no extension to the paranasopharyngeal space, and the internal carotid artery was free of tumor. Although this was a second recurrent tumor, it was still localized in the nasopharynx, thus salvage nasopharyngectomy was planned. As the recurrent tumor was close to the eustachian tube, curative resection should include the resection of the cartilaginous portion of the auditory tube. This could be achieved with the anterolateral approach. The right maxillary antrum together with the hard palate attached to the anterior cheek flap was swung laterally to expose the nasopharynx. Tumor in the right lateral wall of the nasopharynx together with the cartilaginous portion of the eustachian tube was removed *en bloc*. The posterior part of the nasal septum including the rostrum was removed to expose the opposite nasopharynx including the left fossa of Rosenmüller. The anterior wall of the sphenoid sinus was removed to gain additional resection margin. The resection margins were examined with frozen section to ensure complete tumor removal. The inferior turbinate on the side of the swing was removed, and its mucosa was

laid onto the raw area of the nasopharynx to improve healing. The maxilla was returned to its original position and fixed with the rest of the facial skeleton with miniplates and screws. The nasal cavity was packed and a nasogastric tube inserted for feeding in the early postoperative period. The facial and palatal wounds healed well primarily, and the patient was discharged home on the ninth day after operation. The nasal cavity was examined and cleaned at weekly intervals in the first 2 months to ensure complete wound healing. The patient remains well and is free of disease at 5 years after the salvage nasopharyngectomy.

References

1. Sham JS, Choy D, Wei WI. Nasopharyngeal carcinoma: orderly neck node spread. Int J Radiat Oncol Biol Phys 1990;19:929–933
2. Godtfredsen E. On the histopathology of malignant nasopharyngeal tumors. Acta Pathol Microbiol Scand 1944;55(Suppl):38–319
3. Shanmugaratnam K, Sobin LH. Histological typing of upper respiratory tract tumors. In: Shanmugaratnam K, Sobin LH, eds. International Histological Classification of Tumours: No. 19. Geneva: World Health Organization; 1978:32–33
4. Nicholls JM. Nasopharyngeal carcinoma: classification and histological appearances. Adv Anat Path 1997;4:71–84
5. Parkin DM, Whelan SL, Ferlay J, Raymond L, Young J, eds. Cancer Incidence in Five Continents. Vol. VII. Publication No. 143. International Agency for Research on Cancer; 1997:814–815
6. Dickson RI, Flores AD. Nasopharyngeal carcinoma: an evaluation of 134 patients treated between 1971–1980. Laryngoscope 1985;95:276–283
7. Buell P. The effect of migration on the risk of nasopharyngeal cancer among Chinese. Cancer Res 1974;34:1189–1191
8. Fong YY, Chan WC. Bacterial production of di-methyl nitrosamine in salted fish. Nature 1973;243:421–422
9. Yu MC, Ho JH, Lai SH, Henderson BE. Cantonese-style salted fish as a cause of nasopharyngeal carcinoma: report of a case-control study in Hong Kong. Cancer Res 1986;46:956–961
10. zur Hausen H, Schulte-Holthausen H, Klein G, et al. EBV DNA in biopsies of Burkitt tumours and anaplastic carcinomas of the nasopharynx. Nature 1970;228:1056–1058
11. Yu MC, Garabrant DH, Huang TB, Henderson BE. Occupational and other non-dietary risk factors for nasopharyngeal carcinoma in Guangzhou, China. Int J Cancer 1990;45:1033–1039
12. Fang Y, Guan X, Guo Y, et al. Analysis of genetic alterations in primary nasopharyngeal carcinoma by comparative genomic hybridization. Genes Chromosomes Cancer 2001;30:254–260
13. Chen YJ, Ko JY, Chen PJ, et al. Chromosomal aberrations in nasopharyngeal carcinoma analyzed by comparative genomic hybridization. Genes Chromosomes Cancer 1999;25:169–175
14. Cheng Y, Ko JM, Lung HL, Lo PH, Stanbridge EJ, Lung ML. Monochromosome transfer provides functional evidence for growth-suppressive genes on chromosome 14 in nasopharyngeal carcinoma. Genes Chromosomes Cancer 2003;37:359–368
15. Sham JS, Wei WI, Lau SK, Yau CC, Choy D. Serous otitis media. An opportunity for early recognition of nasopharyngeal carcinoma. Arch Otolaryngol Head Neck Surg 1992;118:794–797
16. Lee AW, Foo W, Law SC, et al. Nasopharyngeal carcinoma:presenting symptoms and duration before diagnosis. Hong Kong Med J 1997;3:355–361
17. Ho HC, Ng MH, Kwan HC, Chau JC. Epstein-Barr-virus-specific IgA and IgG serum antibodies in nasopharyngeal carcinoma. Br J Cancer 1976;34:655–660
18. Zeng Y, Zhang LG, Wu YC, et al. Prospective studies on nasopharyngeal carcinoma in Epstein-Barr virus IgA/VCA antibody-positive persons in Wuzhou City, China. Int J Cancer 1985;36:545–547
19. Sham JS, Wei WI, Zong YS, et al. Detection of subclinical nasopharyngeal carcinoma by fibreoptic endoscopy and multiple biopsy. Lancet 1990;335:371–374
20. Chien YC, Chen JY, Liu MY, et al. Serologic markers of Epstein-Barr virus infection and nasopharyngeal carcinoma in Taiwanese men. N Engl J Med 2001;345:1877–1882

21. Henle W, Ho JH, Henle G, Chau JC, Kwan HC. Nasopharyngeal carcinoma: significance of changes in Epstein-Barr virus-related antibody patterns following therapy. Int J Cancer 1977;20:663–672

22. Lo YM, Chan LY, Lo KW, et al. Quantitative analysis of cell-free Epstein-Barr virus DNA in plasma of patients with nasopharyngeal carcinoma. Cancer Res 1999;59:1188–1191

23. Wei WI, Yuen AP, Ng RW, Ho WK, Kwong DL, Sham JS. Quantitative analysis of plasma cell-free Epstein-Barr virus DNA in nasopharyngeal carcinoma after salvage nasopharyngectomy: a prospective study. Head Neck 2004;26:878–883

24. Chong VF, Mukherji SK, Ng SH, et al. Nasopharyngeal carcinoma: review of how imaging affects staging. J Comput Assist Tomogr 1999;23:984–993

25. Emami B, Sethi A, Petruzzelli GJ. Influence of MRI on target volume delineation and IMRT planning in nasopharyngeal carcinoma. Int J Radiat Oncol Biol Phys 2003;57:481–488

26. Sham JS, Cheung YK, Choy D, Chan FL, Leong L. Nasopharyngeal carcinoma: CT evaluation of patterns of tumor spread. AJNR Am J Neuroradiol 1991;12:265–270

27. Chong VF, Fan YF, Khoo JB. Nasopharyngeal carcinoma with intracranial spread: CT and MR characteristics. J Comput Assist Tomogr 1996;20:563–569

28. Fang FM, Leung SW, Wang CJ, et al. Computed tomography findings of bony regeneration after radiotherapy for nasopharyngeal carcinoma with skull base destruction: implications for local control. Int J Radiat Oncol Biol Phys 1999;44:305–309

29. Dillon WP, Mills CM, Kjos B, DeGroot J, Brant-Zawadzki M. Magnetic resonance imaging of the nasopharynx. Radiology 1984;152:731–738

30. Cheng SH, Jian JJ, Tsai SY, et al. Prognostic features and treatment outcome in locoregionally advanced nasopharyngeal carcinoma following concurrent chemotherapy and radiotherapy. Int J Radiat Oncol Biol Phys 1998;41:755–762

31. Ng SH, Chang JT, Ko SF, Wan YL, Tang LM, Chen WC. MRI in recurrent nasopharyngeal carcinoma. Neuroradiology 1999;41:855–862

32. Chong VF, Fan YF. Detection of recurrent nasopharyngeal carcinoma: MR imaging versus CT. Radiology 1997;202:463–470

33. Yen RF, Hung RL, Pan MH, et al. 18-fluoro-2-deoxyglucose positron emission tomography in detecting residual/recurrent nasopharyngeal carcinomas and comparison with magnetic resonance imaging. Cancer 2003;98:283–287

34. Wei WI, Sham JS, Zong YS, Choy D, Ng MH. The efficacy of fiberoptic endoscopic examination and biopsy in the detection of early nasopharyngeal carcinoma. Cancer 1991;67:3127–3130

35. Ho JHC. An epidemiologic and clinical study of nasopharyngeal carcinoma. Int J Radiat Oncol Biol Phys 1978;4:182–198

36. Sobin LH, Wittekind Ch, eds. TNM Classification of Malignant Tumours. 5th ed. New York, NY: Wiley-Liss; 1997;25–30

37. Sham JST, Cheung YK, Choy D, Chan FL, Leong L. Cranial nerve involvement and base of the skull erosion in nasopharyngeal carcinoma. Cancer 1991;68:422–426

38. Chua DTT, Sham JST, Kwong DLW, Choy D, Au GKH, Wu PM. Prognostic value of paranasopharyngeal extension of nasopharyngeal carcinoma. Cancer 1996;78:202–210

39. Teo P, Yu P, Lee WY, et al. Significant prognosticator after primary radiotherapy in 903 nondisseminated nasopharyngeal carcinoma evaluated by computer tomography. Int J Radiat Oncol Biol Phys 1996;36:291–304

40. Fleming ID, Cooper JS, Henson DE, et al, eds. Cancer Staging Manual. 5th ed. Philadelphia, PA: Lippincott-Raven; 1997

41. Cooper JS, Cohen R, Stevens RE. A comparision of staging systems for nasopharyngeal carcinoma. Cancer 1998;83:213–219

42. Özyar E, Yildiz F, Akyol FH, Atahan II. Comparison of AJCC 1988 and 1997 classifications for nasopharyngeal carcinoma. Int J Radiat Oncol Biol Phys 1999;44:1079–1087

43. Lee AW, Sham JS, Poon YF, Ho JH. Treatment of stage I nasopharyngeal carcinoma: analysis of the patterns of relapse and the results of withholding elective neck irradiation. Int J Radiat Oncol Biol Phys 1989;17:1183–1190

44. Kwong D, Sham J, Choy D. The effect of loco-regional control on distant metastatic dissemination in carcinoma of the nasopharynx: an analysis of 1301 patients. Int J Radiat Oncol Biol Phys 1994;30:1029–1036

45. Mesic JB, Fletcher GH, Goepfert H. Megavoltage irradiation of epithelial tumors of the nasopharynx. Int J Radiat Oncol Biol Phys 1981;7:447–453

46. Hoppe RT, Goffinet DR, Bagshaw MA. Carcinoma of the nasopharynx. Eighteen years' experience with megavoltage radiation therapy. Cancer 1976;37:2605–2612

47. Chua DT, Sham JS, Wei WI, Ho WK, Au GK. The predictive value of the 1997 American Joint Committee on Cancer stage classification in determining failure patterns in nasopharyngeal carcinoma. Cancer 2001;92:2845–2855

48. Lee AW, Poon YF, Foo W, et al. Retrospective analysis of 5037 patients with nasopharyngeal carcinoma treated during 1976–1985: overall survival and patterns of failure. Int J Radiat Oncol Biol Phys 1992;23:261–270

49. Wang CC. Improved local control of nasopharyngeal carcinoma after intracavitary brachytherapy boost. Am J Clin Oncol 1991;14:5–8

50. Levendag PC, Lagerwaard FJ, de Pan C, et al. High-dose, high-precision treatment options for boosting cancer of the nasopharynx. Radiother Oncol 2002;63:67–74

51. Ho WK, Wei WI, Kwong DL, et al. Long-term sensorineural hearing deficit following radiotherapy in patients suffering from nasopharyngeal carcinoma: A prospective study. Head Neck 1999;21:547–553

52. Lam KS, Tse VK, Wang C, Yeung RT, Ho JH. Effects of cranial irradiation on hypothalamic-pituitary function–a 5-year longitudinal study in patients with nasopharyngeal carcinoma. Q J Med 1991;78:165–176

53. Pow EH, McMillan AS, Leung WK, Wong MC, Kwong DL. Salivary gland function and xerostomia in southern Chinese following radiotherapy for nasopharyngeal carcinoma. Clin Oral Investig 2003;7:230–234

54. Pow EH, McMillan AS, Leung WK, Kwong DL, Wong MC. Oral health condition in southern Chinese after radiotherapy for nasopharyngeal carcinoma: extent and nature of the problem. Oral Dis 2003;9:196–202

55. Leung SF, Zheng Y, Choi CY, et al. Quantitative measurement of post-irradiation neck fibrosis based on the young modulus: description of a new method and clinical results. Cancer 2002;95:656–662

56. Cheng SW, Ting AC, Lam LK, Wei WI. Carotid stenosis after radiotherapy for nasopharyngeal carcinoma. Arch Otolaryngol Head Neck Surg 2000;126:517–521

57. Lee AW, Kwong DL, Leung SF, et al. Factors affecting risk of symptomatic temporal lobe necrosis: significance of fractional dose and treatment time. Int J Radiat Oncol Biol Phys 2002;53:75–85

58. Lin YS, Jen YM, Lin JC. Radiation-related cranial nerve palsy in patients with nasopharyngeal carcinoma. Cancer 2002;95:404–409

59. Chang YC, Chen SY, Lui LT, et al. Dysphagia in patients with nasopharyngeal cancer after radiation therapy: a videofluoroscopic swallowing study. Dysphagia 2003;18:135–143

60. Lam LC, Leung SF, Chan YL. Progress of memory function after radiation therapy in patients with nasopharyngeal carcinoma. J Neuropsychiatry Clin Neurosci 2003;15:90–97

61. Cheung M, Chan AS, Law SC, Chan JH, Tse VK. Cognitive function of patients with nasopharyngeal carcinoma with and without temporal lobe radionecrosis. Arch Neurol 2000;57:1347–1352

62. Lee PW, Hung BK, Woo EK, Tai PT, Choi DT. Effects of radiation therapy on neuropsychological functioning in patients with nasopharyngeal carcinoma. J Neurol Neurosurg Psychiatry 1989;52:488–492

63. Kwong DL, Sham JS, Au GK, et al. Concurrent and adjuvant chemotherapy for nasopharyngeal carcinoma: a factorial study. J Clin Oncol 2004;22:2643–2653

64. Sham J, Choy D, Kwong PW, et al. Radiotherapy for nasopharyngeal carcinoma: shielding the pituitary may improve therapeutic ratio. Int J Radiat Oncol Biol Phys 1994;29:699–704

65. Waldron J, Tin MM, Keller A, et al. Limitation of conventional two dimensional radiation therapy planning in nasopharyngeal carcinoma. Radiother Oncol 2003;68:153–161

66. Cheng JC, Chao KS, Low D. Comparison of intensity modulated radiation therapy (IMRT) treatment techniques for nasopharyngeal carcinoma. Int J Cancer 2001;96:126–131

67. Wu VW, Kwong DL, Sham JS. Target dose conformity in 3-dimensional conformal radiotherapy and intensity modulated radiotherapy. Radiother Oncol 2004;71:201–206

68. Hsiung CY, Yorke ED, Chui CS, et al. Intensity-modulated radiotherapy versus conventional three-dimensional conformal radiotherapy for boost or salvage treatment of nasopharyngeal carcinoma. Int J Radiat Oncol Biol Phys 2002;53:638–647

69. Lee N, Xia P, Quivey JM, et al. Intensity-modulated radiotherapy in the treatment of nasopharyngeal carcinoma: an update of the UCSF experience. Int J Radiat Oncol Biol Phys 2002;53:12–22

70. Lu TX, Mai WY, Teh BS, et al. Initial experience using intensity-modulated radiotherapy for recurrent nasopharyngeal carcinoma. Int J Radiat Oncol Biol Phys 2004;58:682–687

71. Kwong DL, Pow EH, Sham JS, et al. Intensity-modulated radiotherapy for early-stage nasopharyngeal carcinoma: a prospective study on disease control and preservation of salivary function. Cancer 2004;101:1584–1593

72. Al-Sarraf M, Leblanc M, Giri S, et al. Chemoradiotherapy versus radiotherapy in patients with advanced nasopharyngeal cancer: phase III randomized Intergroup Study 0099. J Clin Oncol 1998;16:1310–1317

73. Lin JC, Jan JS, Hsu CY, et al. Phase III study of concurrent chemoradiotherapy versus radiotherapy alone for advanced nasopharyngeal carcinoma: positive effect on overall and progression-free survival. J Clin Oncol 2003;21:631–637

74. Cheng SH, Jian JJ, Tsai SY, et al. Prognostic features and treatment outcome in locoregionally advanced nasopharyngeal carcinoma following concurrent chemotherapy and radiotherapy. Int J Radiat Oncol Biol Phys 1998;41:755–762

75. Cheng SH, Jian JJ, Tsai SY, et al. Long-term survival of nasopharyngeal carcinoma following concomitant radiotherapy and chemotherapy. Int J Radiat Oncol Biol Phys 2000;48:1323–1330

76. Chua DT, Ma J, Sham JS, et al. Long-term survival after cisplatin-based induction chemotherapy and radiotherapy for nasopharyngeal carcinoma: a pooled data analysis of two phase III trials. J Clin Oncol 2005;23:1118–1124

77. Wang TL, Tan YO. Cisplatin and 5-fluorouracil continuous infusion for metastatic nasopharyngeal carcinoma. Ann Acad Med Singapore 1991;20:601–603

78. Chua DT, Sham JS, Au GK. A phase II study of capecitabine in patients with recurrent and metastatic nasopharyngeal carcinoma pretreated with platinum-based chemotherapy. Oral Oncol 2003;39:361–366

79. Ngan RK, Yiu HH, Lau WH, et al. Combination gemcitabine and cisplatin chemotherapy for metastatic or recurrent nasopharyngeal carcinoma: report of a phase II study. Ann Oncol 2002;13:1252–1258

80. Tan EH, Khoo KS, Wee J, et al. Phase II trial of a paclitaxel and carboplatin combination in Asian patients with metastatic nasopharyngeal carcinoma. Ann Oncol 1999;10:235–237

81. Chua DT, Kwong DL, Sham JS, Au GK, Choy D. A phase II study of ifosfamide, 5-fluorouracil and leucovorin in patients with recurrent nasopharyngeal carcinoma previously treated with platinum chemotherapy. Eur J Cancer 2000;36:736–741

82. Poon D, Chowbay B, Cheung YB, Leong SS, Tan EH. Phase II study of irinotecan (CPT-11) as salvage therapy for advanced nasopharyngeal carcinoma. Cancer 2005;103:576–581

83. Taamma A, Fandi A, Azli N, et al. Phase II trial of chemotherapy with 5-fluorouracil, bleomycin, epirubicin, and cisplatin for patients with locally advanced, metastatic, or recurrent undifferentiated carcinoma of the nasopharyngeal type. Cancer 1999;86:1101–1108

84. Siu LL, Czaykowski PM, Tannock IF. Phase I/II study of the CAPABLE regimen for patients with poorly differentiated carcinoma of the nasopharynx. J Clin Oncol 1998;16:2514–2521

85. Boussen H, Cvitkovic E, Wendling JL, et al. Chemotherapy of metastatic and/or recurrent undifferentiated nasopharyngeal carcinoma with cisplatin, bleomycin, and fluorouracil. J Clin Oncol 1991;9:1675–1681

86. Fandi A, Bachouchi M, Azli N, et al. Long-term disease-free survivors in metastatic undifferentiated carcinoma of nasopharyngeal type. J Clin Oncol 2000;18:1324–1330

87. Cheng LC, Sham JS, Chiu CS, Fu KH, Lee JW, Mok CK. Surgical resection of pulmonary metastases from nasopharyngeal carcinoma. Aust N Z J Surg 1996;66:71–73

88. Kwan WH, Teo PM, Chow LT, Choi PH, Johnson PJ. Nasopharyngeal carcinoma with metastatic disease to mediastinal and hilar lymph nodes: an indication for more aggressive treatment. Clin Oncol (R Coll Radiol) 1996;8:55–58

89. Kao CH, Tsai SC, Wang JJ, Ho YJ, Yen RF, Ho ST. Comparing 18-fluoro-2-deoxyglucose positron emission tomography with a combination of technetium 99m tetrofosmin single photon emission computed tomography and computed tomography to detect recurrent or persistent nasopharyngeal carcinomas after radiotherapy. Cancer 2001;92:434–439

90. Wei WI, Ho CM, Wong MP, Ng WF, Lau SK, Lam KH. Pathological basis of surgery in the management of postradiotherapy cervical metastasis in nasopharyngeal carcinoma. Arch Otolaryngol Head Neck Surg 1992;118:923–929

91. Chua DT, Wei WI, Sham JS, Cheng AC, Au G. Treatment outcome for synchronous locoregional failures of nasopharyngeal carcinoma. Head Neck 2003;25:585–594

92. Huang SC, Lui LT, Lynn TC. Nasopharyngeal cancer: study III. A review of 1206 patients treated with combined modalities. Int J Radiat Oncol Biol Phys 1985;11:1789–1793

93. Sham JS, Choy D. Nasopharyngeal carcinoma: treatment of neck node recurrence by radiotherapy. Australas Radiol 1991;35:370–373

94. Wei WI, Lam KH, Ho CM, Sham JS, Lau SK. Efficacy of radical neck dissection for the control of cervical metastasis after radiotherapy for nasopharyngeal carcinoma. Am J Surg 1990;160:439–442

95. Wei WI, Ho WK, Cheng AC, et al. Management of extensive cervical nodal metastasis in nasopharyngeal carcinoma after radiotherapy: a clinicopathological study. Arch Otolaryngol Head Neck Surg 2001;127:1457–1462

96. Lee AW, Law SC, Foo W, et al. Retrospective analysis of patients with nasopharyngeal carcinoma treated during 1976–1985: survival after local recurrence. Int J Radiat Oncol Biol Phys 1993;26:773–782

97. Xiao J, Xu G, Miao Y. Fractionated stereotactic radiosurgery for 50 patients with recurrent or residual nasopharyngeal carcinoma. Int J Radiat Oncol Biol Phys 2001;51:164–170

98. Yau TK, Sze WM, Lee WM, et al. Effectiveness of brachytherapy and fractionated stereotactic radiotherapy boost for persistent nasopharyngeal carcinoma. Head Neck 2004;26:1024–1030

99. Wang CC, Busse J, Gitterman M. A simple afterloading applicator for intracavitary irradiation of carcinoma of the nasopharynx. Radiology 1975;115:737–738

100. Law SC, Lam WK, Ng MF, Au SK, Mak WT, Lau WH. Reirradiation of nasopharyngeal carcinoma with intracavitary mold brachytherapy: an effective means of local salvage. Int J Radiat Oncol Biol Phys 2002;54:1095–1113

101. Harrison LB, Weissberg JB. A technique for interstitial nasopharyngeal brachytherapy. Int J Radiat Oncol Biol Phys 1987;13:451–453

102. Wei WI, Sham JS, Choy D, Ho CM, Lam KH. Split-palate approach for gold grain implantation in nasopharyngeal carcinoma. Arch Otolaryngol Head Neck Surg 1990;116:578–582

103. Choy D, Sham JS, Wei WI, Ho CM, Wu PM. Transpalatal insertion of radioactive gold grain for the treatment of persistent and recurrent nasopharyngeal carcinoma. Int J Radiat Oncol Biol Phys 1993;25:505–512

104. Kwong DL, Wei WI, Cheng AC, et al. Long term results of radioactive gold grain implantation for the treatment of persistent and recurrent nasopharyngeal carcinoma. Cancer 2001;91:1105–1113

105. Wei WI, Ho CM, Yuen PW, Fung CF, Sham JS, Lam KH. Maxillary swing approach for resection of tumors in and around the nasopharynx. Arch Otolaryngol Head Neck Surg 1995;121:638–642

106. Fee WE Jr, Roberson JB Jr, Goffinet DR. Long-term survival after surgical resection for recurrent nasopharyngeal cancer after radiotherapy failure. Arch Otolaryngol Head Neck Surg 1991;117:1233–1236

107. Morton RP, Liavaag PG, McLean M, Freeman JL. Transcervico-mandibulo-palatal approach for surgical salvage of recurrent nasopharyngeal cancer. Head Neck 1996;18:352–358

108. Fisch U. The infratemporal fossa approach for nasopharyngeal tumors. Laryngoscope 1983;93:36–44

109. Wei WI, Lam KH, Sham JS. New approach to the nasopharynx: the maxillary swing approach. Head Neck 1991;13:200–207

110. Ng RW, Wei WI. Elimination of palatal fistula after the maxillary swing procedure. Head Neck 2005;27:608–612

111. Fee WE Jr, Moir MS, Choi EC, Goffinet D. Nasopharyngectomy for recurrent nasopharyngeal cancer: a 2- to 17-year follow-up. Arch Otolaryngol Head Neck Surg 2002;128:280–284

112. Wei WI. Nasopharyngeal cancer: current status of management. Arch Otolaryngol Head Neck Surg 2001;127:766–769

9

Carcinoma of the Skin of the Head, Face, and Neck

Brian A. Moore, David Rosenthal, Merrill S. Kies, and Randal S. Weber

◆ Epidemiology

Skin cancer, including both melanoma and nonmelanoma cancer, is the most common cancer in the United States, and the incidence continues to rise. Although the biologic behavior of melanoma and nonmelanoma skin cancers differs, the pathogenesis, anatomic considerations, and fundamental techniques employed in the management of these malignancies are similar. Cutaneous melanoma and aggressive nonmelanoma skin cancers of the head and neck require a multidisciplinary approach that involves the judicious application of surgery, radiation, and systemic therapy.

Otolaryngologists and other professionals who care for patients with disorders of the head and neck will be increasingly faced with patients with nonmelanoma skin cancer (NMSC) and cutaneous melanoma. This chapter will provide an overview of the optimal management of these lesions, focusing on their shared, as well as their unique, features. Important differences in the biologic behavior of melanoma versus nonmelanoma skin cancers, with their resultant treatment implications, will be highlighted. By identifying clinical and histopathologic features of aggressive disease, appropriate therapies may be administered, thereby avoiding unnecessary morbidity or toxicity. Surgical techniques that maximize local control with preservation or restoration of function and cosmesis will be described. Contemporary strategies for managing the regional lymphatics and the indications for and types of systemic therapies will be discussed. Because of the increasing frequency of all types of skin cancer of the head and neck, efforts to develop reliable preventive measures and screening programs will also be noted, as the keys to halting the growth and impact of this pandemic lie in prevention and early detection.

Nonmelanoma Skin Cancer

NMSC affects more than 1.3 million people annually in the United States at a total annual cost that exceeds $426 million, and this incidence has risen significantly over the past 30 years.[1-3] Because of the relationship between ultraviolet light exposure and the development of NMSC, these lesions tend to occur on sun-exposed areas of the body, and 75% arise on the head and neck. The impact of ultraviolet light exposure on the development of NMSC is further accentuated by the increasing incidence of NMSC as degrees of latitude converge toward the Equator.[4] Patients, particularly men, over the age of 50 years are generally considered to be at greatest risk of developing NMSC, but recent studies have demonstrated an increase in the incidence of these cancers in women and in younger patients.[5] The rising incidence of NMSC in younger patients is accompanied by evidence that aggressive variants of NMSC are becoming more common in younger patients, especially women.[6]

Basal cell carcinoma accounts for 80% of NMSCs, and squamous cell carcinoma comprises the remaining 20%. Although more than 95% of NMSCs may be cured by a variety of surgical and nonsurgical therapies, aggressive variants of NMSC exist that are characterized by recurrence, metastases, and increased morbidity, leading to at least 2500 deaths per year.[7] The clinical challenge lies in the early identification of these aggressive lesions to deliver appropriate multidisciplinary care, leading to improved disease control and survival. Clinicians can no longer assume that all NMSCs are created equal.

Cutaneous Melanoma

The importance of skin cancer as an emerging public health dilemma is further underscored by the rising incidence and mortality attributed to cutaneous melanoma. Since 1950, reports document an increase of more than 600% in the annual incidence of cutaneous melanoma, with an attendant increase of 165% in annual mortality.[8] Recent estimates indicate that cutaneous melanoma affected more than 55,000 Americans in 2004 and led to more than 7900 deaths, ranking seventh and fifth in cancer incidence among American women and men, respectively.[9] Unlike nonmelanoma skin cancer, cutaneous melanoma tends to afflict a younger population, making it the second leading cause of lost productive years and the most common cancer in women ages 20 to 29 years.[8]

Cutaneous melanoma arises on the skin of the head and neck in up to 30% of cases, making it less common than nonmelanoma skin cancer in this region.[10] Nevertheless, the incidence of cutaneous melanoma of the head and neck remains greater than the relative proportion of total body surface area occupied by craniocervical structures, reflecting the relative impact of sun exposure and melanocyte density on the development of these lesions.[10] The management of cutaneous melanoma provides an excellent example of the importance of a multidisciplinary team in head and neck oncology, as concerns for distant metastases predominate and because many lessons have been learned from the experience of melanoma in other anatomic sites.

◆ Etiology

Ultraviolet Light Exposure

Exposure to ultraviolet light has been identified as the main factor contributing to the development of melanoma and nonmelanoma skin cancer. The impact of early, intermittent, or excessive sun exposure and a history of blistering sunburns cannot be underestimated. The rising incidence of all types of skin cancer may be attributed to societal values on appearance and a tanned complexion arising from sunbathing or the use of artificial tanning beds, in addition to ozone depletion and increased surveillance.[5]

Molecular Biology and Genetics of Nonmelanoma Skin Cancer

The primacy of sun exposure in the development of skin cancer of the head and neck is underscored by its effects at the cellular and ultrastructural levels. Ultraviolet light fosters DNA damage, inflammation, erythema, sunburns, and immunosuppression. The synergistic effects of ultraviolet B (UVB; 290 to 320 nm) and ultraviolet A (UVA; 320 to 400 nm) radiation create mutations in keratinocyte DNA, often through pyrimidine dimer formation in the p53 tumor suppressor gene and through loss of the Fas-Fas ligand interaction.[11] In the usual setting, these mutations are quickly repaired, but inadequate or failed DNA repair mechanisms, as in xeroderma pigmentosum, will allow clonal expansion of the mutated keratinocyte(s) that culminates in the development of cutaneous malignancy.[2]

Chronic ultraviolet light exposure accentuates these acute effects and leads to the accumulation of mutated and dysregulated cells until squamous cell carcinoma develops, further aided by activation of protooncogenes such as *ras* and inactivation of other tumor suppressor genes including *PTCH* and *INK4a/ARF*.[11] Mutations in the *PTCH* tumor suppressor gene, alterations in the pathway of the protein sonic hedgehog, and abnormalities in the nuclear factor kappa B (NF-κB)

signaling pathway have also been linked to the development of sporadic and familial cases of basal cell carcinoma.[12]

The importance of genetics in cutaneous malignancy is epitomized by xeroderma pigmentosum, an autosomal-recessive condition in which defective DNA repair often leads to the development of NMSC or melanoma by age 10 years. Patients with albinism and those with congenital basal cell nevus syndrome also suffer from NMSC at higher rates than does the general population.

Congenital basal cell nevus syndrome is an autosomal dominant condition characterized by multiple pigmented basal cell carcinomas, odontogenic keratocysts, rib anomalies, plantar pits, and calcification of the falx cerebri. Basal cell nevus syndrome has been attributed to a loss of heterozygosity at chromosome 9q22-31, but the condition remains multigenic, with mutations, genetic polymorphisms, and environmental influences all contributing to its pathogenesis.[13,14] Genetic abnormalities predisposing to skin cancer are not restricted to NMSC, however, as mutations are also associated with malignant melanoma.

Molecular Biology and Genetics of Melanoma

Melanoma is thought to arise from a similar interplay of ultraviolet light–induced damage to melanocyte DNA, growth factor release, local immunosuppression, and escape from the controls of normal cell growth. Mutations in the melanocortin-1 receptor (MC1R) gene, cyclin-dependent kinase inhibitor 2a (CDKN2A), CDK4, *NRAS*, and *BRAF* have been linked to malignant melanoma, although aberrations in the latter two do not appear to be causative.[15,16]

Patients with familial melanoma have been shown to develop disease at a younger age than patients with sporadic melanoma, but there remains much debate over potential differences in biologic behavior.[17] Several clinical features have been associated with genetic susceptibility to melanoma: multiple cases of melanoma on the same side of the family, multiple primary cutaneous melanomas in the same individual, earlier age of onset of cutaneous melanoma, multiple nevi, and, possibly, other cancers.[16] In the familial melanoma/dysplastic nevus syndrome (FM/DNS), a pattern of cutaneous melanoma arising in atypical moles has been identified in which the lifetime risk of melanoma for family members with dysplastic nevi approaches 100%. Through linkage analysis, this condition was mapped to chromosome 9p21 at the locus of the p16 gene and CDKN2A.[10,16,18,19] Patients with inactivating mutations in CDKN2A have been reported to have a lifetime risk of melanoma of 50 to 90% by age 90.[20] Unlike cutaneous squamous cell carcinoma, abnormalities in p53 appear to play a less prominent role in the early stages of malignant melanoma.[15]

Precursor Lesions

Preexisting or precursor lesions play a prominent role in the development of both NMSC and cutaneous melanoma of the head and neck. Cutaneous squamous cell carcinoma commonly arises from actinic keratoses (AKs), which are small, scaly lesions that appear pink, brown, or skin-colored. The presence of AKs imparts a cumulative lifetime risk of developing cutaneous squamous cell carcinoma of 6 to 10%, and an individual lesion has an annual risk of progression to invasive cancer of 0.025 to 20%, depending on the duration of the lesion and the total number of AKs present.[2] Cutaneous squamous cell carcinoma has also been described to arise from Bowen's disease, bowenoid papulosis, and epidermodysplasia verruciformis. Similarly, at least 81% of patients with cutaneous melanoma describe a change in a preexisting lesion. Although the presence of numerous freckles or pigmented lesions places an individual at a higher risk of malignant melanoma, large congenital nevi, sporadic dysplastic nevi, and lentigo maligna have been noted to devolve to malignant melanoma at rates of 5 to 33%.[10]

Previous Skin Malignancy

Not surprisingly, a history of cutaneous cancer of the head and neck predisposes individuals to developing additional lesions, and there is a reasonable amount of crossover between NMSC and melanoma. Patients who have been treated for one basal cell carcinoma (BCC) have a 3-year cumulative risk of developing another BCC of 40%, which is 10 times the risk of developing BCC of the general population. Similarly, patients with a history of cutaneous squamous cell carcinoma (SCC) have a 3-year relative risk of a second primary cutaneous SCC of 18%, which is 10 times the risk of initial lesions for the general population.[21] According to surveillance, epidemiology, and end result (SEER) data, patients with a history of cutaneous melanoma are 10 times more likely to develop second primary melanomas than the rate of de novo melanoma in the overall SEER population.[22]

Other Risk Factors

Notwithstanding the importance of ultraviolet light exposure, there are several other patient, environmental, and genetic risk factors for the development of NMSC and melanoma. These associations are summarized in **Table 9–1**.[2,12]

Radiation Exposure

The potential impact of ionizing radiation on skin cancer is underscored by the association between prior radiation treatment and the development of NMSC in survivors. A recent analysis of a cohort of childhood cancer survivors revealed that prior radiotherapy was associated with a 6.3-fold increased risk of developing NMSC, particularly BCC, and the majority of tumors occurred within radiation fields. Survivors were more likely to develop NMSC at a younger age than the general population, and NMSCs have emerged as the most common second malignancy to affect these individuals.[23]

Immune Compromise

Immunosuppression, particularly in the setting of organ transplantation or hematologic malignancy such as chronic

Table 9–1 Risk Factors for Developing Skin Cancer of the Head and Neck

Melanoma and NMSC	Melanoma	NMSC
Childhood sun exposure	Family history of melanoma	Ionizing radiation
Intermittent sun exposure	Preexisting pigmented lesions	Genodermatoses
Severe sunburns	Large congenital nevi	Albinism
Fair complexion	Sporadic dysplastic nevi	Xeroderma pigmentosum
Blond or red hair	Lentigo maligna	Basal cell nevus syndrome
Blue or green eyes		Bazex syndrome
Fitzpatrick class 1–2		Actinic keratoses
		Immunosuppression
		Organ transplantation
		Chronic lymphocytic leukemia
		Lymphoma
		Chemical exposures
		Polycyclic hydrocarbons
		Arsenic
		Coal tar
		Psoralens
		Human papillomavirus infection
		Chronic irritation
		Burn scars
		Prior skin cancer (including melanoma)
		Bowen's disease
		Bowenoid papulosis
		Epidermodysplasia verruciformis

lymphocytic leukemia or lymphoma, constitutes another risk factor for developing cutaneous malignancies. Intensive immunosuppressive regimens for cardiac transplantation have been associated with aggressive cutaneous SCC and melanoma. In this population, cutaneous SCC occurs much more commonly than BCC, and local recurrence, nodal metastases, distant spread, and mortality occur more frequently, reflecting the importance of immune surveillance in the detection and elimination of cutaneous malignancy.[24]

◆ Histopathology

Basal Cell Carcinoma

BCC exists in several histologic subtypes: superficial, nodular, infiltrative, and micronodular. Typically, superficial BCCs (roughly 25% of cases) tend to occur on the trunk and appear as plaque-like lesions, with well-defined borders. Nodular BCCs (60%) present as the characteristic "rodent ulcer," with raised edges around central ulceration, and they exhibit a predilection for the head and neck. Peripheral palisading is the histopathologic hallmark of these subtypes of BCC. Generally, superficial and nodular BCCs are not aggressive neoplasms, and they respond well to a variety of established techniques, including topical interventions.[12,25]

Aggressive Basal Cell Carcinoma

Infiltrative, formerly known as morpheaform, and micronodular BCCs comprise only 2 to 5% and 15% of clinically detected BCCs, but they are regarded as more aggressive variants, with a tendency for local recurrence. Infiltrative lesions demonstrate a significant amount of subclinical spread, due to the existence of tumor islands and ill-defined projections. Micronodular lesions are aptly named due to their appearance as small nodules with peripheral palisading.[12,25] Lesions have been described that demonstrate more than one histologic pattern, and treatment is tailored to the more aggressive pathology. Aggressive BCCs have been defined as lesions with an initial diameter exceeding 1 cm, those that have recurred at least twice despite therapy otherwise deemed to be adequate, and extension into deeper, noncutaneous tissues.[26] BCC rarely metastasizes, with reported incidences of less than 1%, but it tends to be locally aggressive and can result in significant morbidity if neglected (**Fig. 9–1**).

Squamous Cell Carcinoma

The strong association between cutaneous SCC and ultraviolet light exposure predisposes SCC to appear on the head and neck. The lesions commonly appear as firm, pale to pink, textured lesions that may be hyperkeratotic. They frequently arise in the setting of a preexisting AK. Cutaneous SCC must be differentiated from AK and BCC, as well as keratoacanthoma, which is a rapidly growing ulceronodular lesion that resembles SCC histologically but can be differentiated

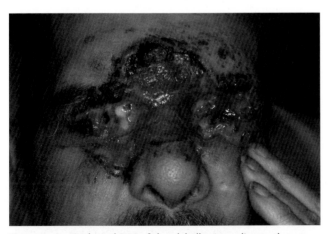

Figure 9–1 Neglected BCC of the glabella. According to the patient, the lesion had been present for ~10 years, but he did not seek medical attention until he lost vision in both eyes. After multidisciplinary evaluation and ethics panel discussion, the patient underwent radical excision of the facial skin, total rhinectomy, and bilateral orbital exenteration with free flap reconstruction. He remains without evidence of recurrent disease after completing adjuvant radiation therapy.

by an experienced dermatopathologist and by its mercurial clinical course. Histologic variants of SCC include verrucous carcinoma, a slow-growing exophytic lesion that can be locally aggressive, spindle cell SCC, desmoplastic SCC, and basosquamous carcinoma.[2]

Spindle Cell Squamous Carcinoma

Spindle cell carcinoma of the skin is an aggressive variant of SCC that is prone to perineural invasion, local recurrence, and regional metastases. Histologically, the hallmark spindle cells are poorly differentiated and surrounded by collagen. Diagnosis may be aided by electron microscopy and immunohistochemical staining for cytokeratins.[27]

Desmoplastic Squamous Cell Carcinoma

Desmoplastic SCC is characterized by fine branches of tumor cells in the periphery and a desmoplastic reaction in the surrounding stroma. Desmoplastic cutaneous SCC demonstrates a predilection for arising on the ear, and it has been noted to be thicker and more advanced at diagnosis compared with typical SCC. These variants have been associated with 6 times the rate of metastasis and 10 times the rate of local recurrence as non–desmoplastic cutaneous SCC in a prospective series.[28]

Basosquamous Carcinoma

Basosquamous carcinoma, also known as basaloid squamous (cell) carcinoma, is another aggressive variant of cutaneous SCC that is characterized by features of both SCC and BCC. Its key features include malignant basal cells with peripheral palisading nuclei and aggregates of squamous cells with eosinophilic cytoplasm without a transition zone between the basal cell and the squamous cell components. Although these lesions account for only 1 to 2% of skin cancers, they often demonstrate lymphatic and perineural invasion. Basosquamous carcinoma of the skin is characterized by local recurrence and metastasis, and adjuvant therapy may be indicated.[29]

Aggressive Nonmelanoma Skin Cancer

Both BCC and SCC of the skin can demonstrate clinically aggressive behavior in which lesions are prone to recurrence and metastasis, with attendant morbidity and mortality. These lesions are of particular importance to the head and neck surgeon, as aggressive NMSCs frequently fail standard ablative or nonablative dermatologic treatments. The clinical and pathologic features of aggressive NMSCs, as described by Lai and colleagues, are summarized in **Table 9–2**.[30,31]

A recent prospective study identified several factors on univariate analysis that were strongly associated with diminished disease-specific survival (DSS) in cutaneous SCC: recurrent lesions, invasion beyond the subcutaneous tissues, perineural invasion, and increasing depth of invasion. Based on statistical models, lesions larger than 4 cm, those with perineural invasion, and invasion beyond the subcutaneous tissues were as-

Table 9–2 Features of Aggressive Nonmelanoma Skin Cancer

Clinical Features	Pathologic Features
Recurrent lesions	Poor differentiation
Regional metastases	Desmoplastic SCC
Size >2 cm	Spindle cell SCC
Rapid growth	Basosquamous carcinoma
Location	Infiltrative BCC
Central H-zone of the face	

sociated with a marked decrease in DSS. In fact, patients with none of these features exhibited a 3-year DSS of 100%, but DSS dropped to 70% when at least one of the high-risk features was present.[32] Other histopathologic features that presage recurrence and metastases include the presence of inflammation and lymphovascular invasion.[33] Fortunately, dermatopathologists now recognize the prognostic import of certain of the above features, and there is increasing documentation of important pathologic features, culminating in the ideal pathology report depicted in **Table 9–3**.[7]

Melanoma

Lentigo Maligna

Lentigo maligna has been described as an atypical proliferation of melanocytes within the epidermis, although it remains unclear if it is a precursor lesion to malignant melanoma. Lentigo maligna frequently occurs on sun-exposed areas of the body in older patients, reflecting the importance of chronic ultraviolet light exposure. Classically, the lesions arise on the cheek, with poorly defined borders and frequent subclinical extension. On histopathologic analysis, there is an increased concentration of atypical melanocytes in the basal layer of the epidermis, appearing as single cells or junctional nests with underlying solar elastosis. Although lentigo maligna has not reached the point of invasion, it merits appropriate

Table 9–3 Components of a Thorough Pathology Report

NMSC	Melanoma
Histologic type	Histologic type
Differentiation	Depth of invasion
Depth of invasion	Clark level
Clark level	Breslow thickness (mm)
Breslow thickness (mm)	Patterns of growth
Perineural invasion	Vertical phase present/absent
Lymphovascular invasion	Radial phase present/absent
Inflammation	Ulceration
Margins	Perineural invasion
Lesion size	Regression
	Margins
	Satellitosis
	Special stains
	S-100
	MART1
	HMB-45

therapy because nearly 20% of lentigo maligna lesions may exhibit features of lentigo maligna melanoma.[34]

Lentigo Maligna Melanoma

Although lentigo maligna melanoma is the least common type of melanoma (5 to 10% of cases), it presents a clinical challenge to head and neck surgeons because 50% of cutaneous malignant melanomas of the head and neck are lentigo maligna melanoma.[34] Patients with lentigo maligna melanoma tend to be older than patients with lentigo maligna, and these lesions are also commonly encountered on the cheek (**Fig. 9–2**). Lentigo maligna melanoma is slowly progressive and exhibits a lengthy radial growth phase, with clustering of neoplastic melanocytes in the epidermal-dermal junction and along skin appendages. The hallmark of lentigo maligna melanoma is invasion into the papillary dermis.[10]

Superficial Spreading Melanoma

Generally regarded as the most common histologic variant of melanoma, superficial spreading melanoma exhibits a radial growth phase that is followed by a vertical growth phase, heralding more aggressive disease. In superficial spreading melanoma, homogeneous neoplastic cells are distributed in all layers of the erpidermis.[10]

Desmoplastic Melanoma

Desmoplastic melanoma is an uncommon histologic subtype that presents a unique clinical challenge because of its atypical appearance and aggressive behavior. The lesions may be nonpigmented and often occur on the head and neck, resembling NMSC as indurated and textured abnormalities. On histopathologic analysis, the lesions are poorly circumscribed, with infiltrates of spindle cells in a fibrous or myxoid stroma.

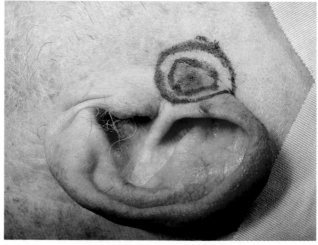

Figure 9–2 Lentigo maligna melanoma of the left preauricular area. This is an intraoperative photograph before planned wide local excision and split-thickness skin graft reconstruction. The borders of the lesion are meticulously marked (inner circle), and 5-mm margins were taken around the lesion.

Special staining for S-100 protein may be required to elucidate the correct diagnosis.[10,35]

Clinically, desmoplastic melanoma is characterized by local recurrence, distant metastases, and a lower than expected risk of regional metastases. Perineural invasion occurs frequently and has been linked to not only the high rate of local failure but also to distant metastases and diminished survival.[35]

Other Variants of Melanoma

Nodular melanoma is characterized by an early vertical growth, leading to deeper lesions at presentation. Fortunately, nodular melanoma has been reported to comprise less than 15% of all melanoma lesions. Although it does not occur on the head and neck, acral lentiginous melanoma merits brief comment. It is encountered on the palms and soles and is marked by large, homogeneous malignant cells in the basal layer of the epidermis.[10]

◆ Diagnosis and Workup

History and Physical Examination

As in all conditions, an adequate history and physical exam holds the clues to the diagnosis in the majority of cases. Patients with risk factors such as fair skin, a history of early or severe sunburns, recreational or occupational exposure to ultraviolet light, family history of skin cancer, previous skin cancers, prior radiation treatment, and immunosuppression should undergo comprehensive cutaneous exams on a regular basis, at least once per year. Early detection of skin cancer, regardless of histology, potentially allows less destructive treatments and promotes improved outcomes.

The most concerning complaint that suggests a diagnosis of skin cancer is growth or change in appearance of an existing cutaneous lesion. Other symptoms such as itching, formication, bleeding, ulceration, and pain may be the harbinger of aggressive disease. Vigilance, from both patient and provider, is required to follow skin lesions and detect significant changes over time. Individual memory and subjective assessment can be augmented by photographic documentation.

"ABCDs" of Melanoma

Following a simple "ABCD" evaluation promotes recognition of suspicious lesions: Asymmetry, Border irregularities, Color variegation, and Diameter greater than 6 mm have been shown to correlate with malignancy, particularly melanoma.[36] In addition to a thorough visual inspection of all cutaneous, lip, and mucosal surfaces, use of a Wood's lamp has been shown to be useful in determining the true clinical extension of pigmented lesions. By preferentially absorbing the UVA black light from the Wood's lamp, the borders of pigmented lesions are depicted in greater contrast.[34]

Care must be taken when examining a patient with melanoma to determine if there are any surrounding abnormalities that could constitute satellite lesions. A comprehensive cutaneous exam should be performed to detect other suspicious lesions and signs of photoaging, including close inspection of the scalp. A careful neurologic exam focusing on motor and sensory function of the cranial nerves should be performed to detect clinical evidence of perineural invasion, although most cases of perineural invasion are asymptomatic. Palpation of the parotid glands and cervical lymphatics should also be performed to detect regional metastases.

Biopsy

Once a suspicious lesion has been identified, a biopsy should be performed to determine the diagnosis. Although many techniques for cutaneous biopsy have been described, the method of choice must allow for an assessment of the depth. Excisional biopsy and incisional techniques such as punch biopsy, with a 2-, 4-, or 6-mm punch, are acceptable methods for lesions on the head and neck. If an excisional biopsy is performed, 1- to 2-mm margins should be taken, and the lesion should be marked and oriented to facilitate subsequent definitive excision, if necessary. If an incisional, or punch, technique is employed, biopsies should be taken from the thickest and most pigmented areas of the lesion.[34] The resultant defect may be allowed to heal by secondary intention, or it may be sutured with absorbable material in either a linear or purse-string fashion. Shave or partial-thickness biopsies are inadequate and should not be performed because they provide no information on the depth of invasion.[10]

Adjuncts

In the majority of cases of BCC and SCC, no additional diagnostic tests are necessary once the pathology has been confirmed. However, once an aggressive NMSC or melanoma has been diagnosed, additional tests may be performed to determine the extent of local disease or the presence of regional or distant metastases. In the setting of aggressive NMSCs, anatomic imaging may be indicated.

Imaging Studies

Evaluation of the extent of a clinically advanced lesion, potential bone involvement, and detection of nodal metastases may be accomplished with computed tomography (CT) scanning. Evidence of advanced perineural invasion may be manifest on CT scan images by enlargement of a neural foramen at the skull base, asymmetry in the pterygomaxillary space, or by asymmetric enhancement of a cranial nerve. Close attention should be paid to the parotid gland, the perifacial nodes, the external jugular chain nodes, and the upper cervical nodes, as these basins are commonly involved with metastatic cutaneous carcinoma.[33]

Because of its improved sensitivity with soft tissue, magnetic resonance imaging (MRI) is a useful adjunct in aggressive NMSC and melanoma, as it can detect perineural invasion, deep extension into subcutaneous tissues, and evidence of involvement of important sensory and neural structures, such as the orbital contents.[37] Both CT and MRI complement each other and together can provide reliable information for tumor staging and treatment planning. For instance, erosion of the calvarium may be detected on a CT scan, but a subsequent MRI will reveal the extent of bone invasion and indicate the presence and degree of intracranial involvement. Other modalities such as ultrasound and positron emission tomography (PET) scanning, as well as emerging techniques that fuse anatomic and metabolic data, demonstrate great potential due to their noninvasive character, but their routine use remains unproved. Detection of systemic metastases in NMSC may be accomplished with simple laboratory tests including a liver panel and a chest radiograph, although this should only be pursued in the setting of advanced disease.

Guidelines for the detection of metastatic disease and follow-up of patients with cutaneous melanoma are determined by the clinical stage of the primary lesion. Algorithms have been developed that are widely accepted and may be obtained from the National Comprehensive Cancer Network (NCCN; www.nccn.gov) and the National Cancer Institute (NCI; www.nci.nih.gov). Patients with lentigo maligna melanoma and those with thin lesions with favorable signs (no ulceration, no extension to the reticular dermis) classified as stage 0 and stage IA do not require additional testing.

In early-stage melanoma, the recommended workup includes a lactate dehydrogenase level (LDH) and a chest radiograph (CXR). These two tests provide the foundation for the workup of a patient with all other stages of cutaneous melanoma, unless there is clinical evidence of metastatic disease. Although there is much interest in PET scan and fusion studies in the initial staging of melanoma, PET scans have not yet been proved to significantly alter the clinical course of patients with early-stage disease, and routine use of PET scans in the initial workup of patients with cutaneous melanoma remains under investigation.[38]

◆ Staging

Accurate clinical staging of head and neck skin cancer is an essential part of treatment planning, and it provides useful, but generalized, prognostic information for both the patient and providers. Widespread use of clinical staging systems for nonmelanoma skin cancer and melanoma facilitates efficient communication between members of the multidisciplinary head and neck cancer team and allows comparison of outcomes between centers. The staging systems proposed by the American Joint Committee on Cancer (AJCC) are designed for use in primary lesions arising on all cutaneous surfaces, potentially underestimating the severity of some skin cancers of the head and neck, particularly nonmelanoma skin cancer. On the other hand, staging of melanoma of the head and neck incorporates contemporary techniques and provides reliable information on the risk of metastasis and disease-specific mortality.

Staging of Nonmelanoma Skin Cancer

The 2002 AJCC staging system for NMSC is delineated in **Table 9–4**.[39] The system focuses on the size of the lesion, its involvement with extracutaneous structures, and the presence or

Table 9–4 Clinical Staging of Nonmelanoma Skin Cancer Adapted from the 2002 American Joint Committee on Cancer System

Primary Tumor (T)	
TX	Primary tumor cannot be assessed
T0	No evidence of primary tumor
Tis	Carcinoma in situ
T1	Tumor 2 cm or less in greatest dimension
T2	Tumor more than 2 cm but not more than 5 cm in greatest dimension
T3	Tumor more than 5 cm in greatest dimension
T4	Tumor invades deep extradermal structures (i.e., cartilage, skeletal muscle, or bone)

Regional Lymph Nodes (N)	
NX	Regional lymph nodes cannot be assessed
N0	No regional lymph node metastases
N1	Regional lymph node metastases

Distant Metastases (M)	
MX	Distant metastases cannot be assessed
M0	No distant metastases
M1	Distant metastases

Stage Grouping	
Stage 0	Tis N0 M0
Stage I	T1 N0 M0
Stage II	T2 N0 M0
	T3 N0 M0
Stage III	T4 N0 M0
	Any T N1 M0
Stage IV	Any T Any N M1

Source: Adapted from Greene F, Page DL, Fleming ID, et al. Cancer Staging Manual. 6th ed. New York: Springer-Verlag; 2002. Adapted with permission.

absence of metastases. Although the clinical staging of NMSC provides an important baseline for prognosis and treatment planning, clinical staging alone may be insufficient, as the ideal histopathology report detailed in **Table 9–3** contains important information. This data may be used to determine the treatment plan for the primary lesion and the regional lymph nodes or it may prompt additional diagnostic tests to seek regional or, less frequently, distant metastases.

The Challenge of Regional Disease in Nonmelanoma Skin Cancer

The limitations of the AJCC system for regional metastases in NMSC are highlighted by the extreme variability in disease that may be classified as N1. A patient could have a small, isolated parotid metastasis or there could be extensive involvement of the parotid and cervical lymphatics, and both patients would be considered to have N1 disease. Recently, O'Brien and colleagues have championed the expansion of the existing AJCC staging system to include more detailed information about parotid and cervical node involvement.[40] This staging system is outlined in **Table 9–5**.

Table 9–5 A New Staging System for Regional Metastases of Cutaneous Squamous Cell Carcinoma

Stage	Features
P1	Single metastatic node in parotid <3 cm in diameter
P2	Single 3–6 cm in diameter parotid metastasis
P3	Parotid mass >6 cm
	Skull base involvement
	Facial nerve involvement
N0	No clinical neck metastases
N1	Single metastatic cervical node <3 cm in diameter
N2	Single metastatic cervical node >3 cm in diameter
	Multiple ipsilateral cervical metastases
	Contralateral cervical metastases

Source: Adapted from O'Brien CJ, McNeil EB, McMahon JD, et al. Significance of clinical stage, extent of surgery, and pathologic findings in metastatic cutaneous squamous cell carcinoma of the parotid gland. Head Neck 2002;24:417–422.

Although expanded staging of regional metastases in NMSC of the head and neck has yet to gain widespread acceptance, early reports indicate that increasing P-stage correlates with diminished locoregional control and survival, increasing N-stage portends diminished survival, and that patients with both parotid and neck disease have a worse prognosis than those with isolated parotid metastases.[40,41] Other authors have noted that the presence of cervical metastases when the parotid remains negative suggests an increased risk of recurrent disease at any site.[33] The issue of regional metastases in NMSC of the head and neck is clearly more complex than is reflected in the current AJCC system. Further investigation into the impact of parotid and cervical metastases on disease control and survival is required so that the TNM staging system provides prognostic information and treatment guidance comparable with the staging of melanoma.

Staging of Melanoma

Reflecting a proactive philosophy for the treatment of cutaneous melanoma, in contrast with the historically reactive treatment of NMSC, clinical staging in melanoma has been subjected to intense and continuous scrutiny and has emerged as a reliable therapeutic and prognostic tool. Although the clinical features used to predict prognosis in cutaneous melanoma have matured over the years, early efforts to stratify risk by location of the lesion and depth of invasion have been substantiated by subsequent work. For instance, lesions arising on the head and neck have been shown to have higher rates of recurrence and lower survival rates than lesions on other anatomic areas.[42] Among head and neck melanomas, patients with lesions arising on the scalp and in the temporal area have worse survival rates than patients with lesions of other subsites.[43] Perhaps the most compelling work into the prognostic features of cutaneous melanoma was performed by Clark and by Breslow, who correlated the depth of invasion or thickness of cutaneous melanoma with biologic behavior.[44,45] Their complementary

depictions of level and depth of invasion, listed in **Table 9–6**, remain important today.

2002 American Joint Committee on Cancer Staging System of Cutaneous Melanoma

The current staging system for cutaneous melanoma was approved by the AJCC and the Union Internationale Contre le Cancer (UICC) in 2002 and reflects an international collaborative effort to accurately depict the biologic behavior of the disease. The 2002 AJCC staging system for cutaneous melanoma relies on contemporary techniques and important clinicopathologic features that have been validated in numerous studies and clinical trials.[46] The new system incorporates clinical staging, which is determined by histologic assessment of the primary lesion plus a clinical and radiographic assessment of metastases, and pathologic staging, which fuses histopathologic detail from both the primary lesion and regional nodes, as determined by sentinel lymph node biopsy (SLNB) or regional lymphadenectomy.[47] The 2002 AJCC staging system for cutaneous melanoma and the stage groupings are listed in **Table 9–7** and **Table 9–8**, respectively.[39]

Classification and Staging of Localized Melanoma

Staging for cutaneous melanoma is based on the TNM system, in which T represents the primary tumor, N depicts regional node metastases, and M indicates distant metastases. In the 2002 AJCC system, tumor thickness and the presence (or absence) of ulceration comprise the key determinants of the T stage because of their strong and independent impact on prognosis. Because of the high predictive value of level of invasion on survival for melanomas thinner than 1.0 mm, the Clark levels of tumor invasion are employed in T1 lesions. For all thicker lesions, the Breslow depth in millimeters correlates more strongly with prognosis and thereby determines the T stage.[46]

Table 9–6 Clark and Breslow Levels of Invasion for Cutaneous Melanoma

Clark Levels	
I	In situ melanoma, lesion confined to the epidermis
II	Invasion of papillary dermis. No extension to papillary-reticular junction.
III	Invasion throughout papillary dermis. No penetration of reticular dermis.
IV	Invasion into reticular dermis but not subcutaneous tissue
V	Invasion into subcutaneous tissue

Breslow Thickness	
Stage I	≤0.75 mm
Stage II	≥0.76 mm, ≤1.50 mm
Stage III	≥1.51 mm, <4.0 mm
Stage IV	≥4.0 mm

Table 9–7 Staging of Cutaneous Melanoma Adapted from the 2002 American Joint Committee on Cancer Melanoma Staging System

Primary Tumor (T)	
TX	Primary tumor cannot be assessed
T0	No evidence of primary tumor
Tis	Melanoma in situ
T1	Tumor ≤1.0 mm thick
a	Without ulceration and Clark level II/III
b	With ulceration or Clark level IV/V
T2	Tumor 1.01–2.0 mm thick
a	Without ulceration
b	With ulceration
T3	Tumor 2.01–4.0 mm thick
a	Without ulceration
b	With ulceration
T4	Tumor >4.0 mm thick
a	Without ulceration
b	With ulceration

Regional Lymph Nodes (N)	
NX	Regional lymph nodes cannot be assessed
N0	No regional lymph node metastases
N1	One positive lymph node
a	Micrometastasis
b	Macrometastasis
N2	Two or three positive lymph nodes
a	Micrometastases
b	Macrometastases
c	In-transit metastases/satellites without metastatic nodes
N3	Four or more positive nodes, matted nodes, or in-transit/satellite nodes with metastatic node(s)

Distant Metastases (M)	
MX	Distant metastases cannot be assessed
M0	No distant metastases
M1	Distant metastases
a	Distant skin, subcutaneous, or lymph node metastasis
b	Lung metastasis
c	All other visceral metastases
	Or any distant metastasis with an elevated serum LDH

Source: From Greene F, Page DL, Fleming ID, et al. Cancer Staging Manual. 6th ed. New York: Springer-Verlag; 2002. Reprinted with permission.

Table 9–8 Clinical and Pathologic Stage Groupings for Cutaneous Melanoma

Stage	Clinical	Pathologic
0	Tis N0 M0	Tis N0 M0
IA	T1a N0 M0	T1a N0 M0
IB	T1b N0 M0	T1b N0 M0
	T2a N0 M0	T2a N0 M0
IIA	T2b N0 M0	T2b N0 M0
	T3a N0 M0	T3a N0 M0
IIB	T3b N0 M0	T3b N0 M0
	T4a N0 M0	T4a N0 M0
IIC	T4b N0 M0	T4b N0 M0
III	Any T N1–N3 M0	
IIIA		T1–T4a N1a M0
		T1–T4a N2a M0
IIIB		T1–T4b N1a M0
		T1–T4b N2a M0
		T1–T4a N1b M0
		T1–T4a N2b M0
		T1–T4a/b N2c M0
IIIC		T1–T4b N1b M0
		T1–T4b N2b M0
		Any T N3 M0
IV	Any T Any N M1	Any T Any N pM1

Source: From Greene F, Page DL, Fleming ID, et al. Cancer Staging Manual. 6th ed. New York: Springer-Verlag; 2002. Adapted with permission.

metastases to the regional lymph nodes (as determined by SLNB) or other sites. Patients with stage I disease are presumed to have a low risk for metastases and mortality from melanoma; whereas patients with stage II disease have an intermediate risk of additional disease-related morbidity or mortality. However, stage II includes patients with ulcerated lesions greater than 4.0 mm thick (T4b) without evidence of regional metastases from sentinel node biopsy, but the high-risk nature of these aggressive lesions is accentuated by its classification as stage IIC.

Classification and Staging of Regional Metastasis

The differences in the clinical and pathologic staging of cutaneous melanoma appear more obvious in the setting of regional metastasis. Patients found to have palpable or radiographic evidence of nodal metastases are classified clinically as stage III, but clinical staging fails to detect occult metastases. With the increasing use of SLNB, pathologic staging of the regional nodes can be performed and is included in the 2002 AJCC system. The status of the regional lymph nodes has emerged as the most powerful indicator of recurrence and survival, and the number of involved nodes, plus the disease burden within the nodes, exerts a significant impact on outcomes of patients with stage III melanoma.[48,49] The number of involved nodes, the disease burden (microscopic vs. macroscopic or clinically detectable), the presence of ulceration in the primary lesion, and the presence of satellite or in-transit metastases are considered in both the N clas-

Within each stage, tumors are further stratified with an "a" or a "b" designation, indicating the presence or absence of ulceration. Tumor ulceration indicates a higher mitotic rate, and ulceration has been associated with increasing tumor thickness and diminished survival. The presence of ulceration independently upstages the tumor compared with nonulcerated lesions of equivalent thickness, as the prognosis of an ulcerated lesion compares with that of a nonulcerated lesion at one higher T stage.[46]

Patients with localized melanoma are classified as stage I or stage II, with various subclassifications, based on the histologic features of the primary lesion and the absence of clinical, radiographic, or histopathologic evidence of

sification and the subcategories of stage III disease.[46] Ulceration is the only feature of the primary lesion that alters the prognosis of patients with regional disease.

Classification and Staging of Distant Metastasis

All patients with distant metastases are classified as having stage IV disease, but there remains some variability in the prognosis of patients with stage IV melanoma. Differences in the survival rates of patients with cutaneous, subcutaneous, distant lymph node, lung, and other visceral metastases prompted the AJCC to subdivide stage IV disease, with 1-year survival rates ranging from 40 to 60%.[46] Detection of an elevated serum lactate dehydrogenase, however, carries the poorest prognosis, signifying hepatic or osseous metastases, and its presence merits the M1c designation.[39,46]

Excluding the importance of lactate dehydrogenase in staging, the search for serum biomarkers of prognosis, disease progression, or response to therapy continues. Several candidates have emerged: S-100B protein, C-reactive protein, tyrosinase, and loss of heterozygosity at tumor suppressor gene loci.[50] Recently, the presence of a 90-kilodalton (kd) glycoprotein antigen called TA90, or an immune complex called TA90-IC in the serum of patients with melanoma, plus the absence of immunoglobulin-M (IgM) antibodies against TA90, has correlated with occult regional and distant metastases, as well as decreased survival, in patients with early and intermediate stage melanoma.[51] Although this work is promising, continued investigation is required before the use of serum biomarkers becomes clinically applicable to detect metastatic or recurrent disease.

◆ Treatment of the Primary Lesion

Diagnosis, staging, treatment of local disease, detection and treatment of regional disease, and prognosis are increasingly intertwined in the multidisciplinary treatment of aggressive NMSC and cutaneous melanoma of the head and neck. In the era of sentinel node biopsy, a procedure commonly performed coincident with extirpation of the primary lesion, important information is gathered that will further impact treatment and the patient's prognosis. Although the diagnosis and treatment of primary and metastatic disease are separated in this chapter to simplify the discussion, one should remember that there is seamless overlap of these concepts in the clinical setting. Finally, the importance of personal appearance demands that any intervention to eradicate the primary cutaneous neoplasm consider the potential reconstructive challenges of the defect and the final aesthetic outcome while strictly adhering to sound oncologic principles.

Treatment of Nonmelanoma Skin Cancer

Regardless of the treatment modality, more than 90% of patients with cutaneous basal cell and squamous cell carcinomas have an excellent prognosis. Because of the high incidence and favorable response to initial therapy, these lesions are treated by a variety of providers, including family physicians,

dermatologists, general surgeons, plastic surgeons, head and neck surgeons, and radiation oncologists. This diverse group of practitioners may choose from an equally diverse armamentarium to treat the majority of BCC and SCC of the head and neck: electrodissection and curettage, cryosurgery, wide local excision, Mohs' micrographic surgery, photodynamic therapy, laser ablation or resection, radiation therapy, and certain topical agents. The challenge in NMSC lies not in eradication of the lesion but in determining in advance which lesions merit more aggressive or multidisciplinary treatment.

Cryotherapy

Cryotherapy has been a reliable method to remove AKs and low-risk NMSC. Cryotherapy involves cooling the lesion with liquid nitrogen, and it is readily performed in the clinic setting. Because general anesthesia is not required, cryotherapy remains a useful method in patients with bleeding diatheses or medical comorbidities that preclude general anesthesia; however, cryotherapy does not provide tissue for pathologic analysis, mandating that it be used with extreme caution in cutaneous malignancy. It is not indicated in cutaneous melanoma.[2]

Electrodissection and Curettage

In electrodissection and curettage, a technique commonly used by dermatologists, a curette is used to scrape the tumor from its bed, which is then cauterized. The process is repeated several times to optimize tumor removal. Although the curetted material may be sent for pathologic analysis, margin assessment is not performed. This technique should be used with caution in NMSC of the head and neck and, like cryotherapy, is not indicated for melanoma.[2,27]

Wide Excision

Wide local excision has been the traditional standard for managing NMSC, and it remains integral to the treatment of aggressive NMSC. Wide excision of a lesion can be accomplished in a circumferential or elliptical fashion without compromising the margins to facilitate reconstruction; however, the primacy of the head and neck in appearance and the importance of neurosensory and functional structures such as the eye, ear, nose, and mouth demand the smallest possible margin that does not compromise oncologic cure.

Surgical Margins Discussion continues about the extent of resection and the required size of the lateral surgical margins, but one should always remember that the pathology and histopathologic features of the tumor ultimately dictate the margin size. Margins of 2.0 to 10 mm and 4.0 to 15 mm have been proffered for BCC and SCC, respectively. A recent prospective effort has determined that local control rates of 96 to 97% can be achieved in BCC and SCC excised with a 4.0-mm margin, but the majority of these lesions were less than 20 mm in diameter.[52] Margins of 6.0 mm have been suggested for SCC larger than 20 mm to achieve comparable cure rates.[53]

Although these recommendations for lateral surgical margin extent result in acceptable rates of local control, the histopathologic assessment of specimens after wide local excision comprises its greatest limitation. Traditional bread-loaf or four-quadrant sectioning techniques do not allow complete assessment of the peripheral margin, and tumor cells may be missed. Tumors with irregular shapes or significant subclinical spread may thereby escape excision, leading to local recurrence.[54] By close collaboration with dermatopathologists, 360-degree margin assessment may be accomplished. Surgical excision constitutes a key component of the management of aggressive NMSC as it allows extirpation of the primary lesion and access to and control of vital subcutaneous structures.

Temporal Bone and Skull Base Involvement Certain situations demand more aggressive multidisciplinary treatment, extending beyond soft tissue extirpation of the cutaneous lesion. Auricular and periauricular NMSCs exhibit a predilection for invading the temporal bone, often requiring sleeve, lateral, subtotal, or total temporal bone resection to achieve gross tumor clearance. Microscopically involved margins, nodal metastases, and perineural invasion are frequently encountered in these patients. Temporal bone invasion presages poor outcomes with overall survival of 63% at a mean follow-up of 26.7 months. Although the rarity of temporal invasion in NMSC precludes large prospective studies, adjuvant radiation therapy may lead to improved survival.[55]

Involvement of the anterior skull base and calvarium also occurs in NMSC, although the true incidence is difficult to compute. The calvarium may be directly invaded by an overlying lesion or it may be secondarily involved as tumor progresses centrifugally along embryonic fusion planes and cranial nerves or through the orbit. If the overlying tumor appears fixed to the pericranium, then bone invasion should be anticipated and appropriate imaging studies obtained. The vast majority of patients with calvarial or skull base invasion suffer from recurrent disease, and many have undergone numerous prior interventions, including radiotherapy. Nevertheless, craniofacial resection may be safely performed by a combined surgical team of head and neck surgeons, neurosurgeons, and reconstructive surgeons, with an acceptable complication rate. Patients requiring craniofacial resection have been shown to have 2-year survival rates of 76% and 92% for SCC and BCC, respectively. These patients benefit from adjuvant radiation therapy and, potentially, concomitant radiation and chemotherapy to maximize disease control and survival. Poorer outcomes are associated with intracranial extension, perineural invasion, and previous radiation therapy.[56]

Mohs' Micrographic Surgery

First devised in the 1930s by a medical student named Frederic Mohs, this increasingly widespread technique involves removal of cutaneous lesions in a staged fashion in the outpatient setting. Margins are processed with horizontal frozen sectioning, theoretically allowing assessment of 100% of the margin. Each specimen is marked and accurately oriented prior to processing, and residual tumor detected on frozen section is then mapped prior to focal re-excision. This process is repeated until margins are cleared. Full details of the surgical technique and processing methods may be found elsewhere.[54]

Although the process is labor intensive, excellent results have been reported in NMSC, with cure rates in primary BCC approaching 99%.[57] Similar results have been noted in recurrent BCC, as well as in primary and recurrent SCC. Mohs' micrographic surgery has demonstrated long-term control rates of 90% in selected, recurrent SCC.[58] Although traditional Mohs' surgery mandates that the extirpative surgeon also serves as the dermatopathologist, the fundamentals of the technique may be applied to a situation in which the surgeon works closely with a dermatopathologist to meticulously map residual disease and achieve tumor clearance.

Meticulous attention should be devoted to detecting the histopathologic features of aggressive NMSC—histology, degree of differentiation, perineural invasion, lymphovascular invasion, invasion to the subcutaneous fat, depth of invasion, and inflammation. However, Mohs' micrographic surgery (MMS) is not indicated in patients with aggressive NMSC and deep invasion beyond the subcutaneous tissues. The presence of major neurovascular structures and the inadequacy of this technique for clearing tumor from bone and muscle, as transected fibers retract, complicate margin assessment and complete resection. Combining MMS with traditional excision may be another surgical philosophy to maximize local control rates in aggressive or deeply invasive lesions. Aggressive lesions require aggressive treatment by a head and neck oncologic surgeon because radical surgery is often required to maximize disease control and survival, dropping tissue preservation to a secondary goal. In aggressive NMSC, it should never be forgotten that multidisciplinary treatment is often required, and the Mohs' surgeon should collaborate regularly with head and neck surgical oncologists, radiation oncologists, and medical oncologists.

Radiation Therapy

Since its introduction in the 20th century, radiation therapy (XRT) has been a popular means of treating cutaneous malignancies, particularly for elderly patients, those deemed to be poor surgical candidates, and in cosmetically important areas such as the eyelids or nose. Although the various methods of radiation therapy are commonly grouped together for assessment, the use of radiation to manage NMSC entails a heterogeneous mix of techniques. Radiation therapy for NMSC includes external beam radiation with orthovoltage x-rays, megavoltage x-rays, electron beam, and interstitial therapy with cesium after-loading catheters.[59] Similarly, delivery techniques continue to evolve, as plain film guidance and wedge pair techniques yield way to intensity-modulated radiation therapy (IMRT) and proton beam therapy. Radiation fractionation has evolved from split-course technique to altered fractionation with acceleration.

Primary Radiation Therapy In general, radiation for cutaneous malignancy attempts to maximize the delivered dose at the skin surface while avoiding deeper structures, so the modern "skin-sparing" techniques used at other body sites are not applicable to cutaneous malignancies. Orthovoltage and electron beam techniques that have limited therapeutic range are the preferred modalities. Orthovoltage irradiation concentrates energies of 100 to 250 keV at the skin surface. The beam can be shaped by the use of relatively thin, custom-shaped lead cut-outs, and intraocular shields can be used to protect the cornea. Because orthovoltage x-rays deliver energy in the diagnostic range that promotes an eightfold relative dose increase in bone compared with soft tissue, this technique must be used with caution in sites adjacent to, or overlying, bone or cartilage. Orthovoltage and appropriate energy electron beams are preferred on the scalp to minimize the risk of brain injury, but special mixed photon-electron "whole scalp" dosimetry setups and IMRT have emerged as viable alternatives due to improved dose homogeneity at the planned tumor volume.[60] Deeply invasive lesions and those lesions requiring treatment of the regional lymphatics require the use of higher-energy electrons, mixed beam electron-photon techniques, or IMRT. Typical cumulative doses range from 40 gray (Gy) for small primary lesions to 65 to 70 Gy for larger or recurrent tumors using a variety of fractionation regimens determined by the size and location of the lesion, as well as its proximity to dose-limiting adjacent structures.[61]

Results from treating NMSC with radiation therapy are comparable with the methods previously discussed. Early BCCs respond well to XRT, with 5-year local control rates of 95%, but local control of larger or more advanced BCC or SCC falls to 56% in some series.[62,63] Similar rates have been reported in the treatment of T4 SCC and BCC, with local control rates slightly higher than 50% in primary disease; local control may be expected in 80 to 90% of patients with T4 lesions after XRT and surgical salvage.[61,64] However, in a randomized, prospective study of patients with BCC smaller than 4.0 cm, XRT was found to be significantly less effective than surgical resection in controlling local disease.[65] Patients who underwent surgical management of their lesions were also found to have notably better cosmetic outcomes than did those treated with XRT, refuting the historical assertions of improved appearance with XRT.[66]

Even in elderly patients or poor surgical candidates, treatment of NMSC with radiation therapy may not be a benign enterprise. Unless modern techniques are employed by experienced operators, the complication rate may be significant. These complications include cutaneous depigmentation, telangiectasias, scar contracture, lipodystrophy, necrosis of bone or soft tissue, atrophy, and ocular injury.[66] Furthermore, the potential to induce a second skin cancer must be considered when making the decision to treat NMSC with XRT for young patients, because of the association between ionizing radiation exposure and the development of skin cancer.[23]

Adjuvant Radiation Therapy Despite the limitations and challenges of treating NMSC with primary XRT, adjuvant radiation therapy plays a significant role in the comprehensive management of aggressive lesions.

Common indications for radiation therapy to the primary lesion after surgical extirpation include positive margins, advanced lesions, lesions located in the central H-zone of the face, temporal bone or skull base involvement, and perineural invasion.[67,68] These efforts to maximize local control may facilitate improved regional control if the clinically negative neck is radiated in the setting of high-risk primary lesions, but additional evidence is required.

Photodynamic Therapy

First introduced in the 1970s, photodynamic therapy (PDT) involves the administration of photosensitive drugs that are activated by light exposure, resulting in selective destruction of malignant cells. A variety of photosensitizing agents has been employed, including benzoporphyrin, 5-aminolevulinic acid, *meta*-tetrahydroxyphenylchlorin (Foscan, Biolitec Pharma, Dublin, Ireland), and porfimer sodium (Photofrin, Axcan Pharma, Quebec, Canada).[69,70] Photodynamic therapy has been used as the sole treatment modality or in conjunction with surgical excision of recurrent or aggressive NMSC in elderly or infirm patients, achieving complete responses in 92% of BCCs and 100% of SCCs in a highly select population.[70] Complications of PDT include delayed wound healing, discomfort, and increased sun sensitivity that persists 4 to 6 weeks after treatment, requiring protective clothing or sun avoidance.[69,70]

Laser Ablation

Although the laser is essentially another surgical tool that can be used to excise skin lesions, there are scattered reports of using the carbon dioxide (CO_2) laser to ablate superficial NMSC. By using a CO_2 laser in a fashion similar to laser skin resurfacing, local control has been achieved in roughly 97% of superficial BCCs.[71] Such applications of the laser, however, are limited by the same shortcoming of other ablative therapies—failure to assess and precisely control tumor margins.

Topical Therapy

The use of topical agents to treat superficial NMSC is increasing in popularity. Topical therapy appears to be useful in treating precursor lesions of NMSC, such as AK, and in managing superficial NMSC in older patients or in those who are not ideal surgical candidates. The most widely used agent is 5-fluorouracil, and it has been used with excellent success for AK.[72] The recent introduction of imiquimod cream (Aldara, Graceway Pharmaceuticals, Bristol, TN) has introduced a new class of agents to the topical armamentarium. These topical immune response modifiers stimulate the immune system, resulting in cytokine and interferon release, increasing cell-mediated immunity.

Imiquimod has demonstrated clinical efficacy in eradicating AK, superficial BCC, Bowen's disease (SCC in situ), extramammary Paget's disease, cutaneous T-cell lymphoma, and the majority of nodular BCCs, although local control rates in nodular BCC are not as high as those in superficial BCC (65% histologic clearance vs. 87% clearance).[73,74] Although increasing the frequency of application may increase the response rates to imiquimod cream, there is an accompanying increase in application-site side effects such as discomfort and pruritus.[72] Other medical interventions for NMSC include intralesional injection of interferon-α and the application of retinoids, which appear to be more beneficial in preventing progression of premalignant conditions than in treating existing lesions.[72]

Treatment of Localized Melanoma

Excision

Surgical excision remains the primary method for treating the primary lesion in cutaneous melanoma. Because of the aggressive behavior of cutaneous melanoma, historical surgical treatment involved wide margins; however, recent clinical trials have revealed that there is little difference in outcome between 3.0- to 5.0-cm margins and 1.0- to 2.0-cm margins, supporting the use of narrower margins in cutaneous melanoma.[75,76] Most of these data are derived from other anatomic sites such as the trunk and extremities where larger margins are less problematic, but surgical margins of 1.0 to 2.0 cm are considered adequate in cutaneous melanoma of the head and neck, with the ultimate width determined by the thickness of the lesion.[10] Lentigo maligna requires a 5.0- to 10.0-mm margin, and lesions less than 1.0 mm can be safely excised with a 1.0-cm margin.[34] Intermediate-thickness lesions (1.0 to 4.0 mm) are typically resected with margins approaching 2.0 cm. Because of the poor prognosis associated with regional and distant metastases in melanomas thicker than 4.0 mm, local recurrence is less of a concern, rendering 2.0-cm margins adequate in these patients as well.

Mohs' Micrographic Surgery

Although debate persists about the reliability of frozen-section analysis of cutaneous melanoma, there is increasing interest within the dermatology community about the application of MMS to cutaneous melanoma. Discordance between *en face* frozen section and permanent section margin assessment has led some dermatopathologists to counsel against the routine use of frozen sections in cutaneous melanoma.[77] On the other hand, experienced dermatopathologists and Mohs' surgeons have achieved 100% sensitivity and 90% specificity with frozen-section evaluation of margins in melanoma.[78] Increasing sophistication in MMS and the use of rapid immunohistochemical stains has led to acceptable local control rates in melanoma in situ and lesions <0.75 mm thick, suggesting a notable incidence of subclinical disease in these early lesions. With final margins that rarely exceeded 1.0 cm but increased with tumor thickness, equivalent local control rates with MMS versus standard excision have been shown, but experience remains limited.[77]

Combination Techniques

The ability to achieve microscopically controlled margins, minimize destruction of normal tissue, and control subclinical disease makes the techniques of MMS attractive in cutaneous melanoma; however, the expertise and experience required to achieve such high success rates in interpreting frozen sections for melanoma are not widespread. The techniques of mapped serial excision and rapid permanent section assessment of melanoma margins theoretically promote comprehensive eradication of cutaneous melanoma by fusing tissue-conserving benefits of MMS with traditional excision and evaluation.[34] Additional investigation is required to determine the optimum method of excision to maximize local control while minimizing morbidity in melanoma.

Radiation Therapy

Despite the historical perception that melanoma is a radioresistant disease, radiation therapy has emerged as a viable component of the multidisciplinary armamentarium. Radiation therapy is frequently given in the adjuvant setting, but it has been used as the primary modality in select patients. Radiation therapy has achieved local control of 93% in patients with lentigo maligna and lentigo maligna melanoma when used as the primary treatment modality.[34] Radiation therapy is currently used as the primary treatment modality only for patients with unresectable disease or for those deemed medically unfit for surgery.

Increasing the dose per fraction and decreasing the number of fractions has resulted in durable locoregional responses.[79] Although some authors advocate the use of radiation therapy in elderly patients or anatomically challenging areas, the hypofractionated schedules should be avoided in proximity to neural or sensory tissues.[10] Postoperative radiation therapy administered to 30 Gy in 5 fractions has resulted in 88% locoregional control in stage II and stage III melanoma, compared with nonirradiated historic controls who had locoregional failure rates of ~50%.[80,81] Common indications include positive margins, recurrent disease at presentation, nodal metastases, perineural invasion, thick primary lesions, ulceration, satellitosis, desmoplastic histology, and for regional control in patients at elevated risk for nodal metastases who have not undergone sentinel node biopsy or regional dissection.[81–83]

Other Techniques in Melanoma

As in NMSC, there are some medical options for the treatment of primary disease in cutaneous melanoma, although the indications are few. Systemic chemotherapy, primarily dacarbazine, has been utilized in advanced disease and in cutaneous metastases, with limited responses.[10] The topical immune response modifier imiquimod and intralesional interferon-α have demonstrated activity against lentigo maligna in anecdotal reports.[34,76] There have been some attempts to eradicate lentigo maligna with cryotherapy and laser ablation, but the inability to accurately determine the margin status and a high recurrence rate have limited their applications.[34] Although it is not recommended for the treatment of primary disease, carbon dioxide laser ablation has been successful in the palliation of cutaneous melanoma metastases.[84]

Reconstruction of Cutaneous Defects of the Head and Neck

Regardless of the histopathology of the lesion and the method used for its excision (i.e., wide excision vs. MMS), extirpation of head and neck skin cancer creates a defect with cosmetic and functional consequences. Like radiation therapy and chemotherapy, reconstructive surgery constitutes an integral component of the multidisciplinary treatment. Potential reconstructive options for an anticipated defect should therefore be considered during thorough surgical planning. Although cosmetic and functional concerns should never alter the oncologic sanctity of a resection, one should never forget that the primary goals in treating skin cancer of the head and neck are achieving the best patient outcome and eliminating disease.

Reconstruction of head and neck cutaneous defects comprises a wide array of techniques that vary according to the involved subsites. The goals of reconstruction are to restore form and function; achieve color, texture, and thickness match; maintain oral competence; minimize ocular distortion; and cover key structures such as the great vessels and the calvarium or dura. Although primary closure and local flaps most closely approximate the tissue characteristics of the defect, vascularized tissue must be incorporated into the treatment field via local, regional, or free flaps in previously radiated areas or in areas likely to be irradiated. Skin grafts, both split thickness and full thickness, may be used for a variety of defects, but the indications for skin grafts are limited by inherent discrepancies in tissue match to the surrounding skin. Nevertheless, skin grafts provide a reliable reconstructive option and may even be employed for short-term wound coverage while awaiting confirmation of surgical margins.

Lip Reconstruction

The challenges of cutaneous reconstruction in the head and neck are epitomized by lip reconstruction. The perioral region comprises a prominent feature in appearance, and abnormalities in the vermilion-cutaneous junction are often readily apparent. The lips function prominently in maintaining oral competence, projecting emotion, and allowing access to the oral cavity for nutrition and insertion of dental appliances. Preservation of these vital functions and aesthetic concerns demands careful planning and meticulous execution. Reconstruction of lip defects with innervated adjacent lip tissue provides the most optimal outcome, unless severe microstomia will arise, as the function of the oral sphincter is preserved and cosmesis is maximized. If residual lip tissue is insufficient to restore oral continuity, then advancement of the adjacent cheek or delivery of vascularized tissue from distant donor sites via pedicled or free flaps may be performed. In all cases, meticulous attention should be paid to placing incisions in the relaxed skin tension lines and closing the wound in multiple layers: mucosa, muscle, subcutaneous tissue, and skin.

For defects up to one quarter of the upper lip and one third of the lower lip, simple wedge excision with V- or W-shaped primary closure may be performed; however, in the multidisciplinary surgical management of lip cancer, lesions should not automatically be excised in a wedge pattern, as this limits the options available to the reconstructive surgeon. The use of V-Y and stair-step techniques, in addition to lip and cheek advancement techniques such as the Karapandzic flap and Webster-Bernard procedure, allow reconstitution of larger red and white lip defects with cheek wounds that frequently occur in tandem.[85-88]

To maintain a functioning oral sphincter, the use of local tissues is preferred in lip reconstruction, and residual lip or cheek tissue is typically sufficient to reconstruct defects of up to 75% of the lip.[85] Lip-switch techniques such as the Abbe or Estlander repairs allow reconstruction of the opposing lip from intact residual lip, although a second stage is frequently required for division of the pedicle or commissuroplasty. Other local options for lip reconstruction include A-T closure for smaller defects, plus the melolabial flap, Gilles' fan flap, and crescentic cheek advancement flap for larger, composite wounds of the cheek and lip.[89]

Free tissue transfer may be employed for more extensive defects when there remains insufficient tissue for local flap repair. Although free flaps provide soft tissue coverage and restore static oral competence, they are limited by the inability to restore dynamic sphincteric function, as well as variations in color, texture, and thickness from native lip tissues. The radial forearm flap has been described most frequently for lower lip repair, and it may be augmented by including the palmaris longus tendon for lateral support of the oral commissures.[85] Free flaps have also been used in conjunction with lip-switch techniques in complex wounds of the lip and mid-face.[90] To maximize the functional and aesthetic outcome, the radial forearm, rectus abdominis, anterolateral thigh, lateral arm, and scapular free flaps may be combined with local flaps for soft tissue, mucosal, and vermilion reconstruction in total or near-total defects.[85]

Nasal Reconstruction

Similar to the lips and perioral region, the nose comprises a prominent feature in appearance and provides a challenge for the reconstructive surgeon due to its delicate interdependence of nasal lining, structural support, and soft tissue cover. An appreciation of nasal anatomy, with recognition of the subunits of the nose, is requisite for proper planning and execution in nasal reconstruction. Based on the work of Burget and Menick, the nose has been divided into aesthetic subunits that provide guideposts for the placement of incisions and scars.[91] The nose was described to consist of nine distinct aesthetic subunits: the dorsum, tip, and columella, plus the paired alae, sidewalls, and soft tissue triangles.[91] Although the subunit concept initially called for the sacrifice of the residual subunit when more than 50% of the subunit had been resected, the desire to conserve uninvolved tissue and tailor the reconstruction to the defect and the individual patient has led several authors to abandon this aggressive philosophy.[92,93]

Nasal reconstruction requires attention to all layers of the nasal framework: the mucosal lining or vestibular skin internally; the bony, soft tissue, and cartilaginous framework; and the overlying skin cover. Because of these complex demands, multiple procedures are frequently required before an acceptable outcome has been achieved.[94] After a thorough assessment of the defect, its components, the location, and the quantity and quality of adjacent nasal skin, reconstruction may proceed. In through-and-through defects, a variety of techniques may be used to re-create the internal lining: skin grafts applied to the undersurface of a soft tissue flap, "turn-over" cutaneous flaps, nasolabial flaps, hinge flaps of septal or turbinate mucosa, pericranial flaps, and even free flaps such as the radial forearm flap, superficial inferior epigastric artery flap, and lateral arm flap have been internalized for this purpose.[95–97]

Cartilage grafts from the nasal septum, conchal bowl, or helical root provide reliable support for the nasal framework, but primary grafting should only be performed when the lining consists of vascularized tissue. Forehead flaps and free flaps may be prelaminated with cartilage grafts prior to definitive harvest and inset, or the framework may be fashioned in a secondary procedure once the lining has been revascularized from adjacent tissues.[98] Full-thickness composite grafts from the base of the helix provide trilaminar coverage in small alar rim defects (less than 1.0 cm), and composite chondrocutaneous grafts from the conchal bowl may be used to provide support plus either internal or external cover.[95]

A variety of local random and axial flaps have been described for coverage in nasal reconstruction. Subcentimeter superficial wounds of the nasal dorsum may be amenable to primary closure after wide undermining, although some structural recontouring may be required. For defects smaller than 1.5 cm in maximum diameter, local flaps such as the banner flap, dorsal nasal flap, and the bilobed flap are useful on the tip and dorsum.[93] The bilobed flap may also be readily employed for sidewall defects <1.5 cm in diameter.[95] Full-thickness skin grafts harvested from the preauricular or post-auricular area or the forehead are useful for small defects of the nasal sidewall. Small, concave wounds near the junction of the ala and tip may be allowed to heal by secondary intention, with acceptable cosmetic results.

For larger defects of the columella, tip, ala, dorsum, and sidewall, reconstruction may be reliably accomplished with a paramedian forehead flap based on the supratrochlear vessels.[93] A superiorly based melolabial flap constitutes a reasonable option to reconstruct medium-sized wounds of the columella, nasal sidewall or ala, although this flap may blunt the nasalfacial angle when used for sidewall defects. The distal aspect of the forehead flap may be primarily defatted to the subdermal plexus, but significant contouring and defatting should be performed with caution in smokers. The paramedian forehead flap requires at least one additional stage for division of the pedicle 3 to 4 weeks later, and it remains the workhouse in complex nasal resurfacing. The patient who requires a subtotal or total rhinectomy for local control may undergo various combinations of the previously noted techniques, but extensive nasal defects may be readily managed by maxillofacial prosthetics on a temporary or permanent basis.[99]

Periorbital Reconstruction

The thin skin and functional demands of the periorbital region, coupled with the proximity to the eye, renders periorbital reconstruction a delicate and demanding task. Poorly executed reconstructions may lead to ectropion and exposure keratopathy, with the potential for visual loss. A logical approach to periorbital reconstruction recognizes the importance of the anterior lamella (skin and muscle) as well as the posterior lamella (tarsus and conjunctiva). Like the nose, the periorbital region is divided into subunits: the upper and lower lids, the medial and lateral canthi, and the eyebrow, and each subunit exhibits unique requirements.[100]

In general, small defects in concave regions such as the medial canthus may be allowed to heal by secondary intention, with acceptable results. For defects of the anterior lamella, full-thickness skin grafts obtained from the ipsilateral or contralateral upper lid provide a reliable and readily accessible option. Because of the inherent laxity of the eyelids, marginal defects up to 50% of one lid may be closed primarily with or without a lateral canthotomy. Care must be taken to ensure proper alignment of the tarsus using meticulous multilayered technique, ensuring that the maximum tension is directed parallel to the eyelid margin. For larger wounds, single or bipedicled transposition flaps, as well as cross-lid techniques such as the Hughes tarsoconjunctival flap or Cutler-Beard composite lid procedure, from the opposing lid may be used.[101] Cervicofacial flaps, as described by Mustarde, constitute other reliable methods for lower eyelid reconstruction.[102,103] These techniques may be performed in concert with free cartilage and mucosal grafts to reconstitute the posterior lamella.[104] Lateral defects may be repaired primarily or with local procedures such as V-Y advancement or rhomboid flaps, with care taken to keep incisions within the relaxed skin tension lines.

Ear Reconstruction

Because of the intricate anatomic detail of the auricle, with its thin skin and closely apposed cartilage, defects of the ear require meticulous surgical planning and execution. Because roughly 50% of auricular cutaneous neoplasms arise on the helix, a variety of techniques have evolved to counter the surgical defect.[105] As with nasal reconstruction, reconstruction is not required, and maxillofacial prosthetics may provide a reasonable alternative in patients who are poor surgical candidates. Nevertheless, superior aesthetic outcomes may be achieved through primary reconstruction.

Although wedge excision of small lesions of the helical rim may be readily accomplished with extension into the antihelix or concha to facilitate closure, primary closure is typically limited to smaller defects, as it can lead to cupping or notching of the ear. Similarly, small lesions may be excised in a star configuration that allows complex primary closure. Larger defects of the helical rim, including some that extend into the scapha and antihelix, may be successfully reconstructed with chondrocutaneous advancement flaps as described by Antia and Buch and by Butler.[106,107] Such advancement flaps allow maintenance of the general shape, appearance, and anatomic detail of the ear, sacrificing size of the auricle and symmetry to the contralateral ear. Small defects of the helical rim may be reconstituted with composite grafts from the other ear, but this creates morbidity at the donor site.

Defects of the conchal bowl may be skin grafted with either full-thickness or split-thickness grafts, and allowances may be made for the anticipated contraction of the graft. The use of postauricular flaps, both cutaneous and myocutaneous, has been advocated for larger wounds of the concha, citing the benefits of less postoperative contraction and deformity.[108,109] If the wound enters the external auditory canal, it may be allowed to heal by secondary intention, provided that it is not circumferential. For extensive defects of the auricle and temporal bone, the temporalis muscle may be transposed into the wound and skin grafted. In previously radiated wounds, vascularized tissue must be transferred into the defect. Common flap choices include the trapezius or latissimus dorsi as pedicled flaps, and the anterolateral thigh, rectus abdominis, and latissimus dorsi as free flaps (**Fig. 9–3**). These patients may be candidates for eventual prosthetic rehabilitation with tissue-borne or osteointegrated implants.

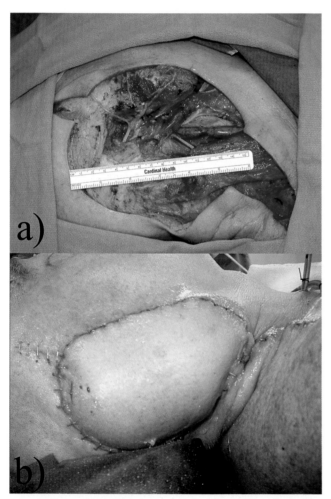

Figure 9–3 Recurrent SCC of the auricle with parotid and cervical metastases. (**A**) The patient underwent auriculectomy, lateral temporal bone resection, parotidectomy, and lateral neck dissection. (**B**) Reconstruction was accomplished with an anterolateral thigh free flap, carrying a cuff of vastus lateralis muscle for placement against the skull base. The anterolateral thigh flap is ideal for temporal bone reconstruction because a broad, large flap may be harvested with reliable vascularity and limited bulk. This fasciocutaneous flap may ultimately serve as a base for an auricular prosthesis.

Cheek Reconstruction

Because of the large relative surface area of the cheek and less complex functional demands, the primary goals of cheek reconstruction are to close the defect and optimize color and texture match. These goals are most efficiently accomplished by primary closure or by using adjacent tissues.

Although small wounds may be allowed to heal by secondary intention, this technique produces the best outcomes in concave areas and has limited applications in the cheek. Both full-thickness and split-thickness skin grafts may be used for temporary or permanent closure of cheek wounds, but the resultant contracture and poor color match render them less than ideal. An array of local rotation or advancement flaps may be used—the choice depends on the size of the defect and its orientation with the relaxed skin tension lines. Banner or note flaps, rhomboid flaps, and bilobed flaps are useful in smaller defects. For larger wounds, medially based rotation flaps of skin, subcutaneous tissue, and platysma (such as the cervicofacial flap) or laterally based composite flaps provide reliable soft tissue coverage.[103,110,111] Wounds in previously radiated patients or that cannot be closed with local tissues may benefit from a thin, fasciocutaneous free flap such as the radial forearm or anterolateral thigh flap, although this technique is limited by a poor color match to the recipient bed. Complex through-and-through wounds demand attention to both the internal and external lining, providing an indication for a free flap used in conjunction with local skin advancement or a folded (or dual skin paddle) free flap.

Scalp and Forehead Reconstruction

Because of its prominent location, the forehead and scalp are frequently involved by skin cancer, and reconstructive surgeons often have the benefit of the full reconstructive ladder. The multilaminar structure of the scalp consists of skin, subcutaneous tissue, the occipitofrontalis muscle and galea aponeurosis, loose areolar connective tissue, and the pericranium of the calvarium. Limitations in the mobility of local tissues, coupled with the challenge of minimizing distortion of hair-bearing skin, have promoted the use of tissue expansion and delay in scalp reconstruction, although the time required for adequate expansion is not always acceptable in aggressive NMSC and melanoma.[112]

Primary closure of forehead and scalp wounds is ideal, with forehead incisions oriented horizontally, parallel to the relaxed skin tension lines. If the pericranium remains intact, then small defects may be allowed to heal by secondary intention or skin grafted, although there will be a resultant hair and skin-thickness deficit. When the pericranium is absent, adjacent pericranium can be rotated to provide a vascularized bed for the graft or the outer table of the calvarium may be burred down to facilitate skin graft take on the vascular diploe.[113] Scalp flaps and local transposition flaps provide excellent cosmetic results, although incisions should respect the theoretical blood supply of the flaps, and a donor site deformity should be anticipated.

Although regional pedicled flaps such as the latissimus dorsi and trapezius have been described for large scalp defects, free tissue transfer provides an excellent method for near-total and total scalp reconstruction, particularly in the setting of prior radiation. Common donor sites include the latissimus dorsi and rectus abdominis anastomosed to the superficial temporal vessels or cervical branches of the external carotid and jugular systems—the muscle flap may then be covered with a large split-thickness skin graft for optimal results (**Fig. 9–4**). The muscle flap will atrophy over time, restoring a natural thickness and appearance.[114]

◆ Diagnosis and Treatment of Regional Disease

Regional metastases to parotid area and cervical lymph nodes indicates aggressive lesions and is associated with diminished disease control and survival in both NMSC and melanoma. Despite the shared predilection for nodal metastases in both NMSC and melanoma, the general management philosophies toward nodal metastases differ. Management of the neck in melanoma has evolved into a proactive endeavor, whereas treatment of regional disease in NMSC remains predominately reactive. Because the lymphatic drainage mechanisms and pathways are not specific to histology, techniques such as SLNB and molecular analysis of nodal specimens that are becoming commonplace in melanoma will be increasingly applied to aggressive NMSC.

Lymphatic Drainage Pathways

Unlike other anatomic regions, lymphatic drainage from cutaneous sites in the head and neck exhibits marked complexity and variability. In general, lesions anterior to a vertical line extending toward the vertex from the auricle will drain to the ipsilateral parotid gland and upper cervical lymph nodes, including lymph nodes along the external jugular chain. More posteriorly located lesions will drain to the post-auricular, occipital, and posterior cervical nodes.[10] Lesions in the mid-face and lower lip may drain to the bilateral anterior cervical nodes, including the superficially located perifacial

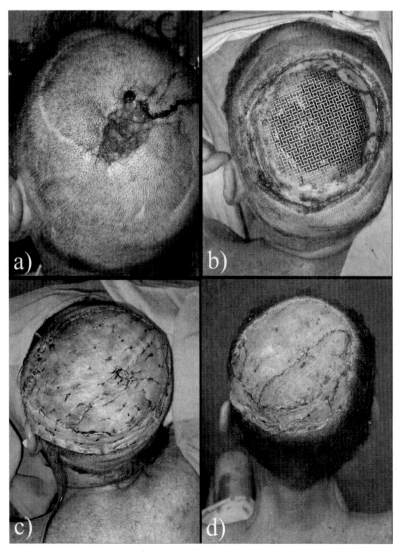

Figure 9–4 (**A**) Recurrent BCC of the vertex of the scalp invading the outer table of the calvarium. (**B**) A radical resection of skin and calvarium was performed, preserving the dura, and the calvarium was reconstructed with wire mesh. (**C**) A latissimus dorsi myofascial flap and skin graft were used for soft tissue reconstruction, with acceptable intraoperative and (**D**) 2-month aesthetic outcome. Atrophy of the skin-grafted muscle flap leads to a more natural scalp contour and thickness than a myocutaneous or fasciocutaneous flap of comparable size.

nodes, submental nodes, and submandibular nodes. Lesions on the neck will likely drain to the closest underlying lymph nodes and those along the external jugular vein, but they are unlikely to involve the parotid gland. A simplified schematic of the lymphatic drainage for cutaneous sites in the head and neck is depicted in **Fig. 9–5**. Within this general framework, there is significant variability, as is evinced by studies that reveal a discordance of up to 34% between the clinical prediction and lymphoscintigraphy.[115]

Risk Factors for Regional Metastases

Nonmelanoma Skin Cancer

The reported incidence of metastatic SCC of the skin ranges from <1% to more than 20%, although the most frequently quoted rate is 5%.[33,58,116] Because of the relative infrequency with which regional metastases are encountered in NMSC, the metastases are generally treated after they are detected;

however, patients with nodal metastases have been found to have diminished overall survival (46.7% vs. 75.7%), disease-free survival (40.9% vs. 65.2%), and disease-specific survival (58.2% vs. 91.5%) at 5 years compared with patients without nodal metastases.[33] As a result, there is a growing appreciation that nodal metastases in NMSC demand aggressive treatment predicated on the early identification of high-risk features in the primary lesion or early detection of regional metastases through SLNB. Risk factors for nodal metastases in NMSC are summarized in **Table 9–9**.[30,33,58,117] Increasing depth of invasion and the histologic presence of lymphovascular invasion have exhibited the strongest correlation with nodal metastases, although additional studies are needed.[33]

Melanoma

As in NMSC, the presence of nodal metastases in cutaneous melanoma portends a worse prognosis. Patients with subclinical lymphatic involvement detected on sentinel node biopsy have a 3-year disease-free survival of roughly 56%, compared with the patients with comparable primary lesions who have negative sentinel nodes and a 3-year disease-free survival of more than 88%. In fact, the presence of lymph node metastases has emerged as a stronger predictor of diminished disease-free survival and disease-specific survival than Clark level, Breslow thickness, and ulceration status.[48]

Much of the recent data on high-risk features for nodal metastases has been gleaned from prospective trials evaluating SLNB. Historically, the depth of the primary melanoma was the most significant determinant of regional metastases, as lesions less than 1.0 mm thick have less than a 5% rate of nodal metastases, and lesions greater than 4.0 mm thick have a 30 to 50% rate of nodal metastases.[49,118] Additional risk factors for regional metastasis in head and neck melanoma are listed in **Table 9–6**.[119] In an interim analysis of the Sun Belt Melanoma Trial, Breslow thickness, Clark level >III, ulceration, and patient age <60 years were independently associated with a positive sentinel node, and patients with these features are at increased risk of occult metastases.[120]

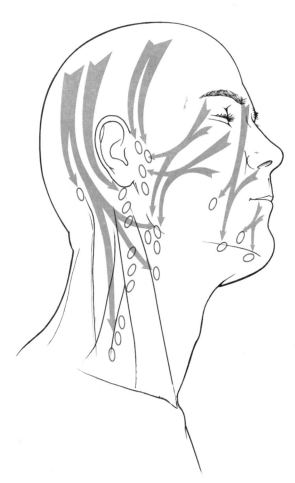

Figure 9–5 Schematic of the lymphatic drainage pathways of the skin of the head and neck. Bilateral drainage to the perifacial nodes and level I is commonly seen in the lower lip and central mid-face. For most other subsites of the face, the parotid gland serves as the primary echelon of drainage, with subsequent drainage to the external jugular chain and levels II to IV. Postauricular lesions commonly drain to occipital and postauricular lymph nodes, as well as level V.

Table 9–9 Risk Factors for Regional Metastases in Skin Cancer of the Head and Neck

NMSC	Melanoma
Recurrent lesion	Breslow thickness (continuous variable)
Size >2.0 cm	
Depth >4.0 mm	Clark level >III
Clark levels IV–V	Ulceration of primary
Invasion to subcutaneous tissues	Patient age <60 years
Poor histologic differentiation	Histologic type other than superficial spreading
Preexisting scar	Lymphovascular invasion
Ear or lip location	Vertical growth phase present
Perineural invasion	Infiltrative tumor strands
Lymphovascular invasion	Single cell infiltration
Inflammation	Acantholysis

Treatment of the Clinically N0 Neck

Intervention in the clinically negative neck remains a highly debatable concept in NMSC, in contrast with the importance placed on histopathologic evaluation of lymph nodes in early-stage and intermediate-stage melanoma. The low rate of nodal metastases in NMSC, combined with a limited appreciation of the risk factors for nodal metastases and a historically conservative approach, has limited the meaningful evaluation of various techniques. As the incidence of NMSC continues to rise and the medical and surgical disciplines gain an improved understanding and appreciation of the risk factors and mechanisms of lymphatic spread, the management of the N0 neck will likely evolve. Because of the importance of histologic assessment of the nodal basins in the staging and prognosis of cutaneous melanoma, the management of the N0 neck has matured through clinical investigation. Regardless of histology, the options for managing the clinically N0 neck in skin cancer of the head and neck include watchful waiting, elective neck dissection, SLNB, and elective radiation.

Watchful Waiting

A conservative initial philosophy toward the parotid and cervical lymphatics has been the mainstay in the management of the clinically negative neck in NMSC. This is evinced by the retrospective nature of the numerous published reviews on parotid and cervical lymphatic metastases in NMSC. Conversely, expectant management of the neck in cutaneous melanoma has been reserved for stage Ia lesions because of their negligible risk of nodal spread.[49] Because of the valuable information obtained from assessment of lymph nodes in melanomas <4.0 mm thick and the perceived lack of clinical benefit for regional treatment in lesions >4.0 mm thick, watchful waiting of the neck has been abandoned in intermediate-thickness melanoma.

Elective Neck Dissection

In aggressive NMSC and melanoma, elective neck dissection may be performed based on clinical assumptions about the pattern(s) of lymphatic metastases. Although this is an imperfect philosophy, clinical projections and pathologically proven metastases correlate in up to 93% of cases.[121] Preoperative lymphoscintigraphy may be useful to target the elective neck dissection to the most likely involved nodal basins because of the potential for unexpected drainage patterns in more than 30% of cases. If elective neck dissection is undertaken in the management of NMSC or melanoma, knowledge of potential lymphatic pathways for a given subsite is required.

Clinicopathologic studies in melanoma and NMSC have delineated typical drainage patterns, although some variability exists. For lesions located on the face and scalp anterior to a vertical line from the external auditory canal, a superficial parotidectomy and lateral neck dissection encompassing levels II to IV should be performed.[10] The parotid contains both paraglandular lymph nodes and intraglandular nodes that are predominantly located lateral to the facial nerve; nearly all lymphoid tissue is located lateral to the retromandibular vein.[122,123] Based on these studies, a superficial parotidectomy is sufficient in the clinically negative gland, reserving a total parotidectomy for those cases with extensive intraglandular metastases. If the facial nerve is uninvolved by tumor and does not demonstrate evidence of perineural invasion, the nerve should be preserved.

For lesions located posterior to the vertical line extending cephalad from the external auditory canal, a thorough posterolateral neck dissection including the postauricular and occipital nodes, in addition to levels II to V, should be performed.[10,124] Lesions of the medial orbit, central mid-face, and lips require at least a unilateral supraomohyoid neck dissection of levels I to III including the perifacial nodes, although bilateral dissection may be indicated in lesions of the central mid-face and lower lip because of the potential for bilateral metastases.[10] Preoperative lymphoscintigraphy may be beneficial in determining the prevailing lymphatic drainage pathways for such lesions.

Although there is little published literature on elective neck dissection in NMSC, it may be considered in aggressive lesions exhibiting one or more of the features outlined in **Table 9–6** and should be performed in lesions directly invading the neck or parotid gland. In patients who have been previously radiated, elective neck dissection should be performed for recurrent lesions exhibiting any of the adverse histologic features.

Elective neck dissection in cutaneous melanoma was a widely accepted practice until the advent of SLNB, based on the theory that early identification and removal of tumor deposits would minimize distant metastases and improve survival. Elective nodal dissection typically identified lymphatic metastases in ~20% of patients with intermediate-thickness melanoma; however, several prospective studies failed to demonstrate a survival benefit of elective nodal dissection over observation in several anatomic sites.[125,126]

A subsequent randomized, controlled surgical trial revealed that patients younger than 60 years with nonulcerated melanomas measuring 1.0 to 2.0 mm thick gained a survival advantage after undergoing elective nodal dissection, although there was no difference in survival with elective dissection for the entire cohort, which was comprised of a minority of head and neck lesions.[127] The importance of early identification of nodal metastases was underscored by another investigation in which patients in the observation arm who later developed regional metastases suffered a significant decrement in survival compared with those who underwent elective dissection and were found to have occult metastases.[128] It remains unclear whether this survival advantage is due to the reduction or elimination of potential foci of distant metastases or the resulting administration of systemic therapy to patients with nodal metastases. Although elective neck dissection for intermediate-thickness melanoma provides valuable staging information, morbidity may be minimized by identifying those patients who truly need a neck dissection.

Sentinel Lymph Node Biopsy

First introduced in 1992 by Morton et al, sentinel lymph node mapping and biopsy is predicated on the premise that metastasizing tumor cells will spread first to the draining lymphatic basin, and an identifiable node within that basin accurately represents the status of the entire basin.[129] Identification of a positive sentinel lymph node (SLN) has emerged as the most important prognostic factor for recurrence and survival in cutaneous melanoma.[48] Conversely, there is little published data on the important of SLNB in NMSC, but its feasibility has been suggested by several case series.[130,131]

According to current clinical practice, SLNB requires both preoperative lymphoscintigraphy and intraoperative lymphatic mapping. Preoperative lymphoscintigraphy involves the intradermal injection of 1.0 to 4.0 µCi of technetium-99m sulfur colloid or technetium-99m antimony trisulfide colloid in the four quadrants of the lesion periphery.[132,133] Immediate and delayed images are then performed to identify the draining lymphatic basins. Intraoperatively, the radiolabeled dye may be augmented by the intradermal injection of isosulfan blue dye to increase the accuracy of the procedure.[48]

After obtaining baseline radioactivity levels with a gamma counter, the primary lesion is excised, and the previously identified basins are inspected with the gamma counter to locate areas of increased radioactivity. Small incisions are made over these areas, and each SLN is identified and removed based on increased radioactivity counts and bluish discoloration. Some authors routinely monitor the facial nerve in cases where the SLNs map to the parotid basin, although this is not a universal practice.[132] Identified SLNs are then analyzed with routine hematoxylin and eosin (H&E) staining, as well as immunohistochemical staining for proteins such as S-100, MART1, Melan-A, and HMB-45. Patients with positive sentinel nodes are then returned to the operating room within 2 to 3 weeks for comprehensive neck dissections.

Identification of the SLN allows the detection of occult regional metastases, promotes accurate staging, and facilitates appropriate delivery of adjuvant therapies. Meticulous serial sectioning of the lymph nodes, augmented by routine analysis and immunohistochemical staining, has identified more patients with positive nodes than elective neck dissection.[134] Limiting formal neck dissections to those patients with positive sentinel nodes spares unnecessary surgical morbidity for the roughly 80% of patients with intermediate-thickness lesions who do not have regional metastases. Subsequently, systemic therapy, with its associated toxicities, may be targeted to those patients who are at the greatest risk of metastases.[48]

Although SLNB has become well-established in other anatomic sites, acceptance has been gradual in the head and neck. The complexity of lymphatic drainage pathways, as well as the intricacy of the anatomy and attendant risk of injury to vital neurovascular structures, has encouraged cautious incorporation of this technique in the head and neck. Some authors advocate lymphoscintigraphy in conjunction with selective dissection of the identified basins, including superficial parotidectomy—the sentinel nodes could be identified in vivo or ex vivo.[135] However, increasing experience with sentinel node biopsy in the head and neck has led to more widespread acceptance.[132]

SLNB is commonly indicated for intermediate-thickness lesions from 0.8 to 4.0 mm thick, as well as for ulcerated lesions of any thickness less than 4.0 mm.[48,136] Because of the high presumed rate of regional metastases in melanoma thicker than 4.0 mm, there is no added benefit to sentinel node biopsy. This technique has been validated in head and neck cutaneous melanoma, with sentinel node identification rates exceeding 92%.[132,137] Because lymphatic drainage in the head and neck may be highly variable, discordant drainage basins should be anticipated and investigated. SLNB in the head and neck remains challenging, because of the variability in lymphatic drainage, the proximity of the basins to the primary (which complicates differentiation of both radioactivity and color change between the primary and the nodal basin), and the higher number of sentinel nodes per basin.[133]

Reported rates of positive sentinel nodes in the head and neck range from 10 to 18%, which is comparable with rates in other anatomic sites.[132,137] As in elective neck dissection, increasing Breslow thickness, Clark level >III, and ulceration of the primary tumor demonstrated a significant relationship with positive sentinel nodes. Interestingly, younger patients may be more likely to develop regional metastases, as there is a decrease of 20% in the probability of nodal metastases with each 10-year increase in age.[134] Frequently, the SLN contains the only evidence of metastases, although involved non-SLNs have been identified in at least 15% of patients—the likelihood of involved non-SLNs increases with male gender, increasing Breslow thickness, extracapsular spread, and more than three positive sentinel nodes.[138] Early identification of involved SLNs, followed by comprehensive nodal dissection, has been shown to improve overall survival compared with delayed nodal dissection after the clinical appearance of regional metastases in melanoma of other body sites (80.7% vs. 67.6% 5-year overall survival), but this potential survival benefit remains controversial.[139]

Complications are uncommon, and they include seroma, hematoma, sialocele formation, cranial nerve injury to the spinal accessory nerve or the facial nerve, and adverse reactions to the blue dye that range from erythema to anaphylaxis.[133,135,137] In addition to these potential complications, some procedural and oncologic limitations of the technique have been proposed. Concerns about the potential increase in in-transit metastases from entrapped melanoma cells among patients undergoing SLNB have been refuted by subsequent reports.[140–142]

Although there is an acknowledged learning curve for sentinel node biopsy, false-negative results have been documented in up to 10% of cases and have been attributed to surgical failure or insufficient histopathologic detection.[132,133] By adhering to the "10% rule" proposed by McMasters and colleagues, detection of occult metastases may be optimized by removing all blue lymph nodes, all clinically suspicious nodes, and all nodes that are ≥10% of the ex vivo radioactive count of the most radioactive sentinel node.[120] A false-negative result may lead to delayed detection and treatment of regional metastases, which could negatively impact survival.[128]

Horizons in the Detection of Regional Metastases

Using reverse transcriptase–polymerase chain reaction (RT-PCR) techniques to identify a battery of molecular markers of melanoma may increase the sensitivity of SLNB in detecting occult metastases. Potential markers include tyrosinase, MART1, Mage3, and gp100.[35,50] Continued evolution of the laboratory techniques, such as electrophoresis-based PCR and PCR on previously paraffin-embedded specimens, may further increase sensitivity and accuracy in detecting micrometastases. Additionally, identification of the events that promote lymphatic invasion and increased tumor vascularity may identify patients who would benefit from systemic treatment strategies, with potential markers of metastasis including NF-κB and activating transcription factor-2 (ATF-2).[50]

The survival benefit of these advanced diagnostic techniques, as well as SLNB itself, remains debatable, and further investigation, or prolonged follow-up in ongoing studies, is required.[120] In the absence of other minimally invasive tests with comparable sensitivity and specificity, lymphatic mapping and SLNB (or selective dissection), augmented by molecular diagnostics, comprises the best available means to assess the regional lymph nodes for occult metastases, provides reliable staging and prognostic information, and facilitates targeted application of comprehensive neck dissection, radiation therapy, and adjuvant therapy in cutaneous melanoma of the head and neck.

Management of the Positive Neck

Given the common drainage mechanism and pathways for cutaneous malignancies of the head and neck, the type of therapeutic neck dissection performed will be the same, regardless of pathology. Comprehensive neck dissection with preservation of vital neurovascular structures, when possible, is indicated for clinical nodal metastases or those detected by SLNB. The type of dissection performed must be tailored to the location of the primary and the metastatic focus and all intervening lymphatics addressed.[10] In general, selective neck dissections may be performed if adjuvant radiotherapy is planned that will encompass undissected areas, but modified radical neck dissections or comprehensive neck dissections of all at-risk levels should be executed when postoperative radiation is not an option.[33]

Multimodality Therapy of Neck Metastases

Nonmelanoma Skin Cancer In both NMSC and melanoma, the clinical or histologic detection of regional metastases demands aggressive treatment to maximize locoregional control and survival. Patients with lymphatic metastases from cutaneous SCC have demonstrated significant improvements in locoregional control (80% vs. 57%) and 5-year disease-free survival (74% vs. 54%) with surgery and radiation compared with neck dissection alone.[143] Therefore, postoperative radiation therapy is recommended in patients with parotid or cervical metastases from NMSC after either comprehensive or therapeutic selective neck dissection. At-risk, undissected levels are included in the radiation portals, thereby minimizing potential surgical morbidity in levels with a low likelihood of involvement.[33]

Extrapolating from the success of concomitant chemoradiotherapy in cervical metastases from SCC of the upper aerodigestive tract (UADT), patients with metastatic NMSC exhibiting high-risk features may benefit from postoperative concomitant chemotherapy and radiation therapy. Patients who demonstrated more than two positive lymph nodes, extracapsular spread, or positive margins of resections achieved significant improvements in local and regional control, as well as disease-free survival, with concomitant cisplatin and radiotherapy compared with radiotherapy alone in a recent Intergroup trial.[144] A similar European study supports these findings, in addition to noting improved progression-free survival and overall survival in patients receiving combined-modality therapy.[145] Although the combined regimens lead to increased toxicity, concomitant chemoradiotherapy may be beneficial in aggressive and metastatic NMSC.

Melanoma The administration of radiation therapy in metastatic cutaneous melanoma after comprehensive neck dissection has been shown to promote regional control of 94% at 10 years. Postoperative radiation therapy, delivered to 30 Gy in 5 fractions, is associated with 10-year disease-specific survival and distant metastasis-free survival of 48% and 43%, respectively in patients with clinical stage III disease. Common indications for adjuvant radiation therapy include extracapsular spread, lymph nodes larger than 3.0 cm, multiple involved lymph nodes, recurrent disease, and less than radical or modified radical neck dissection.[146]

Radiation Therapy as the Sole Means of Regional Treatment

In an effort to capitalize on the benefits of postoperative neck irradiation in metastatic cutaneous melanoma and to minimize the potential morbidity of parotidectomy or neck dissection, some authors have investigated the use of radiation therapy in the elective treatment of regional metastases. Using the hypofractionation schedule outlined previously, 5-year rates of local control, regional control, locoregional control, disease-specific survival, and disease-free survival of 94%, 89%, 86%, 68%, and 58%, respectively, were achieved with elective neck irradiation. Although there was not a formal control group, these rates were deemed to be better than historical controls, and elective neck irradiation has been proposed as an alternative in patients who are poor candidates for systemic adjuvant therapy or neck dissection.[147] Because of its effectiveness in achieving regional control after removal of nodal metastases, radiation therapy may prove to be a reasonable alternative to SLNB or comprehensive neck dissection in patients with positive sentinel nodes, although additional study is needed.[148]

Management of the Unknown Primary with Neck Metastases

In both NMSC and melanoma, the development of regional metastases in the absence of a primary lesion presents a clinical challenge. Patients should be queried as to their history of skin cancer or skin lesions that have been removed previously. Often, an index lesion can be identified, but an exhaustive search for potential lesions should be undertaken in the absence of a clear history. Mucosal and ocular sources of metastatic melanoma should be investigated in melanoma of unknown primary. Importantly, patients with parotid or cervical involvement by SCC should be evaluated for primary lesions of the UADT.

Patients with regional metastases and no identifiable primary should be treated aggressively with neck dissection followed by XRT for NMSC. Concomitant chemotherapy may be beneficial in SCC with adverse features, as previously discussed. Patients with melanoma of unknown primary should undergo neck dissection, with the possibility of postoperative XRT to optimize regional control, and they should be evaluated for systemic therapy, as they have stage III disease. Although some authors have asserted that patients with only regional metastases from melanoma have improved outcomes compared with patients with known primary lesions, additional studies have not demonstrated a difference in survival.[149,150]

◆ Treatment of Advanced and Systemic Disease

Nonmelanoma Skin Cancer

Because the rarity of advanced or widely metastatic NMSC, very little data exist to guide its management. A few isolated case series demonstrate the potential benefit of decreasing tumor burden in patients with unresectable skin cancers, but no randomized studies exist to support the routine use of neoadjuvant chemotherapy in NMSC or to provide concise guidelines for systemic therapy.[151,152] The success of newer, taxane- and platinum-based regimens in the treatment of SCC of the UADT, particularly the oropharynx and larynx, may be applied to disfiguring or otherwise unresectable NMSC of the head and neck.

At the present time, surgery with or without postoperative radiation therapy remains the mainstay for managing aggressive NMSC. The role of chemotherapy is predominately limited to concomitant therapy for high-risk regional metastases, distant metastases, and palliation; however, phase II studies have demonstrated overall responses and complete responses of 34% and 17%, respectively, in patients with locally advanced or metastatic NMSC with combinations of interferon-α (IFN-α), retinoic acid, and cisplatin. Although the results were better in patients with locally advanced rather than metastatic disease, the median response duration was 9 months, and the toxicities were deemed acceptable. The addition of cisplatin to an earlier regimen of IFN-α and retinoic acid appears to increase the efficacy of the combination.[153,154] These results are promising, but novel approaches are needed in advanced, aggressive NMSC.

Melanoma

Despite advances in the detection and treatment of primary melanoma, distant metastases will develop in roughly 30% of patients.[155] Patients with stage IIB, IIC, and III melanoma are at high risk of systemic metastases and subsequent death. Treatment strategies have evolved to minimize the likelihood of distant metastases, but survival rates remain poor for patients who progress to stage IV disease.

Adjuvant Systemic Therapy for Stage IIB to III Disease

The 2002 AJCC staging system for cutaneous melanoma identifies those patients who are at an increased risk of recurrent or metastatic disease. Although the potential for local and/or regional recurrence may be mitigated by appropriate therapy of the primary and regional lymphatics, the possibility of distant metastases has greater import for survival—the only outcome that truly matters. Because melanoma is an immunogenic tumor, many strategies have attempted to improve the body's immune response to melanoma, with resultant investigations of biologic response modifiers, vaccines, and immune stimulants.[10]

Despite vigorous research, high-dose interferon α-2b (IFNα-2b) is the only adjuvant treatment approved by the U.S. Food and Drug Administration (FDA) to minimize the chance of recurrence and metastasis in stage IIB to III melanoma. Although the benefit of IFNα-2b for overall survival remains controversial, it has demonstrated significant improvements in relapse-free survival (20 to 30%) in several trials.[156–158] The high-dose IFNα-2b regimen consists of an induction period of 20 million units m^{-2} day^{-1} subcutaneously 5 days per week for 4 weeks, followed by 10 million units m^{-2} day^{-1} subcutaneously 3 times per week for 48 weeks. The high-dose regimen also is effective in salvaging recurrent disease in high-risk patients who initially did not receive adjuvant therapy.[157] Unfortunately, the high-dose regimen is associated with significant toxicities including constitutional symptoms, fatigue, headache, nausea, weight loss, depression, hepatic injury, and myelosuppression, but, with dose modification, most patients are able to complete the proscribed course.[8,159]

The toxicity of high-dose IFNα-2b, coupled with its modest response rates, has engendered an ongoing search for other, more effective therapies. Intermediate- and low-dose regimens have been investigated, with suboptimal results for the low-dose regimens. The adjuvant therapy of high-risk cutaneous melanoma remains an area of intense research, and patients with stage IIB to III disease should be encouraged to participate in clinical trials if they are not candidates for, or refuse, high-dose IFNα-2b. Combinations of interferon with melanoma vaccines, other biologic response modifiers such as interleukin-2 (IL-2), gene therapy, and chemotherapeutics such as dacarbazine, cisplatin, and vinblastine are currently undergoing stage I to III trials.[8,10]

Treatment of Stage IV Disease

In general, patients with stage IV disease have a poor prognosis, with ~5 to 20% 5-year survival.[155] Common sites for metastases include the lung, skin and subcutaneous tissues, brain, gastrointestinal tract, adrenal glands, bone, and liver. Patients with cutaneous melanoma of the head and neck may have a higher incidence of brain metastases than patients with primaries in other anatomic sites.[160] Patients with distant skin, subcutaneous, and nodal metastases have a better prognosis than do patients with lung or visceral metastases.

To counter the dire prognosis in patients with stage IV disease, aggressive chemotherapy regimens have evolved, with minimal success. High-dose IL-2 has demonstrated some efficacy, with overall response rates around 15%, and the response is often durable, potentially justifying the severe toxicities of treatment that include hypotension, capillary leak, myocarditis, renal insufficiency, and sepsis.[8] Surgical resection of isolated metastases may be effective, particularly in patients with an earlier primary tumor stage, no history of regional metastasis, and a prolonged interval between treatment of the primary and the detection of distant metastases.[155] Dacarbazine has been the mainstay of cytotoxic therapy, with response rates ranging from 15 to 20%. Newer agents such as temozolomide, plus combinations of drugs including tamoxifen, taxanes, and cisplatin, have been investigated.[8] The desire for synergistic therapies has encouraged combinations of cytotoxic agents with IL-2 and IFNα-2b in a concept entitled biochemotherapy, but the severe toxicities have limited their acceptance.[161] As in NMSC, the poor prognosis for patients with advanced melanoma of the head and neck demands novel therapies and treatment approaches, including prevention.

◆ Prevention

Common strategies to minimize sun and ultraviolet radiation exposure include wearing protective clothing while in direct sunlight, avoiding sun exposure during the midday hours, and wearing sunscreen. Epidemiologic studies have indicated that sunscreen use can effectively prevent cutaneous melanoma[162]; however, there is also evidence that sunscreen does not prevent skin cancer, potentially due to the limitations of early sunscreen formulations against UVA or to a sense of false confidence sunscreens may impart to the user that promotes prolonged sun exposure.[163]

Despite an improved awareness of skin cancer in the United States, increased knowledge has translated poorly into an increased use of skin-protective behaviors and has not improved skin cancer prevention. Failure to employ skin-protective behaviors such as sun avoidance, sunscreens, and protective clothing has been shown to correlate with other high-risk behaviors like smoking, not wearing seat belts in the front seat of vehicles, and avoiding regular general physical examinations.[1] Conversely, educational programs in Australia have increased public awareness, leading to earlier detection of lesions and a decrease in the incidence of cutaneous melanoma.[164] Additional time is needed to determine if advocacy of sun-protective behaviors and skin cancer awareness beginning in childhood will corral the rising incidence skin cancer in the United States.

There is growing interest in preventative strategies for individuals with genetic, occupational, or recreational risk factors for developing skin cancer. Retinoids have shown reasonable promise in prohibiting the progression of AKs to invasive carcinoma. Much interest has been generated in the potential benefits of nonsteroidal anti-inflammatory drugs (NSAIDs) and inhibitors of cyclooxygenase (COX) in cancer prevention, given the overexpression of COX-2 in numerous cancers, including skin cancer. Similarly, the benefits of a low-fat diet, β-carotene, vitamins C and E supplementation, extracts from green tea and grape seeds, and analogues of 1,25-dihydroxyvitamin D3 suggest a role for dietary modification in the prevention of skin cancer of the head and neck, but further investigation is required.[72]

◆ Clinical Cases

Case 1   Recurrent squamous cell carcinoma of the lip.

Presentation   Patient 1 is a 49-year-old man who underwent resection of an SCC of the left lower lip 1 year ago. He developed persistent swelling of the left lower lip, left-sided facial pain followed by focal paresthesias, and a slowly evolving, partial left facial paralysis.

Physical Examination   The patient has brow ptosis with poor eye closure and decreased activity of the marginal mandibular nerve. Function of the buccal branch remains intact and symmetric. He has a paramedian incision on the lip with a 1.5-cm area subcutaneous and submucosal fullness in the midportion of the left lower lip. The oral commissure is not involved (**Fig. 9–6A**). Additionally, there is a 1.5-cm, firm, mobile level Ia lymph node.

Diagnosis and Workup   To obtain a tissue diagnosis, either an incisional biopsy of the lip mass (through the previous scar) or a fine-needle aspiration biopsy of the lip or neck mass could be performed. After determining that the lesion and node represent recurrent SCC, a CT scan of the head and neck, from the skull base to the clavicles, should be obtained to evaluate for additional lymphadenopathy and perineural invasion. Because of the high probability of perineural invasion, an MRI may be complementary. Consultations will be placed with plastic and reconstructive surgery, radiation oncology, and medical oncology because this patient with aggressive, metastatic SCC of the lip will require multidisciplinary care.

Options for Treatment   Although radiotherapy with or without chemotherapy may provide locoregional control in patients who are not reasonable surgical candidates, wide excision of the subcutaneous recurrence in conjunction with parotidectomy and supraomohyoid neck dissection will facilitate clearance of gross perineural disease and regional metastases. Concomitant postoperative chemoradiotherapy will likely be indicated, given the recurrent nature of the neoplasm and the presence of perineural invasion.

Treatment of the Primary Lesion   Wide local excision of the lower lip recurrence with 1.5-cm margins may be readily performed, with preservation of the oral commissure if possible. The mental nerve was grossly abnormal in appearance, prompting dissection of mental nerve through the mandible to achieve microscopic clearance of the nerve at the mandibular foramen (**Fig. 9–6B**). The result-

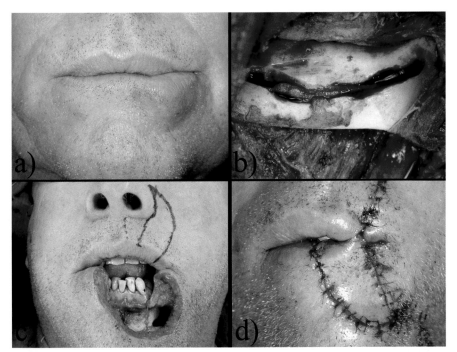

Figure 9–6 Patient 1 of case 1. (**A**) The lesion is evident as a subtle subcutaneous fullness of the left lateral lip. The lesion does not extend into the oral commissure. (**B**) With the intraoperative identification of perineural invasion into the mental nerve, the nerve was dissected through its canal until frozen-section clearance was achieved at the mandibular foramen. (**C**) The surgical defect after mucosal advancement of the left lateral lip—an Abbe flap was selected for soft tissue reconstruction and preservation of oral competence. (**D**) The immediate postoperative view after Abbe flap reconstruction. The pedicle was divided 4 weeks later, and the patient went on to receive postoperative concomitant chemotherapy and radiation therapy.

ant defect will require complex reconstruction to restore the continuity of the oral sphincter to maximize postoperative function. Local and regional tissues provide the best color and texture match, with the potential to maintain innervation. In this case, we elected to advance the ipsilateral cheek and reconstruct the lip defect with an Abbe flap (**Fig. 9–6C,D**).

Treatment of the Regional Lymphatics Because of the presence of gross perineural invasion of the facial nerve, a superficial parotidectomy was performed to expose the entire nerve, and gross clearance was achieved at the stylomastoid foramen. Because of the aggressive nature of this neoplasm and the need for postoperative radiation therapy to the primary, a therapeutic selective neck dissection of levels I to IV was performed.

Adjuvant Therapy In the presence of a recurrent lesion, extracapsular spread in the submental lymph node, multiple positive nodes, close margins, and perineural invasion to the skull base, this patient will require postoperative XRT. The primary bed and ipsilateral involved neck should receive at least 60 Gy, with 50 to 60 Gy delivered to the lower-risk contralateral neck and ipsilateral supraclavicular fossa via IMRT techniques. Based on experience in UADT SCC with aggressive features, there may be a role for postoperative concomitant chemotherapy and XRT in high-risk patients.

Summary of Treatment For recurrent SCC of the head and neck with perineural invasion and regional metastases, aggressive multimodality therapy is required to maximize the chances for locoregional control. Local tissues provide the best match for facial defects, particularly in the lip so that a functional oral sphincter may be preserved. The presence of adverse histologic features such as extracapsular spread and multiple positive nodes justifies the use of concomitant chemoradiotherapy, which has proved effectiveness in regional metastases of SCC of the UADT.

Case 2 A 3.5-mm melanoma of the posterior scalp.

Presentation Patient 2 is a 38-year-old woman who noticed a rapidly growing pink nodule on the vertex of her scalp.

Physical Examination On close inspection, there is 1.0-cm nodule on the vertex of her scalp. Palpation of the neck reveals no lesions.

Diagnosis and Workup A punch biopsy of the lesion was performed, revealing a 3.5-mm-thick nodular melanoma invading to Clark level V, perineural invasion, but no lymphovascular invasion, regression, vertical growth phase, or satellitosis. She underwent a contrast CT scan of the head and neck, as well as a chest radiograph and an LDH level—all of which were normal. The lesion is therefore staged as T3a N0 M0 (stage IIA) melanoma of the scalp.

Treatment of the Primary Lesion Because the patient has no contraindications to surgery, she should undergo wide local excision of this lesion, with 1.5-cm margins. Although a variety of rotation flaps and scalp flaps are available for reconstruction, a split-thickness or full-thickness skin graft provides a reliable means of immediate reconstruction. Once the final margins are determined to be negative on permanent section analysis, a definitive reconstruction may be performed, although the benefits of such a procedure should be weighed against the patient's overall prognosis.

Treatment of the Neck Because of the risk of regional metastasis in this intermediate-thickness melanoma, this patient is a candidate for SLNB. After preoperative lymphoscintigraphy to localize the primary drainage basin(s), intraoperative lymphatic mapping followed by SLNB should be performed. In this patient's case, the sentinel nodes mapped to the postauricular region, and two nodes exhibited microscopic foci of disease. Because of the involved nodes, she should undergo comprehensive posterolateral neck dissection (**Fig. 9–7**) and postoperative radiotherapy to the primary and neck to 30 Gy in 5 fractions twice weekly.

Adjuvant Therapy After completing locoregional therapy, the patient requires close follow-up, according to the protocols established by the National Comprehensive Cancer Network. Because she has stage IIIA disease, she would potentially benefit from high-dose therapy with interferon α-2b or inclusion in a clinical trial of adjuvant therapy.

Summary of Treatment This case outlines the routine management for intermediate-thickness melanoma, including wide local excision of the primary lesion with immediate reconstruction and SLNB. The presence of mi-

crometastatic disease demands comprehensive treatment of the neck, which can be accomplished with neck dissection or, potentially, radiation therapy. For patients with multiple positive nodes, nodes larger than 3.0 cm, and extracapsular spread, and in those patients who undergo less than a modified radical neck dissection, adjuvant irradiation may be beneficial to maximize locoregional control. Because she is at high risk of recurrence and metastases, she is a candidate for systemic adjuvant therapy.

References

1. Santmyire BR, Feldman SR, Fleischer AB Jr. Lifestyle high-risk behaviors and demographics may predict the level of participation in sun-protection behaviors and skin cancer primary prevention in the United States: results of the 1998 national health interview survey. Cancer 2001;92:1315–1324

2. Alam M, Ratner D. Primary care: cutaneous squamous cell carcinoma. N Engl J Med 2001;344:975–983

3. Chen JG, Fleischer AB Jr, Smith ED, et al. Cost of nonmelanoma skin cancer treatment in the United States. Dermatol Surg 2001;27:1035–1038

4. Johnson TM, Rowe DE, Nelson BR, Swanson NA. Squamous cell carcinoma of the skin (excluding lip and oral mucosa). J Am Acad Dermatol 1992;26:467–484

5. Christenson LJ, Borrowman TA, Vachon CM, et al. Incidence of basal cell and squamous cell carcinomas in a population younger than 40 years. JAMA 2005;294:681–690

6. Leffell DJ, Headington JT, Wong DS, Swanson NA. Aggressive-growth basal cell carcinoma in young adults. Arch Dermatol 1991;127:1663–1667

7. Khanna M, Fortier-Riberdy G, Dinehart SM, Smoller B. Histopathologic evaluation of cutaneous squamous cell carcinoma: results of a survey among dermatopathologists. J Am Acad Dermatol 2003;48:721–726

8. Tsao H, Atkins MB, Sober AJ. Medical progress: management of cutaneous melanoma. N Engl J Med 2004;351:998–1012

9. Jemal A, Tiwari RC, Murray T, et al. Cancer statistics, 2004. CA Cancer J Clin 2004;54:8–29

10. Lentsch EJ, Myers JN. Melanoma of the head and neck: current concepts in diagnosis and management. Laryngoscope 2001;111:1209–1222

11. Melnikova VO, Ananthaswamy HN. Cellular and molecular events leading to the development of skin cancer. Mutat Res 2005;571:91–106

12. Tilli CMLJ, Van Steese IMAM, Krekels GAM, et al. Molecular aetiology and pathogenesis of basal cell carcinoma. Br J Dermatol 2005;152:108–112

13. Gailani MR, Bale SJ, Leffell DJ, et al. Developmental defects in Gorlin syndrome related to a putative tumor suppressor gene on chromosome 9. Cell 1992;69:111–117

14. High A, Zedan W. Basal cell nevus syndrome. Curr Opin Oncol 2005;17:160–166

15. Thompson JF, Scolyer RA, Kefford RF. Cutaneous melanoma. Lancet 2005;365:687–701

16. Kefford RF, Newton Bishop JA, Bergman W, et al. Counseling and genetic testing for individuals perceived to be genetically predisposed to melanoma: a consensus statement of the melanoma genetics consortium. J Clin Oncol 1999;17:3245–3251

17. Florell SR, Boucher KM, Garibotti G, et al. Population-based analysis of prognostic factors and survival in familial melanoma. J Clin Oncol 2005;23:7168–7177

18. Green MH, Clark WH Jr, Tucker MA, et al. High risk of malignant melanoma in melanoma-prone families with dysplastic nevi. Ann Intern Med 1985;102:458–465

19. Cannon-Albright LA, Goldgar DE, Meyer LJ, et al. Assignment of a locus for familial melanoma, MLM, to chromosome 9p13–22. Science 1992;258:1148–1152

20. Bishop DT, Demenais F, Goldstein AM, et al. Geographical variation in the penetrance of CDKN2A mutations for melanoma. J Natl Cancer Inst 2002;94:894–903

21. Marci II, Stern RS. Risk of developing a subsequent nonmelanoma skin cancer in patients with a history of nonmelanoma skin cancer:

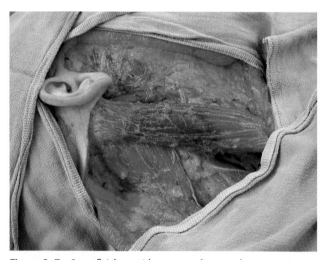

Figure 9–7 Superficial parotidectomy and comprehensive posterolateral neck dissection for micrometastatic melanoma of the vertex of the scalp. Note the comprehensive removal of all fibrofatty lymph node–bearing tissue of the occipital and postauricular region, as well as levels II to V and the superficial parotid specimen. Cranial nerve was preserved and is visible in the posterior triangle. Because of extensive dissection, postoperative physical therapy is mandatory in these patients to prevent shoulder syndrome.

a critical review of the literature and meta-analysis. Arch Dermatol 2000;136:1524–1530

22. Goggins WB, Tsao H. A population-based analysis of risk factors for a second primary cutaneous melanoma among melanoma survivors. Cancer 2003;97:639–643

23. Perkins JL, Liu Y, Mitby PA, et al. Nonmelanoma skin cancer in survivors of childhood and adolescent cancer: a report from the childhood cancer survivor study. J Clin Oncol 2005;23:3733–3741

24. Veness MJ, Quinn DI, Ong CS, et al. Aggressive cutaneous malignancies following cardiothoracic transplantation: the Australian experience. Cancer 1999;85:1758–1764

25. Wong CSM, Strange RC, Lear JT. Basal cell carcinoma. BMJ 2003;327: 794–798

26. Vico P, Fourez T, Nemec E, et al. Aggressive basal cell carcinoma of head and neck areas. Eur J Surg Oncol 1995;21:490–497

27. Rudolph R, Zelac DE. Squamous cell carcinoma of the skin. Plast Reconstr Surg 2004;114:82e–94e

28. Breuninger H, Schaumberg-Lever G, Holzschuh J, Horny H-P. Desmoplastic squamous cell carcinoma of the skin and vermilion surface. Cancer 1997;79:915–919

29. Martin RCG II, Edwards MJ, Cawte TG, et al. Basosquamous carcinoma: analysis of prognostic factors influencing recurrence. Cancer 2000;88:1365–1369

30. Lai SY, Weinstein GS, Chalian AA, et al. Parotidectomy in the treatment of aggressive cutaneous malignancies. Arch Otolaryngol Head Neck Surg 2002;128:521–526

31. Panje WR, Ceilley RI. The influence of the mid-face on the spread of epithelial malignancies. Laryngoscope 1979;89:1914–1920

32. Clayman GL, Lee JJ, Holsinger FC, et al. Mortality risk from squamous cell skin cancer. J Clin Oncol 2005;23:759–765

33. Moore BA, Weber RS, Prieto V, et al. Lymph node metastases from cutaneous squamous cell carcinoma of the head and neck. Laryngoscope 2005;115:1561–1567

34. Arlette JP, Trotter MJ, Trotter T, Temple CLF. Management of lentigo maligna and lentigo maligna melanoma: seminars in surgical oncology. J Surg Oncol 2004;86:179–186

35. Lens MB, Newton-Bishop JA, Boon AP. Desmoplastic malignant melanoma: a systematic review. Br J Dermatol 2005;152:673–678

36. Friedman RJ, Rigel DS, Kopf AW. Early detection of malignant melanoma: the role of physician examination and self-examination of the skin. CA Cancer J Clin 1985;35:130–151

37. Ginsberg LE. MR imaging of perineural tumor spread. Neuroimaging Clin N Am 2004;14:663–677

38. Wagner JD, Schauwecker D, Davidson D, et al. Inefficacy of F-18 fluorodeoxy-D-glucose-positron emission tomography scans for initial evaluation in early-stage cutaneous melanoma. Cancer 2005;104:570–579

39. Greene F, Page DL, Fleming ID, et al. Cancer Staging Manual. 6th ed. New York: Springer-Verlag; 2002

40. O'Brien CJ, McNeil EB, McMahon JD, et al. Significance of clinical stage, extent of surgery, and pathologic findings in metastatic cutaneous squamous carcinoma of the parotid gland. Head Neck 2002;24:417–422

41. Palme CE, O'Brien CJ, Veness MJ, et al. Extent of parotid disease influences outcome in patients with metastatic cutaneous squamous cell carcinoma. Arch Otolaryngol Head Neck Surg 2003;129:750–753

42. Morton DL, Wen DR, Wong JH, et al. Technical details of intraoperative lymphatic mapping for early stage melanoma. Arch Surg 1992;127:392–399

43. Ballantyne AJ. Malignant melanoma of the skin of the head and neck: an analysis of 405 cases. Am J Surg 1970;120:425–431

44. Clark WH Jr, From L, Bernardino EA, Mihm MC. The histogenesis and biologic behavior of primary human malignant melanomas of the skin. Cancer Res 1969;29:705–727

45. Breslow A. Thickness, cross-sectional areas and depth of invasion in the prognosis of cutaneous melanoma. Ann Surg 1970;172:902–908

46. Balch CM, Buzaid AC, Soong S-J, et al. New TNM melanoma staging system: linking biology and natural history to clinical outcomes. Semin Surg Oncol 2003;21:43–52

47. Petro A, Schwartz J, Johnson T. Current melanoma staging. Clin Dermatol 2004;22:223–227

48. Gershenwald JE, Thompson W, Mansfield PF, et al. Multi-institutional melanoma lymphatic mapping experience: the prognostic value of sentinel lymph node status in 612 stage I or II melanoma patients. J Clin Oncol 1999;17:976–983

49. Balch CM, Soong S-J, Gershenwald JE, et al. Prognostic factors analysis of 17,600 melanoma patients: validation of the American Joint Committee on Cancer melanoma staging system. J Clin Oncol 2001;19:3622–3634

50. Torabian S, Kashani-Sabet M. Biomarkers for melanoma. Curr Opin Oncol 2005;17:167–171

51. Litvak DA, Gupta RK, Yee R, et al. Endogenous immune response to early- and intermediate-stage melanoma is correlated with outcomes and is independent of locoregional relapse and standard prognostic factors. J Am Coll Surg 2004;198:27–35

52. Thomas DJ, King AR, Peat BG. Excision margins for nonmelanoma skin cancer. Plast Reconstr Surg 2003;112:57–63

53. Brodland DG, Zitelli JA. Surgical margins for excision of primary cutaneous squamous cell carcinoma. J Am Acad Dermatol 1992;27:241–248

54. Nelson BR, Railan D, Cohen S. Mohs' micrographic surgery for nonmelanoma skin cancer. Clin Plast Surg 1997;24:705–718

55. Gal TJ, Futran ND, Bartels LJ, Klotch DW. Auricular carcinoma with temporal bone invasion: outcomes analysis. Otolaryngol Head Neck Surg 1999;121:62–65

56. Backous DD, DeMonte F, El-Naggar A, et al. Craniofacial resection for nonmelanoma skin cancer of the head and neck. Laryngoscope 2005;115:931–937

57. Rowe DE, Carroll RJ, Day CL Jr. Long-term recurrence rates in previously untreated (primary) basal cell carcinoma: implications for patient follow-up. J Dermatol Surg Oncol 1989;15:315–328

58. Rowe DE, Carroll RJ, Day CL Jr. Prognostic factors for local recurrence, metastasis, and survival rates in squamous cell carcinoma of the skin, ear, and lip. J Am Acad Dermatol 1992;26:976–990

59. Mendenhall WM, Parsons JT, Mendenhall NP, Million RP. T2–T4 carcinoma of the skin of the head and neck treated with radical irradiation. Int J Radiat Oncol Biol Phys 1987;13:975–981

60. Bedford JL, Childs PJ, Hansen VN, et al. Treatment of extensive scalp lesions with segmental intensity-modulated photon therapy. Int J Radiat Oncol Biol Phys 2005;62:1549–1558

61. Mendenhall WM, Kalbaugh KJ, Mendenhall NP, Parsons JT. Radiotherapy as definitive treatment and as a surgical adjunct. In: Weber RS, Miller MJ, Goepfert H, eds. Basal and Squamous Cell Cancers of the Head and Neck. Philadelphia, PA: Williams & Wilkins; 1996:331–350

62. Wilder RB, Kittelson JM, Shimm DS. Basal cell carcinoma treated with radiation therapy. Cancer 1991;68:2134–2137

63. Shimm DS, Wilder RB. Radiation therapy for squamous cell carcinoma of the skin. Am J Clin Oncol 1991;14:383–386

64. Al-Othman MOF, Mendenhall WM, Amdur RJ. Radiotherapy alone for clinical T4 skin carcinoma of the head and neck with surgery reserved for salvage. Am J Otolaryngol 2001;22:387–390

65. Avril M-F, Auperin A, Margulis A, et al. Basal cell carcinoma of the face: surgery or radiotherapy? Results of a randomized study. Br J Cancer 1997;76:100–106

66. Petit JY, Avril MF, Margulis A, et al. Evaluation of cosmetic results of a randomized trial comparing surgery and radiotherapy in the treatment of basal cell carcinoma of the face. Plast Reconstr Surg 2000;105:2544–2551

67. Morrison WH, Garden AS, Ang KK. Radiation therapy for nonmelanoma skin cancers. Clin Plast Surg 1997;24:719–729

68. Fowler BZ, Crocker IR, Johnstone PAS. Perineural spread of cutaneous malignancy to the brain: a review of the literature and five patients treated with stereotactic radiotherapy. Cancer 2005;103:2143–2153

69. Schweitzer VG. Photofrin-mediated photodynamic therapy for treatment of aggressive head and neck nonmelanomatous skin tumors in elderly patients. Laryngoscope 2001;111:1091–1098

70. Kubler AC, Haase T, Staff C, et al. Photodynamic therapy of primary nonmelanomatous skin tumours of the head and neck. Lasers Surg Med 1999;25:60–68

71. Iyer S, Bowes L, Kricorian G, et al. Treatment of basal cell carcinoma with the pulsed carbon dioxide laser: a retrospective analysis. Dermatol Surg 2004;30:1214–1218

72. Chakrabarty A, Geisse JK. Medical therapies for non-melanoma skin cancer. Clin Dermatol 2004;22:183–188

73. Sterry W, Herrera E, Takwale A, et al. Imiquimod 5% cream for the treatment of superficial and nodular basal cell carcinoma: randomized studies comparing low-frequency dosing with and without occlusion. Br J Dermatol 2002;147:1227–1236

74. Urosevic M, Dummer R. Role of imiquimod in skin cancer treatment. Am J Clin Dermatol 2004;5:453–458

75. Balch CM, Soong SJ, Smith T, et al. Long-term results of a prospective trial comparing 2 cm vs. 4 cm excision margins for 740 patients with 1–4 mm melanomas. Ann Surg Oncol 2001;8:101–108

76. Khayat D, Rixe O, Martin G, et al. Surgical margins in cutaneous melanoma (2 cm versus 5 cm for lesions measuring less than 2.1 mm-thick. Cancer 2003;97:1941–1946

77. Prieto VG, Argenyi ZB, Barnhill RL, et al. Are en face frozen sections accurate for diagnosing margin status in melanocytic lesions? Am J Clin Pathol 2003;120:203–208

78. Zitelli JA, Brown CD, Hanusa BH. Surgical margins for excision of primary cutaneous melanoma. J Am Acad Dermatol 1997;37:422–429

79. Ang KK, Byers RM, Peters LJ, et al. Regional radiotherapy as adjuvant therapy for head and neck melanoma: preliminary results. Arch Otolaryngol Head Neck Surg 1990;116:169–172

80. Ang KK, Peters LJ, Weber RS, et al. Postoperative radiotherapy for cutaneous melanoma of the head and neck region. Int J Radiat Oncol Biol Phys 1994;30:795–798

81. Stevens G, Thompson JF, Firth I, et al. Locally advanced melanoma: results of postoperative hypofractionated radiation therapy. Cancer 2000;88:88–94

82. Ballo MT, Ang KK. Radiotherapy for cutaneous malignant melanoma: rationale and indications. Oncology 2004;18:99–107

83. Vongtama R, Safa A, Gallardo D, et al. Efficacy of radiation therapy in the local control of desmoplastic malignant melanoma. Head Neck 2003;25:423–428

84. Gibson SC, Byrne DS, McKay AJ. Ten-year experience of carbon dioxide laser ablation as treatment for cutaneous recurrence of malignant melanoma. Br J Surg 2004;91:893–895

85. Langstein HN, Robb GL. Lip and perioral reconstruction. Clin Plast Surg 2005;32:431–445

86. Pelly AD, Tan E-P. Lower lip reconstruction. Br J Plast Surg 1981;34:83–86

87. Johanson B, Aspelund E, Breine U, Holmstrom H. Surgical treatment of non-traumatic lower lip lesions with special reference to the step technique. Scand J Plast Reconstr Surg 1974;8:232–240

88. Karapandzic M. Reconstruction of lip defects by local arterial flaps. Br J Plast Surg 1974;27:93–97

89. Hamilton MM, Branham GH. Concepts in lip reconstruction. Otolaryngol Clin North Am 1997;30:593–606

90. Cordeiro PG, Santamaria E. Primary reconstruction of complex midfacial defects with combined lip-switch procedures and free flaps. Plast Reconstr Surg 1999;103:1850–1856

91. Burget GC, Menick FJ. The subunit principle in nasal reconstruction. Plast Reconstr Surg 1985;76:239–247

92. Singh DJ, Bartlett SP. Aesthetic considerations in nasal reconstruction and the role of modified nasal subunits. Plast Reconstr Surg 2003;111:639–648

93. Rohrich RJ, Griffin JR, Ansari M, et al. Nasal reconstruction—beyond aesthetic subunits: a 15-year review of 1334 cases. Plast Reconstr Surg 2004;114:1405–1416

94. Menick FJ. A 10-year experience in nasal reconstruction with the three-stage forehead flap. Plast Reconstr Surg 2002;109:1839–1855

95. Chang JS, Becker SS, Park SS. Nasal reconstruction: the state of the art. Curr Opin Otolaryngol Head Neck Surg 2004;12:336–343

96. Winslow CP, Cook TA, Burke A, Wax MK. Total nasal reconstruction: utility of the free radial forearm fascial flap. Arch Facial Plast Surg 2003;5:159–163

97. Murakami CS, Kriet JD, Ierokomos AP. Nasal reconstruction using the inferior turbinate mucosal flap. Arch Facial Plast Surg 1999;1:97–100

98. Walton RL, Burget GC, Beahm EK. Microsurgical reconstruction of the nasal lining. Plast Reconstr Surg 2005;115: In press

99. Teichgraeber JF, Goepfert H. Prosthetic rehabilitation following major nasal resection. Otolaryngol Head Neck Surg 1990;102:362–369

100. Spinelli HM, Jelks JW. Periocular reconstruction: a systematic approach. Plast Reconstr Surg 1993;91:1017–1024

101. Renner G, Kang T. Periorbital reconstruction: brows and eyelids. Facial Plast Surg Clin North Am 2005;13:253–265

102. Mustarde JC. Reconstruction of the lower eyelid. In: Mustarde JC, ed. Repair and Reconstruction in the Orbital Region. 3rd ed. New York: Churchill Livingstone; 1991:125–190

103. Moore BA, Wine T, Netterville JL. Cervicofacial and cervicothoracic flaps in head and neck reconstruction. Head Neck 2005;27:1092–1101

104. Fante RG. Reconstruction of the eyelids. In: Baker S, ed. Local Flaps in Facial Reconstruction. Philadelphia: Mosby; 2007:387–414

105. Leferink VJ, Nicolai JP. Malignant tumors of the external ear. Ann Plast Surg 1988;21:550–554

106. Antia NH, Buch VI. Chondrocutaneous advancement flap for the marginal defect of the ear. Plast Reconstr Surg 1967;39:472–477

107. Butler CE. Reconstruction of marginal ear defects with modified chondrocutaneous helical rim advancement flaps. Plast Reconstr Surg 2003;111:2009–2013

108. Talmi YP, Horowitz Z, Bedrin L, Kronenberg J. Auricular reconstruction with a postauricular myocutaneous island flap: flip-flop flap. Plast Reconstr Surg 1996;98:1191–1199

109. Azaria R, Amir A, Hauben DJ. Anterior conchal reconstruction using a posteroauricular pull-through transpositional flap. Plast Reconstr Surg 2004;113:2071–2075

110. Menick FJ. Reconstruction of the cheek. Plast Reconstr Surg 2001;108:496–504

111. Boutros S, Zide Z. Cheek and eyelid reconstruction: the resurrection of the angle rotation flap. Plast Reconstr Surg 2005;116:1425–1430

112. Campbell BH, Sanger JR, Yousif NJ, et al. Basal and squamous cell skin cancer of the forehead and scalp. In Weber RS, Miller MJ, Goepfert H, eds. Basal and Squamous Cell Skin Cancers of the Head and Neck. Baltimore: Williams & Wilkins; 1996:195–210

113. Leedy JE, Janis JE, Rohrich RJ. Reconstruction of acquired scalp defects: an algorithmic approach. Plast Reconstr Surg 2005;116:54e–72e

114. Lipa JE, Butler CE. Enhancing the outcome of free latissimus dorsi muscle flap reconstruction of large scalp defects. Head Neck 2004;26:46–53

115. O'Brien CJ, Uren RF, Thompson JF, et al. Prediction of potential metastatic sites in cutaneous head and neck melanoma using lymphoscintigraphy. Am J Surg 1995;170:461–466

116. Lund HZ. How often does squamous cell carcinoma of the skin metastasize? Arch Dermatol 1965;92:635–637

117. Cherpelis BS, Marcusen C, Lang PG. Prognostic factors for metastasis in squamous cell carcinoma of the skin. Dermatol Surg 2002;28:268–273

118. Slingluff CL Jr, Stidham KR, Ricci WM, Stanley WE, Seigler HF. Surgical management of regional lymph nodes in patients with melanoma: experience with 4682 patients. Ann Surg 1994;219:120–130

119. McMasters KM, Wong SL, Edwards MJ, et al. Factors that predict the presence of sentinel lymph node metastasis in patients with melanoma. Surgery 2001;130:151–156

120. McMasters KM, Noyes RD, Reintgen DS, et al. Lessons learned from the Sunbelt Melanoma Trial. J Surg Oncol 2004;86:212–223

121. Pathak I, O'Brien CJ, Petersen-Schaeffer K, et al. Do nodal metastases from cutaneous melanoma of the head and neck follow a clinically predictable pattern? Head Neck 2001;23:785–790

122. Conley J, Arena S. Parotid gland as a focus of metastasis. Arch Surg 1963;87:757–764

123. McKean ME, Lee K, McGregor IA. The distribution of lymph nodes in and around the parotid gland: an anatomical study. Br J Plast Surg 1985;38:1–5

124. Goepfert H, Jesse RH, Ballantyne AJ. Posterolateral neck dissection. Arch Otolaryngol 1980;106:618–620

125. Veronesi U, Adamus J, Bandiera DC, et al. Inefficacy of immediate node dissection in Stage I melanoma of the limbs. N Engl J Med 1977;297:627–630

126. Sim FH, Taylor WF, Pritchard DJ, Soule EH. Lymphadenectomy in the management of stage I malignant melanoma: a prospective randomized study. Mayo Clin Proc 1986;61:697–705

127. Balch CM, Soong S-J, Bartolucci AA, et al. Efficacy of elective regional lymph node dissection of 1 to 4 mm thick melanomas for patients 60 years of age and younger. Ann Surg 1996;224:255–266

128. Cascinelli N, Morabito A, Santinami M, et al. Immediate or delayed dissection of regional nodes in patients with melanoma of the trunk: a randomized trial. Lancet 1998;351:793–796

129. Morton DL, Wen DR, Wong JH, et al. Technical details of intraoperative lymphatic mapping for early stage melanoma. Arch Surg 1992;127:392–399

130. Weisberg NK, Bertagnolli MM, Becker DS. Combined sentinel Lymphadenectomy and Mohs micrographic surgery for high-risk cutaneous squamous cell carcinoma. J Am Acad Dermatol 2000;43:483–488

131. Michl C, Starz H, Bachter D, Balda B-R. Sentinel lymphonodectomy in nonmelanoma skin malignancies. Br J Dermatol 2003;149:763–769

132. Schmalbach CE, Nussenbaum B, Rees RS, et al. Reliability of sentinel lymph node mapping with biopsy for head and neck cutaneous melanoma. Arch Otolaryngol Head Neck Surg 2003;129:61–65

133. de Wilt JHW, Thompson JF, Uren RF, et al. Correlation between preoperative lymphoscintigraphy and metastatic nodal disease sites in 362 patients with cutaneous melanomas of the head and neck. Ann Surg 2004;239:544–552

134. Doubrovsky A, de Wilt JHW, Scolyer RA, et al. Sentinel node biopsy provides more accurate staging than elective lymph node dissection in patients with cutaneous melanoma. Ann Surg Oncol 2004;11:829–836

135. Eicher SA, Clayman GL, Myers JN, Gillenwater AM. A prospective study of intraoperative lymphatic mapping for head and neck cutaneous melanoma. Arch Otolaryngol Head Neck Surg 2002;128:241–246

136. Zapas JL, Coley HC, Beam SL, et al. The risk of regional lymph node metastases in patients with melanoma less than 1.0 mm thick: recommendations for sentinel lymph node biopsy. J Am Coll Surg 2003;197:403–407

137. Shpitzer T, Segal K, Schachter J, et al. Sentinel node guided surgery for melanoma in the head and neck region. Melanoma Res 2004;14:283–287

138. Sabel MS, Griffith K, Sondak VK, et al. Predictors of nonsentinel lymph node positivity in patients with a positive sentinel node for melanoma. J Am Coll Surg 2005;201:37–47

139. Kretschmer L, Hilgers R, Mohrle M, et al. Patients with lymphatic metastases of cutaneous malignant melanoma benefit from sentinel lymphonodectomy and early excision of their nodal disease. Eur J Cancer 2004;40:212–218

140. Estourgie SH, Nieweg OE, Valdes Olmos RA, et al. Review and evaluation of sentinel node procedures in 250 melanoma patients with median follow-up of 6 years. Ann Surg Oncol 2003;10:681–688

141. Kang JC, Wanek LA, Essner R, et al. Sentinel lymphadenectomy does not increase the incidence of in-transit metastases in primary melanoma. J Clin Oncol 2005;23:4764–4770

142. Kretschmer L, Beckmann I, Thoms KM, et al. Sentinel lymphonodectomy does not increase the risk of loco-regional cutaneous metastases of malignant melanomas. Eur J Cancer 2005;41:531–538

143. Veness MJ, Morgan GJ, Palme CE, Gebski V. Surgery and adjuvant radiotherapy in patients with cutaneous head and neck squamous cell carcinoma metastatic to lymph nodes: combined treatment should be considered best practice. Laryngoscope 2005;115:870–875

144. Cooper JS, Pajak TF, Forastiere AA, et al. Postoperative concurrent radiotherapy and chemotherapy for high-risk squamous cell carcinoma of the head and neck. N Engl J Med 2004;350:1937–1944

145. Bernier J, Domenge C, Ozsahin M, et al. Postoperative irradiation with or without concomitant chemotherapy for locally advanced head and neck cancer. N Engl J Med 2004;350:1945–1952

146. Ballo MT, Bonnen MD, Garden AS, et al. Adjuvant irradiation for cervical lymph node metastases from melanoma. Cancer 2003;97:1789–1796

147. Bonnen MD, Ballo MT, Myers JN, et al. Elective radiotherapy provides regional control for patients with cutaneous melanoma of the head and neck. Cancer 2004;100:383–389

148. Ballo MT, Garden AS, Myers JN, et al. Melanoma metastatic to cervical lymph nodes: can radiotherapy replace formal dissection after local excision of nodal disease? Head Neck 2005;27:718–721

149. Nasri S, Namazie A, Dulguerov P, Mickel R. Malignant melanoma of cervical and parotid lymph nodes with an unknown primary site. Laryngoscope 1994;104:1194–1198

150. Katz KA, Jonasch E, Hodi FS, et al. Melanoma of unknown primary: experience at Massachusetts General Hospital and Dana-Farber Cancer Institute. Melanoma Res 2005;15:77–82

151. Denic S. Preoperative treatment of advanced skin carcinoma with cisplatin and bleomycin. Am J Clin Oncol 1999;22:32–34

152. Sadek H, Azli N, Wendling JL, et al. Treatment of advanced squamous cell carcinoma of the skin with cisplatin, 5-fluorouracil, and bleomycin. Cancer 1990;66:1692–1696

153. Lippman SM, Parkinson DR, Itri LM, et al. 13-cis-retinoic acid and interferon-alpha-2a: effective combination therapy for advanced squamous cell carcinoma of the skin. J Natl Cancer Inst 1992;84:235–241

154. Shin DM, Glisson BS, Khuri F, et al. Phase II and biologic study of interferon alfa, retinoic acid, and cisplatin in advanced squamous skin cancer. J Clin Oncol 2002;20:364–370

155. Essner R, Lee JH, Wamek LA, Itakura H, Morton DL. Contemporary surgical treatment of advanced-stage melanoma. Arch Surg 2004;139:961–967

156. Kirkwood JM, Strawderman MH, Ernstoff MC, et al. Interferon alfa-2b adjuvant therapy of high-risk resected cutaneous melanoma: the Eastern Cooperative Oncology Group trial EST 1684. J Clin Oncol 1996;14:7–17

157. Kirkwood JM, Ibrahim JG, Sondak VK, et al. High and low-dose interferon alfa-2b in high risk melanoma: first analysis of Intergroup trial E1690/S9111/C9190. J Clin Oncol 2000;18:2444–2458

158. Kirkwood JM, Ibrahim JG, Sosman JA, et al. High-dose interferon alfa-2b significantly prolongs relapse-free and overall survival compared with the GM2-KLH/QS-21 vaccine in patients with resected stage IIB-III melanoma: results of Intergroup trial E1694/S9512/C509801. J Clin Oncol 2001;19:2370–2380

159. Muggiano A, Mulas C, Fiori B, et al. Feasibility of high-dose interferon alpha-2b adjuvant therapy for high-risk resected cutaneous melanoma. Melanoma Res 2004;14(Suppl 1):S1–S7

160. Daryanani D, Plukker JT, de Jong MA, et al. Increased incidence of brain metastases in cutaneous head and neck melanoma. Melanoma Res 2005;15:119–124

161. Chapman PB, Panageas KS, Williams L, et al. Clinical results using biochemotherapy as a standard of care in advanced melanoma. Melanoma Res 2002;12:381–387

162. Rodenas JM, Delgado-Rodriguez M, Herrantz MT, et al. Sun exposure, pigmentary traits, and risk of cutaneous malignant melanoma: a case-control study in a Mediterranean population. Cancer Causes Control 1996;7:275–283

163. Autier P, Dore JF, Schifflers E, et al. Melanoma and use of sunscreens: an EORTC case-control study in Germany, Belgium, and France. Int J Cancer 1995;61:749–755

164. Marks R. Two decades of the public health approach to skin cancer control in Australia: why, how and where we are now? Australas J Dermatol 1999;40:1–5

10

Carcinoma of Unknown Primary Site

Eric M. Genden, Johnny Kao, Stuart H. Packer, and Adam S. Jacobson

◆ Etiology

Carcinoma of unknown primary site (CUP) is defined as a biopsy-proven cancer of the neck that, after a complete clinical and radiographic workup, yields no demonstrable primary tumor. Previously referred to as an undetected primary, the etiology of this clinical entity has been the subject of much debate. Some suggest that CUP is a result of an undetected primary tumor that often is detected later in the clinical course, whereas others believe that the primary tumor undergoes an immune-mediated spontaneous regression while the metastatic tumor escapes immune surveillance. Irrespective of the etiology, it is interesting to note that the Surveillance, Epidemiology, and End Results (SEER) program cancer registry demonstrates that the rate of CUP is declining. This likely represents the identification of more unknown primary tumors as a result of improved imaging and clinical evaluation. High-resolution imaging has undoubtedly been instrumental in identifying more primary carcinomas leading to a decline in the prevalence of CUP.

Development

There has been an interesting evolution in the understanding of CUP of the head and neck. One of the earliest explanations was introduced by Volkmann in 1882,[1] who hypothesized that the neck mass was the result of a branchiogenic cyst that had degenerated into a carcinoma. Volkmann's explanation was widely accepted until the 1940s when Martin and Morfit reexamined Volkmann's hypothesis.[2–4] Studying 55 patients, Martin and Morfit demonstrated that only eight patients met the Volkmann criteria. Subsequently, the Volkmann explanation for an undetectable primary tumor originating within a branchiogenic cyst has been dismissed. A second hypothesis suggested that the disease develops in an embryologic remnant of epithelial tissue that resided within a normal lymph node. Although benign rests of thyroid along with salivary tissue have been documented within normal lymph nodes, squamous epithelium has never been reported to occur in normal lymph node tissue. Therefore, this theory seems unlikely. Finally, it has been suggested that spontaneous regression of the primary tumor may occur while the metastatic cancer continues to grow. It is believed that the regression of the primary is due to the cellular and humoral host immune response that for an ill-defined reason leads to regression of the primary site without affecting the growth of the metastatic tumor. This concept seems to represent the most plausible explanation for head and neck CUP; however, there is little evidence to confirm this theory. Whereas spontaneous regression has been documented in primaries outside of the head and neck, it is rare that such an event occurs in the upper aerodigestive tract.

The possibility that the neck metastasis may arise from an infraclavicular primary is supported by several studies including a review of 267 cases in which 11% were determined to be a result of an infraclavicular primary.[4] This highlights the importance of a careful evaluation of the lung, the most common infraclavicular site for a misdiagnosed CUP. The most contemporary hypothesis accounting for undetectable primary malignancies in the head and neck is the "subclinical primary tumor" theory. This theory suggests that an occult primary malignancy acquiring a metastatic capability early in its development metastasizes to a cervical lymph node. The primary tumor is present but undetectable because of its occult location and small size. Interestingly, even though these tumors acquire an aggressive biological behavior regionally, locally these tumors remain dormant. The primary tumor may remain occult and stable, evolve into a clinically apparent primary tumor, or it can regress spontaneously. When investigating a patient with CUP, however, there is no substitute for a detailed knowledge of the lymphatic drainage patterns of the head and neck.

◆ Anatomy of the Lymphatic Drainage of the Upper Aerodigestive Tract

A comprehensive understanding of the lymphatic pathways of the upper aerodigestive tract is essential to evaluating a patient with a CUP. The cervical lymphatic network is divided into superficial and deep networks that communicate and drain the head and neck. The superficial network drains into the deep network, and the deep network in turn drains into the paired jugular lymphatic ducts that empty into the circulatory system at the junction of the internal jugular vein and subclavian vein. Each anatomic area of the upper aerodigestive tract has its own drainage pathway originally described in 1938 by Rouvierre and further refined in 1972 by Lindberg.[5,6]

The lymphatic anatomy of the neck is well organized and divided into six discrete levels (**Fig. 10–1**). The drainage pathways have been well documented. In general, carcinoma of the oral cavity drains into the submental (level IA), submandibular (level IB), upper jugular (level II), and mid-jugular (level III) lymph nodes, whereas carcinomas of the oropharynx, larynx, and hypopharynx drain most commonly in to the jugular chain (levels II, III, and IV). Palatal and nasopharyngeal carcinoma may drain into the retropharyngeal basin in addition to the upper jugular chain.

Oral Cavity

The lymphatic drainage of the floor of the mouth and mandibular gingiva is divided into anterior and posterior systems.[5–7] Malignancy of the anterior floor of the mouth first drains into the anterior system composed of the submental lymph nodes (level IA). More advanced disease drains posterior along the floor of mouth into the level IB lymph nodes, and the posterior two-thirds of the floor of the mouth drains into the posterior system, which drains into level II lymph nodes (**Fig. 10–2**). Lymphatic drainage may bypass the level II and directly drain into the level III lymph nodes. This highlights the possibility of "skip metastasis" in malignancy of the oral cavity. Equally important, the lymphatic system of the floor of the mouth has bilateral drainage patterns, therefore, both sides of the neck are at risk in floor of mouth carcinoma.

The oral tongue is composed of a dense lymphatic network that is divided into superficial and deep lymphatic systems. The superficial system runs from the tip of the tongue to the circumvallate papillae and drains into the deep lymphatic system. There are three components of the deep lymphatic system. The first, the anterior pathway, drains the tip of the tongue primarily into level III nodes. The second and more common pathway, the lateral pathway, drains the lateral one-third of the dorsum of the tongue from the tip to the circumvallate papillae into lymph node levels II and III (**Fig. 10–3**). The final pathway, the central pathway, drains the central two-thirds of the tongue into lymph node levels I and III. Although rare, "skip metastases" from oral cancer may occur in level IV without the involvement of levels I, II, or III.[7,8] Similar to the floor of the mouth, the oral tongue drains bilaterally.

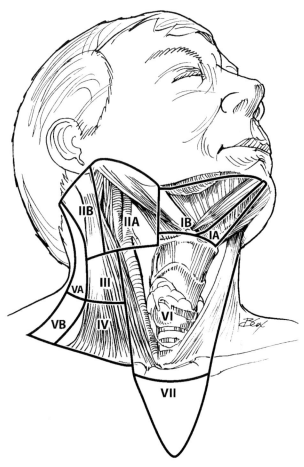

Figure 10–1 Lymphatics of the neck. (*IA*) Lymph nodes that lie within a triangle defined by anterior bellies of the digastric muscles and the hyoid bone (previously classified as submental nodes). (*IB*) Lymph nodes that lie within the triangle formed by the anterior belly of the digastric muscle, the stylohyoid muscle, and the body of the mandible (previously classified as submandibular nodes). (*II*) Level II lymph nodes are located adjacent to the upper third of the jugular vein and spinal accessory nerve. They exist in the area of the neck extending from the skull base and to the lower body of the hyoid bone. The anterior medial boundary is the stylohyoid muscle, and the posterior boundary is the sternocleidomastoid muscle. Radiographically, level II nodes lie anterior to a transverse line drawn on each axial image through the posterior edge of the sternocleidomastoid muscle and lie posterior to a transverse line drawn on each axial scan through the posterior edge of the submandibular gland. *IIA* refers to lymph nodes anterior to the spinal accessory nerve. *IIB* refers to lymph nodes posterior to the spinal accessory nerve. (*III*) Level III lymph nodes are adjacent to the middle third of the internal jugular vein extending from the hyoid bone to the lower margin of the cricoid cartilage. The medial border is the lateral border of the sternohyoid muscle, and the posterior border is the posterior border of the sternocleidomastoid muscle. (*IV*) Level IV lymph nodes are located around the lower third of the internal jugular vein extending from the inferior border of the cricoid cartilage to the clavicle. (*V*) Level V lymph nodes are located in the posterior triangle of the neck located along the spinal accessory nerve. The superior boundary is the convergence of the trapezius muscle and the sternocleidomastoid muscle. The inferior boundary is the clavicle. The anterior boundary is the posterior border of the sternocleidomastoid muscle. The posterior boundary is the anterior border of the trapezius. (*VI*) Level VI lymph nodes include pretracheal and paratracheal lymph nodes. The superior border is the hyoid bone, and the inferior border is the suprasternal notch. The lateral borders are the common carotid arteries.

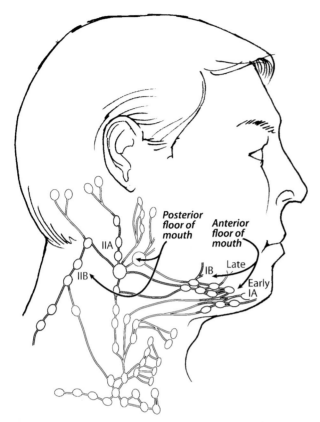

Figure 10–2 Lymphatic drainage of the floor of the mouth. Malignancy of the anterior floor of the mouth first drains into level IA. More advanced disease drains posterior along the floor of the mouth into the level IB lymph nodes. The posterior two-thirds of the floor of the mouth drains into the posterior system, which drains into level II lymph nodes.

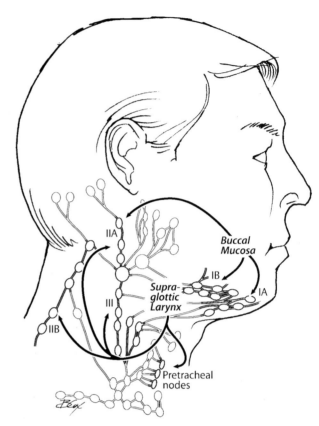

Figure 10–4 The supraglottic larynx is drained through the thyrohyoid membrane into the pretracheal lymph nodes and levels II and III. Anterior lesions of the buccal mucosa drain into levels IA and IB. Posterior buccal lesions drain into the level II lymph nodes.

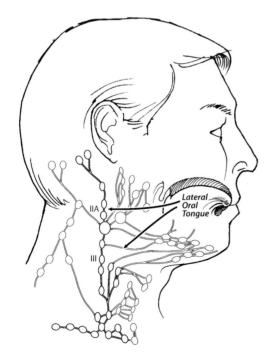

Figure 10–3 The primary drainage pattern of the lateral oral tongue. Lymphatic drainage is primarily into levels II and III.

The buccal mucosa primarily drains into the submandibular space, therefore depending on the location of the tumor, metastasis may occur in level IA, IB, and/or level IIA (**Fig. 10–4**).

Nasopharynx

The nasal septum and nasopharynx drains via a lateral pathway and medial pathway[5–7]; however, the primary direction of drainage is laterally into the lateral retropharyngeal lymph nodes and levels II and V (**Fig. 10–5**). The medial pathway drains the posterior wall and roof of the nasopharynx and the nasal septum into the medial retropharyngeal lymph nodes. The nasopharyngeal drainage is usually bilateral, therefore both sides of the neck are at risk for cervical metastasis.

Oropharynx

The base of the tongue is drained by a superficial and deep lymphatic network. The superficial network is continuous with the superficial oral tongue network and ultimately drains into levels II and III (**Fig. 10–6**). The deep lymphatic network has significant crossover and can therefore drain bilaterally.

The palatine tonsils primarily drain into the ipsilateral level II nodes as well as retropharyngeal nodes (**Fig. 10–7**).

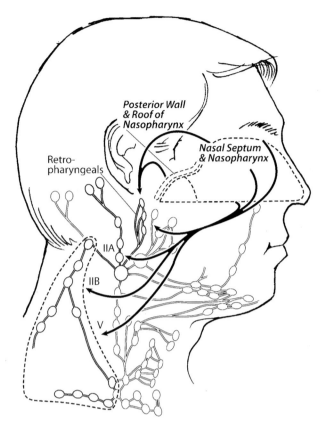

Figure 10–5 Lymphatic drainage of the nose and nasopharynx. The primary direction of drainage from the nasopharynx is laterally into the lateral retropharyngeal lymph nodes and levels II and V.

Less commonly, the palatine tonsils can drain directly into the ipsilateral level III nodes.

The soft palate lymphatic drainage system is subdivided into a anterior, middle, and posterior networks (**Fig. 10–6**). All three networks have the potential to drain bilaterally. The anterior network primarily drains to level I nodes, the middle pathway primarily drains to level II nodes, and the posterior network primarily drains to the lateral retropharyngeal nodes. According to Mukherji, the middle pathway is the most constant and has crossed lymphatic drainage.[8]

Larynx

The supraglottic larynx is drained by a superficial mucosal network of lymphatics that drains into the deep lymphatic network. The deep network combines with the inferior pharyngeal network of lymphatics and exits the larynx through the thyrohyoid membrane into the pretracheal lymph nodes and levels II and III (**Fig. 10–8**). In contrast, the glottic larynx has minimal lymphatic drainage. Within the true vocal cords, there is a paucity of lymph vessels and instead the glottic larynx serves as a natural barrier between the supraglottic and subglottic larynx.

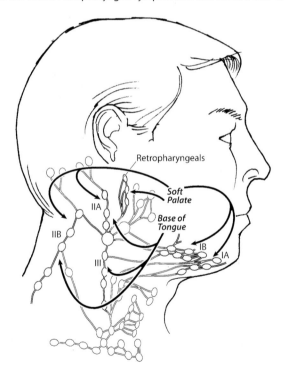

Figure 10–6 Lymphatic drainage for the soft palate and the base of the tongue. The soft palate drains both anterior into levels IA and IB and posterior into levels IIA and IIB, and the base of the tongue drains into levels IIA and IIB.

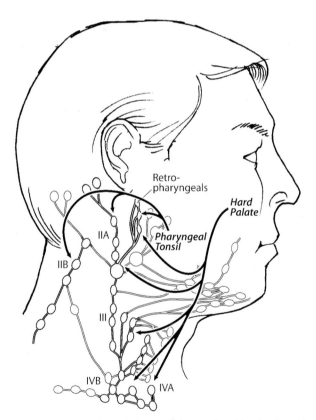

Figure 10–7 Lymphatic drainage of the tonsil and hard palate. The tonsil drains into level II and the hard palate drains into levels II, III, and IV.

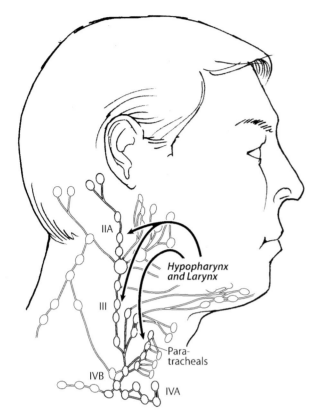

Figure 10–8 Lymphatic drainage of the hypopharynx. The hypopharynx and larynx drain to levels II, III, and IV.

The Hypopharynx

The lymphatic network of the hypopharynx and piriform sinus is divided into an anterior and a posterior group. The anterior system exits the laryngopharynx along with the lymphatics of the supraglottic larynx via the thyrohyoid membrane draining primarily into levels II and III (**Fig. 10–6**). The posterior group drains the inferior hypopharynx into the paratracheal lymph nodes, lateral retropharyngeal nodes, and the jugular chain nodes. Bilateral drainage occurs from the superficial lymphatic system along the midline of the posterior pharynx. The most frequently involved lymph nodes are level II, and unilateral lymph node involvement is more common than bilateral disease.

◆ Presentation

Patients who present with CUP are typically between the ages of 50 and 70 years and present with a unilateral level II painless neck mass. Eighty percent of patients are men, and commonly patients have a history of alcohol and tobacco use, although some may not. The incidence of CUP of the head and neck ranges from 3 to 5%, with squamous cell carcinoma representing ~75% of all reported cases.[9–13] To be considered a CUP, an exhaustive search demonstrating no evidence of a primary tumor must be completed. Fundamental to this workup, all patients must have a thorough head and neck examination including panendoscopy. The patient must have no medical history of a

prior malignancy, including a cutaneous malignancy or ablation of an undefined lesion. The neck mass must be a confirmed malignancy by either cytology or histology without radiologic evidence of a primary lesion. Additionally, there can be no history of symptoms related to a specific organ system.

When a neck mass is identified, it is important to establish a history regarding the duration of the neck mass, the progression of the mass, and any fluctuation in size. All that is a neck mass in not necessarily CUP, and therefore it is important to rule out congenital, infectious, and benign neck masses before establishing the diagnosis of CUP. The neck mass may represent one of a variety of tumors including primary malignancies of the neck such as malignant lymphoma or sarcoma or metastasis from another primary site (**Table 10–1**). Patients with malignant lymphoma often present with multiple soft "rubbery" lymph nodes. Additionally, patients may relate a history of constitutional symptoms including weight loss, night sweats, and/or fever. More advanced disease may be heralded by mucosal petechiae or gingival bleeding as a result of bone marrow replacement. Head and neck sarcomas are relatively rare tumors, accounting for only about 2% of all head and neck malignancies and 4 to 10% of all sarcomas.[14] Patients generally present with a palpable neck mass, skin changes most commonly noted on the scalp or face, or subsite-specific symptoms such as hoarseness or dysphagia.

A cystic neck mass may represent a unique challenge because it is most commonly attributed to a congenital malfor-

Table 10–1 Differential Diagnosis of Cervical Mass

Malignant metastasis to cervical lymph node
    Squamous cell carcinoma
    Adenocarcinoma
    Undifferentiated carcinoma
    Melanoma
    Thyroid carcinoma
    Adenoid cystic carcinoma
    Mucoepidermoid carcinoma
    Lymphoma
Rhabdomyosarcoma
Malignant peripheral nerve sheath tumors
Paraganglioma
Schwannomas
Neurofibromas
Lipoma
Lymphadenitis
    Viral (HIV)
    Bacterial
    Granulomatous (typical and atypical mycobacteria, actinomycosis, sarcoid, *Bartonella*)
Congenital
    Branchial cleft cyst (2nd and 3rd)
    Lymphangioma
    Cystic hygroma
    Hemangioma
    Dermoid cyst
    Epidermal and sebaceous cysts

mation such as a brachial cleft cyst, thyroglossal duct cyst, or a lymphangioma. A congenital cyst may be present but small and undetectable for years prior to presentation. Tenderness and erythema may suggest an infectious component; however, malignancy may also present as a cystic neck mass. A cystic neck mass at level II in an adult patient with risk factors of squamous cell carcinoma should be considered a tonsil primary until proved otherwise. For reasons not understood, metastasis from a tonsil primary commonly presents as a level II cystic neck mass. Although uncommon, papillary thyroid and squamous cell carcinoma of the upper aerodigestive tract may present as a cystic neck mass. It is not uncommon that a clinician will perform an excisional neck biopsy of a presumed congenital neck cyst only to find that the pathology demonstrates a malignancy. Therefore, it is important to discuss with the patient the possibility of a neck dissection and panendoscopy in the event that the frozen section reveals squamous cell carcinoma. Fine-needle aspiration (FNA) can be helpful in identifying as many as three quarters of cystic malignancies and prevent such a scenario.[15]

◆ Diagnosis and Workup

History and Physical Examination

The character and location of a neck mass may provide important information regarding the site of the primary tumor. Supraclavicular lymph nodes more likely represent an infraclavicular primary site such as the breast or lung, whereas jugular chain lymphadenopathy is more commonly associated with an upper aerodigestive tract primary. Once the initial evaluation has been performed and the origin of the neck mass remains occult, a FNA of the neck mass will usually confirm the diagnosis and rule out a congenital or infectious etiology. We routinely submit a sample for cytology, culture, and flow cytometry to evaluate for malignant lymphoma. Although blood tests have a limited role in the workup, a complete blood count (CBC) may be useful to rule out infection, and an Epstein-Barr titer may identify an occult nasopharyngeal carcinoma.

The physical examination should include a careful survey of the skin of the scalp and neck to rule out a cutaneous malignancy. Light-skinned individuals or those with a history of excessive sunburns as a child are at higher risk for cutaneous malignancy. In such patients, a careful survey of the skin and the scalp may be fruitful. Irregular or ulcerated lesions should be evaluated, and a dermatology consultation may be warranted. The sinonasal mucosa and mucosa of the upper aerodigestive tract should be meticulously evaluated using a fiberoptic endoscope.

Office nasopharyngoscopy is an important first step in evaluating the aerodigestive tract; however, a small lesion can easily hide within a mucosal fold of Waldeyer's ring and escape detection (**Fig. 10–9**). For this reason, every patient should undergo panendoscopy including esophagoscopy, nasopharyngoscopy, direct laryngoscopy, and tracheobronchoscopy under general anesthesia. The popularity of

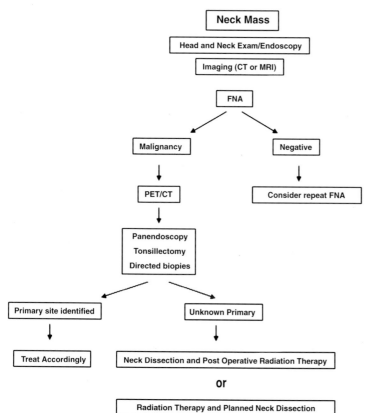

Figure 10–9 Algorithm for management of a neck mass.

office-based transnasal esophagoscopy and nasopharyngoscopy has led some to consider office-based panendoscopy; however, this technique does not allow the surgeon to distend the mucosal folds of the pharynx or palpate the tissue for submucosal lesions. Intraoperative panendoscopy can be valuable in identifying a subtle lesion, and therefore an office panendoscopy is not a substitute for an examination under general anesthesia.

Imaging

Imaging plays an important role in the CUP workup. Chest x-ray, computed tomography (CT), and magnetic resonance imaging (MRI) have all been extensively used for detection of a CUP; however, coregistered positron emission tomography and computed tomography (PET-CT) has emerged as the most popular tool for evaluating CUP. Functional imaging such as PET represents a very attractive option for detection of an unknown primary tumor, especially in the case of negative CT or MRI scans. PET is based on the concept that tumors maintain a higher level of metabolic activity than surrounding normal aerodigestive mucosa. Fluorodeoxyglucose (FDG)-PET uses a glucose analogue [^{18}F]fluoro-2-deoxy-D-glucose that enters into cells and is shunted into the normal metabolic cycle where ATP is produced. The analogue is able to enter into the glucose metabolism cycle but cannot complete the cycle and therefore accumulates in the cells. Because glucose metabolism is increased in malignant cells, these cells accumulate larger quantities of the radiolabeled analogue than do normal cells. When the scan is then performed, the areas of increased metabolic activity are localized. The data evaluating the utility of PET for CUP has been divided. Whereas several studies demonstrate that FDG-PET can detect a primary lesion in 21 to 47% of cases,[16–18] there is evidence to the contrary suggesting that FDG-PET does not significantly improve the rate of CUP detection.[19] Our group has not found PET-CT useful in the workup of CUP.

Recently, the fusion of PET imaging with coregistered CT imaging has improved the ability to correlate these areas of increased uptake with definable anatomic structures. This fusion imaging has produced a more accurate image that has been helpful in identifying the location of an occult primary malignancy. A recent study by Miller et al examined the use of PET imaging in the setting of an occult primary tumor. Twenty-six patients who had cervical metastasis with an occult primary tumor were enrolled. All the patients had a complete history and physical examination, flexible nasopharyngoscopy, CT or MRI imaging, PET imaging, and panendoscopy with directed biopsies. Of the 26 patients studied, eight occult malignancies were found via PET imaging, resulting in a detection rate of 30.8%, and four occult tumors were identified during panendoscopy despite negative PET imaging findings. This resulted in a sensitivity of 66% and specificity of 92.9%.[20] Currently, the ability to detect small areas of increased activity is limited to ~5 mm. The areas most difficult to diagnose with FDG-PET include the supraglottic region and Waldeyer's ring. Occult tumors of Waldeyer's ring are especially difficult to interpret because tumors are commonly superficial and surrounded by an abundance of lymphoid tissue and salivary gland tissue that characteristically concentrates FDG making interpretation difficult.

Endoscopy

The panendoscopy, including direct operative laryngoscopy, esophagoscopy, nasopharyngoscopy, and bronchoscopy, remains the gold standard for evaluating patients with CUP. By performing a complete head and neck examination under anesthesia, the surgeon is able to palpate and visualize the entire upper aerodigestive tract for areas of induration, asymmetry, and firmness. There is no substitute for deep palpation of the neck and base of the tongue under general anesthesia. During operative endoscopy, areas that are difficult to evaluate in the office, such as the esophageal inlet can be thoroughly examined. Furthermore, if a suspicious area is noted, a directed biopsy should be performed with frozen-section analysis of the specimen. If no lesions are identified, random biopsies can be performed of the base of the tongue, nasopharynx, tonsils, and piriform sinus. These sites are often evaluated because they represent the sites with the highest likelihood of harboring an occult primary carcinoma. There is controversy regarding the role for blind directed biopsies of the upper aerodigestive tract; however, there is literature to suggest that directed biopsies may reveal an occult carcinoma in nearly 20% of cases.[21]

Tonsillectomy

As the primary component of Waldeyer's ring, the tonsils are the most common location of an occult primary malignancy. There has been controversy regarding the optimal method to assess the tonsillar region for malignancy. Random tonsil biopsies or a formal tonsillectomy is a topic of great debate. More recently, it has been demonstrated that microscopic or submucosal disease can be missed on a random tonsil biopsy.[22] The tonsil can harbor small lesions deep within its crypts that can be missed on biopsy making it difficult to rule out the tonsil as the primary site of malignancy. Fortunately, unlike other potential sites of origin of the primary malignancy, the tonsil can be removed *en bloc* by formal tonsillectomy with minimal morbidity and avoiding the sampling error of a random biopsy. In 1998, McQuone et al demonstrated that the detection rate of occult tonsillar carcinoma is increased by performing a formal tonsillectomy rather than a focal tonsillar biopsy.[22] They found that only 13% of the tonsil biopsy specimens were positive for squamous cell carcinoma but 39% of the patients undergoing bilateral tonsillectomy were found to have squamous cell carcinoma within a tonsil.

The importance of bilateral versus unilateral tonsillectomy is less clear. Although there is minimal morbidity associated with tonsillectomy, it is important to justify the necessity for performing a bilateral tonsillectomy during the investigation of a unilateral occult metastasis. It has been demonstrated that as many as 10% of the patients with an occult malignancy may possess either bilateral or contralateral tonsillar malignancy.[23] Based on this finding and the low risk associated with tonsillectomy, we advocate a bilateral tonsillectomy during the CUP workup in all patients if a primary lesion is not identified at the time of panendoscopy.

Evaluation of Distant Disease

An evaluation for distant disease is usually completed during the initial workup and therefore no further workup should be necessary. While a variety of laboratory tests including CBC, SMA-20, and liver function tests (LFTs) may be ordered, they are usually low yield. Abnormal LFTs may be abnormal in as many as 50% of patients with a history of head and neck cancer but no detectable liver metastasis.

◆ Staging and Prognostic

By definition, CUP is T0 and N+. Therefore, all CUP patients are considered stage III if they have N1 disease and stage IV if they have N2 or N3 disease. The American Joint Committee on Cancer (AJCC) staging system serves as the primary tool for staging cancer of the head and neck worldwide (**Table 10–2**). Because the AJCC staging system is largely based on the surface dimensions of the primary tumor, the ability to categorize a cervical malignancy with an undetected primary tumor is limited. The only change in staging with the introduction of the 6th edition of the AJCC *Cancer Staging Manual* is that a designation of "U" or "L" may be used to indicate metastasis above the lower border of the cricoid (U) or below the lower border of the cricoid (L).

Extracapsular Spread

The survival and prognosis of a patient with a cervical mass of an undetectable primary tumor is affected by a variety of factors including patient comorbidity, performance status, nutritional status, and the patient's intact immune response. Unlike cases of a known primary, CUP provides minimal histopathologic information that can be used for prognosis with the exception of number of lymph nodes and extracapsular spread. Like all other head and neck squamous cell carcinomas, the prognosis seems equivalent to that observed in patients with overt primary and similar nodal stage. Extracapsular spread increases the risk for both regional and distant recurrence[24,25] and in one study tripled the risk of distant metastasis as the first site of failure.[26] As expected, extracapsular spread is a significant predictor of poor disease-free and overall survival. These findings have prompted several trials using adjuvant chemotherapy in patients with documented extracapsular spread. In the combined analysis of the Radiation Therapy Oncology Group (RTOG) 95-01 and European Organization for Research on Treatment of Cancer (EORTC) postoperative trials, patients with extracapsular extension had an improved locoregional control and overall survival with adjuvant chemoradiation compared with radiation alone.[27]

Nodal Location

There are several studies that demonstrate that pathologic lymph nodes located low in the cervical chain (level IV) are associated with an increased risk of regional recurrence, distant recurrence, and decreased survival.[28,29] Furthermore, the presence of low cervical chain disease is associated with an increased risk of concomitant pulmonary metastasis.[30] Supraclavicular disease should be considered a separate entity from jugular chain disease because of its high association with infraclavicular malignancy. Breast, prostate, and gastric cancer have been documented to present with supraclavicular malignant adenopathy; however, lung cancer is the most common infraclavicular site. When CUP presents in the supraclavicular region, 5-year survival is less than 15%.[31,32]

Patterns of Failure and Management of Recurrent Disease

The pattern of failure largely depends on the initial treatment regimen. Following radiotherapy, the predominant

Table 10–2 The American Joint Committee on Cancer Staging System for Carcinoma of Unknown Primary Site

Regional Lymph Nodes (N)
• N1: Metastasis in a single ipsilateral lymph node, 3 cm or less in greatest dimension*
• N2: Metastasis in a single ipsilateral lymph node, more than 3 cm but not more than 6 cm in greatest dimension, or in multiple ipsilateral lymph nodes, none more than 6 cm in greatest dimension, or in bilateral or contralateral lymph nodes, none more than 6 cm in greatest dimension*
N2a: Metastasis in a single ipsilateral lymph node more than 3 cm but not more than 6 cm in greatest dimension*
N2b: Metastasis in multiple ipsilateral lymph nodes, none more than 6 cm in greatest dimension*
N2c: Metastasis in bilateral or contralateral lymph nodes, none more than 6 cm in greatest dimension*
• N3: Metastasis in a lymph node more than 6 cm in greatest dimension*

Distant Metastasis (M)
• MX: Distant metastasis cannot be assessed
• M0: No distant metastasis
• M1: Distant metastasis

Note: There is no tumor classification (T) for occult primary cancer metastatic to neck lymph nodes.
*A designation of "U" or "L" may be used to indicate metastasis above the lower border of the cricoid (U) or below the lower border of the cricoid (L).

patterns of recurrence include regional and distant metastases.[33–35] Regional recurrence often represents a difficult problem because the recurrence is often invasive and advanced. This likely reflects that recurrence is often difficult to detect on physical exam. The radiated neck is often firm and woody making palpation difficult. CT and MRI have been important tools for surveillance however the use of PET/CT has become the preferred method for identifying recurrence.[36,37]

When distant metastasis is identified, it usually occurs within a year following completion of therapy. Pulmonary metastasis is the most common site for distant recurrence, occurring in one-third of patients. The location and volume of disease will guide therapy. Peripherally located pulmonary metastasis may be managed surgically while more advanced and unresectable disease may be managed with chemoradiation with the intent to cure or palliative chemotherapy depending on the disease status.

Emergence of the primary tumor may occur in as few as 0% to as many as 66% of patients originally diagnosed with CUP and occurs most commonly in those treated initially with surgery alone.[38,39] Emergence of a primary tumor usually occurs within 24 months and will likely present in the oral cavity, oropharynx, and nasopharynx.[39] Some have observed poor prognosis following detection of the primary lesion however the data is conflicting because in some series tumor emergence later than 5 years after primary treatment was classified as a second primary, whereas in others studies tumor emergence was considered to be the site of origin.[40] As a result the significance of an emergence of a primary tumor is unclear.

Outcome and Survival

Unlike CUP of the infraclavicular region, where the prognosis is poor, CUP of the head and neck is unique with 5-year disease-specific survival rates as high as 74%,[41,42] and overall survival rates range from 40 to 66%.[41–45] The outcome and survival of patients with CUP is variable largely because the outcomes are derived from several retrospective studies with a diverse patient population (**Table 10–3**). Several studies have reported favorable results with combined surgery and

Table 10–3 Summary of Outcomes for Occult Primary Carcinoma

First Author/ Institution/Reference	No of Patients and Percent Stage IV	Treatment Modalities and Percent	5-Year OS (%)	Mucosal Failure (%)	Neck Failure (%)	Distant Failure (%)
Jesse, M.D. Anderson[31]	104 (N/A)	S only (100%)	57*	20	16†	N/A
Jesse, MD Anderson[31]	52 (N/A)	RT only (100%)	48*	6	0†	N/A
Jesse, MD Anderson[31]	28 (N/A)	S + RT (100%)	46*	14	0†	N/A
Erkal, University of Florida[71]	126 (90%)	RT only (44%)				
		S + RT (56%)	47	13	22	14
Reddy, Loyola[53]	32 (89%)	Bilateral RT + S (75%)	53	8	14	~15
		Bilateral RT only (25%)				
Reddy, Loyola[53]	16 (69%)	Ipsilateral RT + S (75%)	47	44	44	~15
		Ipsilateral RT only (25%)				
Argiris, University of Chicago[47]	25 (100%)	S + CRT (88%)				
		CRT only (12%)	75	0	4	8
Colletier, M.D. Anderson[41]	136 (77%)	S + RT (100%)	60	10	9	18
Grau, Danish Multi-institutional[33]	277 (83%)	S only (8%) RT only (81%)	36	54 (S only) 15 (RT or S + RT)	~44 (S only) 50 (RT only)	N/A
		S + RT (9%)			38 (RT +S)	N/A
Maulard, University of Paris[72]	113 (73%)	S + RT (100%)	38	10	14	16
Marcial-Vega, Washington University[32]	72 (83%)	RT (57%) S + RT (43%)	45*	12	N/A	N/A
Weir, Princess Margaret Hospital[38]	144 (85%)	Neck only RT (60%)	41	7 (neck only)	49	23
		Bilateral RT (40%)		2 (bilateral)		
Nieder, literature review[35]	4 papers (N/A)	S (100%)	~66	~25	~34	N/A
Nieder, literature review[35]	6 papers (N/A)	Ipsilateral RT (100%)	37 median	8 median (range, 5 to 44)	52 median	N/A (only report 38)
Nieder, literature review[35]	12 papers (N/A)	Bilateral RT (100%)	50 median	10 median (range, 2 to 13)	19 median	19 median

Abbreviations: CRT, chemotherapy and radiation; N/A, nonapplicable; RT, radiation therapy; S, surgery.
*Disease-free survival.
†Contralateral neck failure.

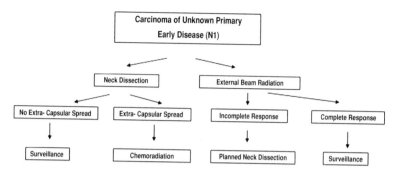

Figure 10–10 Management of early CUP (N1).

radiation therapy[39,41,46]; however, there are only two smaller studies utilizing chemoradiation that have demonstrated promising results.[10,47]

◆ Treatment

Surgical Treatment

Early Disease

The management principles of CUP can be organized into early disease (N1) and advanced disease (any disease with extracapsular spread, N2 and N3). Less than 30% of patients presenting with CUP will have early disease. Following the diagnosis of early CUP, the options for therapy include ipsilateral neck dissection with radiation reserved for high-risk pathologic features or ipsilateral neck dissection with planned postoperative radiation (**Fig. 10–10**). Surgical staging is important for directing therapy. There is often significant disparity between clinical staging and pathologic staging.[48] Lefebre et al found that as many as 57% of patients who were clinically staged N1 had multiple pathologic lymph nodes at the time of dissection. In addition to a disparity in staging, the rate of extracapsular spread in N1 disease without radiographic evidence of extracapsular spread has been reported as high as 35% highlighting the limitations of clinical and radiographic staging.[43,45] For this reason, it is indicated to perform the neck dissection prior to radiotherapy to gain information regarding the pathologic stage and the presence of extracapsular spread. This information can be used to determine the necessity for postoperative radiation and chemotherapy.

In most cases, early disease can be managed with a neck dissection alone or in combination with postoperative radiation therapy. In such cases, the extent of the neck dissection has been a point of controversy. Traditionally, a radical or modified radical neck dissection has been indicated for management of the N+ neck; however, patients should be carefully selected.[49] It is clear that the selective neck dissection is an effective operation for the management of the N+ neck.[50] If there is evidence of extracapsular spread, however, we recommend a modified neck dissection with removal of any effected structures.

The American Head and Neck Society and the American Academy of Otolaryngology–Head and Neck Surgery proposed a definition of the types of neck dissection that have been classified into four different operations and a series of subtype operations based on the structures removed during surgery (**Table 10–4**). The radical neck dissection (RND) is the standard operation wherein the lymph nodes of levels I to V are removed with the sternocleidomastoid muscle (SCM), internal jugular vein (IJV), and the accessory nerve (cranial nerve XI). A modified radical neck dissection (MRND) suggests that one or more nonlymphatic structures are preserved. A selective neck dissection includes removal of the lymph-bearing tissue in fewer than all five regions of the neck with preservation of the SCM, IJV, and cranial nerve XI. An extended neck dissection involves removal of any lymph nodes or nonlymphatic structures not routinely removed.

When a planned neck dissection is performed after full-course radiation, we recommend performing surgery within 3 weeks after the final radiation treatment to limit the risk of postoperative wound complications and reduce the risk associated with excessive scaring.

Radiation Therapy

In the multidisciplinary approach to squamous cell carcinoma of unknown primary, the clinician must consider both the neck and potential mucosal sites. When the radiation oncologist considers whether to irradiate a given volume,

Table 10–4 Classification of Neck Dissection

Dissection Type	Lymph Nodes Removed	Structures Removed
Radical neck dissection	I–V	SCM, IJV, cranial nerve XI
Modified	I–V	
Type I	I–V	SCM, IJV
Type II	I–V	SCM
Type III	I–V	None
Selective neck dissection (SND)		
SND I–III/IV	I–III/IV	None
SND II–IV (lateral)	I–IV	None
SND II–V (posterolateral)	II–V	None
SND VI	IV	None
Extended neck dissection	Any neck dissection that is extended to include either lymph node groups or structures in the neck not routinely removed	

the marginal benefit must be carefully weighed against the added toxicity. Unfortunately, there are no published randomized controlled trials available to guide treatment policies. Therefore, treatment recommendations are based on retrospective analyses.

For squamous cell carcinomas of the head and neck, the N1 neck can be treated with either radiation therapy or surgery alone with 85 to 93% neck control.[51,52] Therefore, the modality selected will be determined by the approach to the primary mucosal sites. For a well-differentiated N1 submandibular node with no extracapsular extension, the most likely source of a primary lesion is the oral cavity. Electively irradiating the oral cavity and oropharynx would result in significant acute mucositis. A subsequent oral cavity primary would likely be detected at an early stage with careful clinical examination. Therefore, a level I to V neck dissection followed by careful observation of the oral cavity would be a rational approach to this presentation. When reserved for carefully selected patients, this approach can be effective.[42] The mucosal recurrence rate for selected patients treated with surgery alone is ~25%, the nodal recurrence rate is ~34%, and the 5-year overall survival rate is ~66%.[35]

Elective Mucosal and Nodal Irradiation

For all other N1 presentations, the benefits of irradiating the neck and primary mucosal sites in reducing neck and mucosal failure appear to outweigh the risks of elective radiation (**Table 10–1**). A study from M.D. Anderson treated 210 patients with squamous cell carcinoma of unknown primary with surgery, irradiation, or both.[31] Patients treated with combined surgery and radiation tended to have more advanced disease. The 3-year disease-free survival was ~50% in all three treatment groups. Compared with surgery alone, radiation to the mucosal sites reduced the risk of a failure at the primary site from 20 to 6%.[31] The 3-year overall survival was 58% when the primary site was controlled versus 31% when a primary manifested. Additionally, comprehensive neck irradiation reduced the risk of contralateral failure from 16% to 0. Among the cohort treated with surgery (excisional biopsy or neck dissection) and postoperative radiation, the 5-year risk of regional recurrence was 9%, with all recurrences occurring in patients with extracapsular extension.[41] The distant metastasis rate was 18%, and the 5-year overall survival rate was 60%.

In an effort to reduce toxicity, several investigators have evaluated the efficacy of ipsilateral neck irradiation without elective treatment of the contralateral neck or mucosal sites. A study from Loyola University compared ipsilateral neck irradiation with comprehensive neck and mucosal irradiation in a cohort of 52 patients with occult primary carcinoma.[53] Elective radiation dramatically reduced the likelihood of subsequent mucosal failure from 44 to 8% and contralateral failure from 44 to 14%.[54] Ipsilateral neck control was similar in both groups (69% vs. 81%, N = 0.4). The 5-year overall survival was ~50% in both treatment groups. In the largest reported study from the Danish Society for Head and Neck Oncology, comprehensive neck irradiation was associated with a higher 5-year locoregional control than ipsilateral neck ir-

radiation (51% vs. 27%, P = 0.05).[32] This difference translated into a trend toward higher 5-year disease-specific survival for comprehensive neck irradiation (45% vs. 28%, P = 0.1).[33]

The University of Florida treated 69 patients with radical irradiation with or without neck dissection.[44] There was a 10% mucosal failure at 5 years and 25% mucosal failure at 10 years. The 10-year mucosal failure rate was identical to a historical control of patients with known primary tumors that were locally controlled (P = 0.49), suggesting that radiation successfully controlled the unknown primary but did not prevent second primary cancers. In a recent update of the Florida series, the 5-year nodal failure rate was 22%, 5-year distant failure rate was 14%, and the 5-year overall survival was 47%.[54] Most patients received comprehensive neck irradiation, but patients with N1 disease with no extracapsular extension received only ipsilateral irradiation. The likelihood of neck control after excisional biopsy of a single positive node and postoperative radiation is 95%.[54] These patients are at high risk of failure if radiotherapy is omitted.[55]

Although comprehensive irradiation is consistently associated with a lower risk of neck relapse than ipsilateral radiation, in some studies the difference in mucosal failure is small. Depending on the technique of ipsilateral irradiation, the pharyngeal axis may receive a clinically significant dose of radiation. Taken together, these data indicate that radiation alters the natural history of occult primary carcinoma by preventing contralateral nodal recurrences and mucosal recurrences, but a survival benefit has not been demonstrated. Comprehensive radiation is associated with higher locoregional control than is ipsilateral radiation, but overall survival appears similar because of the significant competing risks of distant failure and neck failure.

Radiation Techniques: Determination of Target Volume and Dose

Elective mucosal radiation for the most common presentations (level II, III, and upper V) requires coverage of the nasopharynx, oropharynx, hypopharynx, supraglottic larynx, and bilateral neck. This large-volume field is historically associated with significant xerostomia when treated with the conventional technique of opposed laterals matched to a lower anterior neck field.[56] Intensity-modulated radiation therapy (IMRT) allows the radiation oncologist to deliver higher doses to the target volume than to adjacent avoidance structures. This technology allows preferential sparing of the spinal cord, brain stem, parotid glands, and oral cavity. Although clinical data with this approach have not yet matured, it appears that the improved dose distributions with IMRT translate into less long-term toxicity and better locoregional control than conventional radiation.[57–59] In the interim, this approach is recommended when treatment is at centers with expertise in head and neck IMRT to reduce the toxicity associated with large-field radiotherapy.

Elective mucosal radiation may be tailored depending on the location of the involved node(s). For a level I node, only the oral cavity and oropharynx should be irradiated. For a metastasis to the low neck (level IV or low level V), the nasopharynx may be excluded.

Radiation dose levels consisting of 50 Gy to the low-risk neck, 60 to 66 Gy to high-risk microscopic disease, and 70 to 75 Gy to gross disease has largely been determined empirically.[60] The impact of radiation dose to electively treated mucosal sites was investigated in a small study from the University of Florida. Although retrospective and underpowered, there was a positive trend between dose and mucosal site control. The mucosal control rate was 91% for patients receiving 50.1 to 60.0 Gy versus 81% for patients receiving 45.1 to 50.0 Gy.[44]

Radiation Toxicity

Xerostomia is the most common late complication of elective mucosal irradiation. Based on comparison with historical controls, this may be markedly reduced by IMRT. The risk of severe late complications with elective radiation of the neck is relatively low. The most common toxicities from neck irradiation are subcutaneous fibrosis and submental edema. Osteoradionecrosis, permanent gastrostomy tube dependence, severe arytenoid edema, and esophageal stricture were rare and occurred in less than 2% of patients receiving radiation.[61] During radiation, mucositis, increased pharyngeal secretions, and dermatitis are the most common acute toxicities resulting from comprehensive radiation. The incidence and severity of mucositis, weight loss, and xerostomia are lower with ipsilateral radiation only.[53] These acute discomforts associated with radiation generally resolve within 1 month of completing radiation and are managed with supportive care. If chemoradiation is used, approximately half of the patients will require a gastrostomy tube for nutritional support.[47] The long-term rate of gastrostomy tube dependence may be higher with the use of chemoradiation compared with that of radiation alone.

Chemotherapy

Systemically administered chemotherapy has become an integral part of the multimodality treatment of squamous cell carcinoma of the head and neck. Indeed, in many patients with locoregionally advanced squamous cell cancer of the head and neck, concurrent chemoradiotherapy has become the standard of care. Unfortunately, owing to the rarity, clinical and biologic heterogeneity, and lack of randomized controlled studies in this group of patients, the exact role of chemotherapy in the management of CUP is unclear. Nevertheless, treatment paradigms can be developed utilizing principles that have been established in the treatment of locally advanced squamous cell cancer of the head and neck.

The rationale for concomitant chemoradiotherapy is that it can improve local tumor control by radiosensitization while also providing systemic antitumor activity. Consequently, treatment strategies have evolved utilizing concurrent chemoradiotherapy in the management of locoregionally advanced disease and in organ preservation. This approach has been substantiated in single-institution trials, multi-institutional studies, as well as in meta-analysis. Concurrent chemoradiotherapy has become the standard of care

in locoregionally advanced unresectable cancer and in selected patients with nasopharyngeal and laryngeal cancer. In the postoperative adjuvant setting, two randomized trials showed an improvement in overall survival and local control with the use of combined chemoradiation when compared with radiation alone in high-risk patients.

There are no randomized controlled studies specifically addressing the issue of integrating chemotherapy into the management of CUP. Given the rationale that CUP represents metastatic disease in the form of lymphatic spread and therefore by definition locoregionally advanced disease, concurrent chemoradiotherapy is appropriate in patients with good performance status.

Single-institution studies have shown encouraging results with the use of chemoradiotherapy when compared with historical controls. Several groups have used CRT protocols reporting good outcomes; however, the patients suffered extensive treatment-related morbidity.[10,62,63] Assuming there are no comorbid conditions or poor performance status that would preclude the use of chemotherapy; we recommend that patients with N2 or N3 disease be treated with chemoradiotherapy and surgery. Outside of a clinical trial, use of standard-dose cisplatin, either on a 3-week (100 mg/m^2) or weekly (40 mg/m^2) schedule, is reasonable. Taxanes, either as single agents or in combination with platinum drugs, have been shown to be effective when used concurrently with radiotherapy. Whether treatment with more aggressive regimens will result in improved results awaits further study. The use of concomitant chemoradiotherapy is unavoidably associated with an increase risk of mucosal complications as well as the need for intensive nutritional support. These toxicities can be successfully managed by dedicated caregivers primarily involved with the management of patients with head and neck cancer.

Targeted Therapy

Targeted therapy refers to the use of agents that are specifically directed against tumor cells and as a consequence mitigate the toxicities usually seen with standard cytotoxic chemotherapy. Several different classes of targeted agents have been investigated including epidermal growth factor receptor (EGFR) inhibitors, antiangiogenic agents, Ras inhibitors, proteasome inhibitors and immune modulators. The best studied and the two that have entered clinical practice in the treatment of head and neck cancer are the EGFR and vascular endothelial growth factor (VEGF) inhibitors.

EGFR is involved in several critical pathways and regulates cell growth. Overexpression of EGFR is associated with cell proliferation and is an independent predicator of locoregional relapse and survival. Two major classes of EGFR inhibitors have been developed and have undergone phase II or III trials in patients with head and neck cancer.

Gefitinib and erlotinib are oral, small-molecule tyrosine kinase inhibitors that have been tested as single agents in recurrent or metastatic squamous cell cancer of the head and neck. Gefitinib has also been evaluated in a phase II trial integrated into a program of concurrent chemoradiotherapy. The only significant toxicities seen in these trials were skin rash and diarrhea. There was no synergistic toxicity when added to chemotherapy.

Cetuximab is humanized monoclonal antibody directed against the extracellular domain of EGFR. It has been studied in recurrent or metastatic disease both as a single agent in platinum refractory patients as well as in combination with cisplatin. Bonner et al have reported a study comparing radiation alone to cetuximab plus radiation in patients with locoregionally advanced squamous cell carcinoma of the head and neck.[64] They found that the addition of cetuximab to radiation increased both the duration of local control and survival.

There are currently no studies utilizing targeted therapy in the management of patients with CUP. Whether the addition of these agents to radiation will improve local control and survival compared with chemoradiotherapy is unknown. The results of the Bonner study suggest that it would not be unreasonable to consider the addition of cetuximab to radiation in patients unwilling or unable to tolerate chemotherapy.

Advanced Neck Disease

Trimodality Approach

For patients with N2a to N3 neck disease, radiation or surgery alone is inadequate therapy (**Fig. 10–11**). Neck failure occurs in 20 to 35% of patients with N2 disease treated with radiation alone and in 35 to 65% of patients with N3 disease treated with radiation alone.[51,52] Neck failure occurs in 30% of patients with N2a disease and 70 to 75% of patients with N2b to N3 disease treated with surgery alone. Combined surgery and radiation reduces the rate of neck failure to ~15%. Based on these data, multidisciplinary management of the N2 to N3 neck is indicated, although the added benefit of combined therapy for N2a disease is small.[52]

Although there are no randomized trials specifically addressing the role of chemoradiation for patients with an N2 to N3 unknown primary cancer, multiple phase III randomized trials demonstrate a locoregional control advantage for concurrent chemoradiation compared with radiation therapy alone for stage III to IVA/B head and neck cancer in the potentially resectable, unresectable, and postoperative

settings.[65,66] This translated into an overall survival advantage in several of these trials.

Despite the improved locoregional control conferred by chemoradiation, the addition of a selective neck dissection appears beneficial for patients with N2 to N3 disease.[47,67–69] We advocate planned neck dissection after chemoradiation for patients with N2 to N3 disease. Unlike early disease, we recommend a planned neck dissection after combined chemoradiation. Advanced disease is commonly associated with extension into the deep musculature, nerves, and, in some cases, the overlying skin. Additionally, chemoradiation may reduce the disease extension and free up vital structures like the carotid artery making the surgery more technically feasible.

Therefore, for patients that can tolerate this aggressive approach, trimodality therapy consisting of chemoradiation followed by selective neck dissection is associated with the highest locoregional control and overall survival rates reported in the literature. Investigators at the University of Chicago reported a highly promising 87% 5-year progression-free survival rate and 75% 5-year overall survival rate by using a trimodality approach to patients with N2 to N3 disease. This approach is associated with significant acute toxicity, so patients selected for this aggressive strategy should be carefully selected.[47,70] For patients with advanced disease with poor performance status and motivation or distant metastases, palliative radiotherapy alone is often the most appropriate course of action. A regimen of 30 Gy in 10 fractions results in durable symptomatic improvement in ~60% of patients.[63]

Treatment of Recurrence

The pattern of failure largely depends on the initial treatment regimen. After radiotherapy, the predominant patterns of recurrence include regional and distant metastases.[33–35] Regional recurrence often represents a difficult problem because the recurrence is often invasive and advanced. This likely reflects that recurrence is often difficult to detect on physical exam. The radiated neck is often firm and woody making palpation difficult. CT and MRI have been important tools for surveillance; however, the use of PET-CT has become the preferred

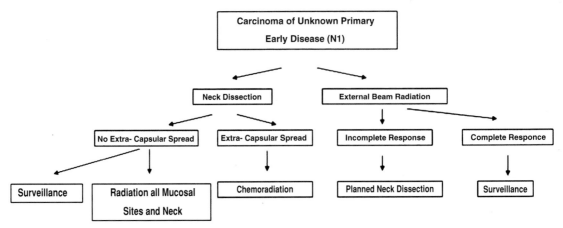

Figure 10–11 Management of advanced CUP (N2 and N3).

method for identifying recurrence.[36,37] When distant metastasis is identified, it usually occurs within a year after completion of therapy. Pulmonary metastasis is the most common site for distant recurrence, occurring in one third of patients. The location and volume of disease will guide therapy. Peripherally located pulmonary metastasis may be managed surgically, and more advanced and unresectable disease may be managed with chemoradiation with the intent to cure or palliative chemotherapy depending on the disease status.

Emergence of the primary tumor may occur in as few as 0 to as many as 66% of patients originally diagnosed with CUP and occurs most commonly in those treated initially with surgery alone.[38,39] Emergence of a primary tumor usually occurs within 24 months and will likely present in the oral cavity, oropharynx, and nasopharynx.[39] Some have observed poor prognosis after detection of the primary lesion; however, the data are conflicting because in some series, tumor emergence later than 5 years after primary treatment was classified as a second primary, whereas in other studies, tumor emergence was considered to be the site of origin.[40] As a result, the significance of an emergence of a primary tumor is unclear.

◆ Adenocarcinoma

When adenocarcinoma occurs as a CUP, it most commonly occurs in the supraclavicular region and is associated with a significantly worse outcome than that of squamous cell carcinoma.[21,71] The addition of radiation may prolong disease-free survival but has no documented impact on overall survival. When an adenocarcinoma CUP is identified, the routine workup should be complemented with a prostate-specific antigen (in men), mammogram (in women), and a CT of the abdomen.

◆ Malignant Melanoma

Malignant melanoma of the head and neck is not uncommon, and as many as 4% of malignant melanomas will present as a CUP. In addition to a complete head and neck examination, a retinal exam is mandatory. In one study, it was shown that the extent of surgical resection and the use of adjuvant radiation had no impact on survival.[72] Interestingly, patients with an unknown primary experienced an improved outcome when compared with those with a known primary tumor.

◆ Conclusions

For a mobile, well-differentiated level I node with no extracapsular extension, we recommend a neck dissection followed by careful observation of the oral cavity. For all other presentations of N1 disease, we recommend neck dissection followed by comprehensive neck and primary site irradiation (nasopharynx, oropharynx, and hypopharynx). A dose of 54 Gy to mucosal sites and clinically uninvolved nodal stations is appropriate. We recommend 60 Gy to suspected primary site and 60 to 66 Gy to the excised node (higher doses for microscopic positive margins). If the appropriate technology and clinical expertise are available, IMRT is recommended. If IMRT is not available, ipsilateral neck irradiation is an option for reducing acute and late toxicity.

For patients with N2 to N3 or extracapsular extension, both neck dissection and chemoradiation are indicated. Therefore, the neck dissection may be performed before or after radiation. Neck dissection should be limited to the side(s) with clinical involvement because radiation can effectively sterilize the clinical N0 neck. We recommend concurrent chemoradiation with the goal of improving locoregional control and possibly overall survival. We recommend a dose of 50 to 54 Gy to mucosal sites and clinically uninvolved nodal stations, 60 Gy to suspected primary site and involved nodal stations, and 70 to 72 Gy to grossly involved nodes. For N3 nodes, doses as high as 75 Gy may be required. If performed postoperatively, we recommend a dose of 63 to 66 Gy to areas of extracapsular extension or microscopic positive margins. Selective neck dissection should be performed after chemoradiation irrespective of response to therapy.

◆ Clinical Cases

Case 1 Solitary neck mass in otherwise healthy male.

Clinical Presentation   A 47-year-old man presented to his primary care physician with a right-sided neck mass after a 2-week course of antibiotics. The patient was subsequently referred to an otolaryngologist for assessment. The patient had no history of malignancy but had a 30 pack-year history of smoking tobacco.

Examination   On examination, the patient was a malnourished male with a right-sided level II neck mass measuring 2×2.5 cm. The mass was firm but mobile. Examination of the oral cavity failed to reveal a mass or ulcer, and the endoscopic examination was normal and revealed no masses or ulcers.

Diagnosis and Workup   After a thorough physical examination and fiberoptic examination, FNA was performed. The patient was then scheduled for a coregistered PET-CT scan with emphasis on the neck (**Fig. 10–12**). The patient was scheduled for a diagnostic laryngoscopy, biopsy, and bilateral tonsillectomy. The preoperative imaging failed to reveal a primary site, and the tonsils and directed biopsies of the ipsilateral base of the tongue and the nasopharynx were negative for malignancy.

Options for Treatment   Once the diagnosis of CUP was made, the patient was evaluated by the dentist for carious dentition and fluoride therapy. The patient was also seen by a nutritionist, and because of his malnourished presentation, a percutaneous gastrostomy tube (PEG) was placed.

Surgical Treatment of the Neck   The patient's physical exam and imaging suggested N1 disease without evidence of extracapsular spread, therefore a selective neck dissection was performed during the initial operation. The neck dissection pathology demonstrated one positive lymph node with extracapsular spread.

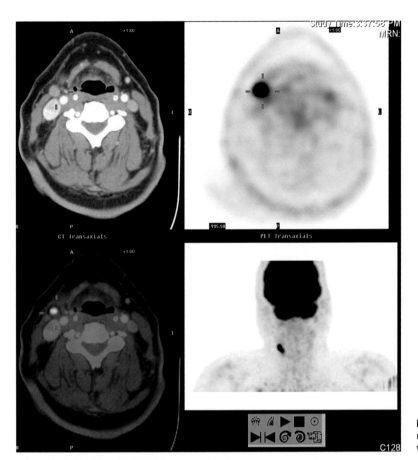

Figure 10–12 Coregistered PET-CT demonstrating a right neck mass with intense uptake (serum uptake value [SUV] = 11).

C128

Adjuvant Therapy   Elective comprehensive neck and primary site irradiation results in improved locoregional control for patients with CUP and is indicated in most patients. The finding of extracapsular extension makes adjuvant radiation mandatory, and concurrent chemotherapy should be considered. Because this patient was young and able to tolerate aggressive therapy, we recommend concurrent chemoradiation with the goal of improving locoregional control and possibly overall survival.

Summary of Treatment   When a CUP presents with N1 disease, a neck dissection offers information that is key to the treatment planning. When a patient presents with a single pathologic lymph node without evidence of extracapsular spread, a neck dissection will provide useful information regarding the presence of multiple pathologic lymph nodes or extracapsular spread that may influence the choice of adjuvant therapy.

Case 2 Solitary cystic neck mass.

Clinical Presentation   A 68-year-old woman presented with a left-sided level III cystic neck mass. The patient had a 34 pack-year history of tobacco use and no prior history of malignancy. The patient denied pain or irritation in the mouth or oropharynx, and the patient denied hoarseness or otalgia.

Examination   On examination, the patient had a firm left-sided level III neck mass measuring 4 × 6 cm. Examination

of the oral cavity and endoscopic examination was normal and revealed no masses or ulcers.

Diagnosis and Workup   FNA had been performed on two separate occasions and revealed "nondiagnostic" pathology. Because of the prior negative FNAs, the patient was sent for an ultrasound-guided FNA of the solid component of the mass. A straw-colored fluid was obtained but no diagnostic cells were obtained. The MRI that was performed at an outside hospital demonstrated a well-circumscribed cystic neck mass with no other abnormalities (**Fig. 10–13**).

Surgical Treatment of the Neck   The patient consented to an excision of the left-sided neck mass with frozen-section evaluation and possible selective neck dissection, diagnostic laryngoscopy, biopsies, and tonsillectomy in the event that the frozen-section pathology analysis demonstrated malignancy. Although the FNA was nondiagnostic, the advanced age of the patient represents a rare presentation for a branchial cleft cyst. At the time of surgery, the cystic neck mass was excised and the frozen-section pathology demonstrated squamous cell carcinoma. A selective neck dissection was performed. After the neck dissection, a diagnostic laryngoscopy with directed biopsies and bilateral tonsillectomy was performed. The pathology revealed one cystic lymph node positive for squamous cell carcinoma. There was no evidence of extracapsular spread.

Adjuvant Therapy   For the pN2 neck, combined surgery and radiation results in superior regional control. Therefore,

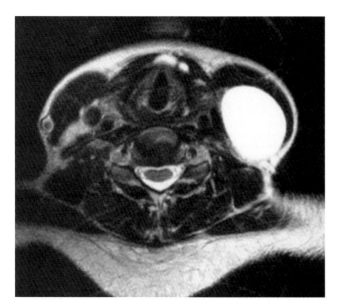

Figure 10–13 MRI demonstrating a well-circumscribed cystic neck mass with no other abnormalities.

comprehensive neck and primary site irradiation is recommended. Because the patient has stage IVa disease, systemic therapy either in the form of chemotherapy or targeted therapy should be considered. The decision to treat is based primarily on performance status and comorbid conditions.

Summary of Treatment Although rare, squamous cell carcinoma may present as a cystic neck mass. The surgeon should be prepared to manage such a situation. It is the surgeon's responsibility to prepare the patient for the possibility of a diagnostic laryngoscopy, biopsies, and surgical management of the neck at the time of the open neck biopsy.

Case 3 Fixed neck mass.

Clinical Presentation A 62-year-old woman presented to an otolaryngologist with a firm, fixed, left-sided neck mass. The patient has no history of malignancy. The patient has a 10 pack-year history of smoking tobacco and drinks alcohol occasionally.

Examination On examination, the patient had a left-sided level IV neck mass measuring 4 × 6 cm. The mass was firm and fixed to the underlying tissue. Physical examination revealed no mass or ulcer in the upper aerodigestive tract. Endoscopic examination was normal and revealed no masses or ulcers.

Diagnosis and Workup The physical examination and fiberoptic examination were negative. FNA was positive for adenocarcinoma. A colonoscopy was performed in addition to high resolution CT scan of the chest and abdomen and a bronchoscopy with bronchial washings. A mammography was performed and the patient was scheduled for a coregistered PET-CT scan with emphasis on the neck. The patient was also scheduled for a diagnostic laryngoscopy, biopsy, and bilateral tonsillectomy. Directed biopsies of

the upper aerodigestive tract were performed in addition to the tonsillectomy, however no primary site was identified.

Options for Therapy Prior to the management of metastatic adenocarcinoma, it is imperative that a thorough surveillance be completed to identify the primary site. Identification of a primary site may significantly change the approach to therapy. When no primary site is discovered, therapy is focused on management of the neck disease.

Surgical Treatment of the Neck Management of the neck entails a therapeutic neck dissection. The neck dissection will also provide histologic information that may be used in directing therapy.

Adjuvant Therapy The only role of radiation for a neck adenocarcinoma of unknown origin is for local control of the neck. Radiation to the ipsilateral neck only is indicated for close or positive margins and/or extracapsular extension. The role of chemotherapy in the management of patients with a solitary focus of adenocarcinoma from an unknown primary is unclear. Assuming that immunohistochemical staining is nondiagnostic, some clinicians are treating poorly differentiated adenocarcinomas with empiric chemotherapy, generally consisting of a platinum and taxane combination.

Summary of Management A level IV CUP is highly suggestive of an infraclavicular origin. Therefore, great attention should be given to pulmonary and gastrointestinal workup.

Case 4 Metastatic melanoma of unknown primary site.

Clinical Presentation A 21-year-old, light-skinned woman presented with a firm, fixed, left-sided neck mass. The patient was a healthy college student with no history of malignancy, tobacco, or alcohol use.

Examination On examination, the patient had a left-sided level III neck mass measuring 1 × 2 cm. The mass was firm and mobile. Physical examination revealed no masses or ulcer in the upper aerodigestive tract, and the endoscopic examination was normal.

Diagnosis and Workup FNA revealed malignant melanoma. The patient then underwent a thorough examination of the skin including the scalp and auricles. A repeated nasal endoscopy was performed to identify any abnormality, and the patient was referred to an ophthalmologist and dermatologist for examination. A PET-CT scan demonstrated a single focus at the site of the left neck mass with no evidence of a primary lesion.

Options for Therapy The approach to management of regional metastasis of melanoma is directed at controlling the disease. The morbidity of therapy must be weighed against the impact on outcome—management of the neck metastasis has not been shown to improve the rate of cure.

Surgical Treatment of the Neck The patient was taken to the operating room, and again an examination under anesthesia was performed followed by a diagnostic laryngoscopy, esophagoscopy, and a left modified neck dissection was performed. The final pathology demonstrated 1 of 37 lymph nodes positive for malignant melanoma.

Adjuvant Therapy There is no standard adjuvant therapy for the management of malignant melanoma; however, a large study from M.D. Anderson demonstrated improved locoregional control (88% at 5 years) in patients with head and neck melanoma with the addition of hypofractionated irradiation to a dose of 30 Gy in 5 fractions delivered over 2.5 weeks to the tumor bed and ipsilateral neck. There was no observed benefit in overall survival compared with historical controls. Because the patient had only a single positive node with no extracapsular extension and had an adequate neck dissection, the patient is at relatively low risk for locoregional failure after surgery alone. Unfortunately, melanomas of the head and neck are associated with a poor prognosis with survival rates of 10 to 45% at 5 years. Postoperative treatment with interferon-α is an option for patients with resected node-positive melanoma with no medical contraindications; however, the results have been disappointing.

Summary of Treatment In the rare event of a malignant melanoma CUP, the role of neck dissection with or without radiation therapy serves to control regional recurrence. There is no evidence to suggest that surgical management of the neck affects survival, but it does improve regional control.

References

1. Volkmann R. Das tiefe branchiogenge Halscarcinom. Zbl Chirurgie 1882;9:49–51
2. Martin H, Morfit HM. Cervical lymph node metastasis as the first symptom of cancer. Surg Gynecol Obstet 1944;78:133–159
3. Martin H, Morfit HM, Ehrlich H. The case for branchiogenic cancer (malignant branchioma). Ann Surg 1950;132(5):867–887
4. Issing WJ, Taleban B, Tauber S. Diagnosis and management of carcinoma of unknown primary in the head and neck. Eur Arch Otorhinolaryngol 2003;260(8):436–443
5. Lindberg R. Distribution of cervical lymph node metastases from squamous cell carcinoma of the upper respiratory and digestive tracts. Cancer 1972;29(6):1446–1449
6. Rouvierre H. Lymphatic Systems of the Head and Neck. 1938
7. Mukherji SK, Armao D, Joshi VM. Cervical nodal metastases in squamous cell carcinoma of the head and neck: what to expect. Head Neck 2001;23(11):995–1005
8. Byers RM, Wolf PF, Ballantyne AJ. Rationale for elective modified neck dissection. Head Neck Surg 1988;10(3):160–167
9. Talmi YP, Wolf G, Hazuka M, et al. Unknown primary of the head and neck. J Laryngol Otol 1996;110(4):353–356
10. de Braud F, Heilbrun LK, Ahmed K, et al. Metastatic squamous carcinoma of an unknown primary localized to the neck. Advantages of an aggressive treatment. Cancer 1989;64(2):510–515
11. Lee DJ, Rostock RA, Harris A, et al. Clinical evaluation of patients with metastatic squamous carcinoma of the neck with occult primary tumor. South Med J 1986;79(8):979–983
12. Fried MP, Diehl WH, Brownson RJ, et al. Cervical metastasis from an unknown primary. Ann Otol Rhinol Laryngol 1975;84(2 Part 1):152–157
13. Comess MS, Beahrs OH, Dockerty MB. Cervical metastasis from occult carcinoma. Surg Gynecol Obstet 1957;104(5):607–617
14. Kraus DH, Dubner S, Harrison LB, et al. Prognostic factors for recurrence and survival in head and neck soft tissue sarcomas. Cancer 1994;74(2):697–702
15. Sheahan P, O'Leary G, Lee G, et al. Cystic cervical metastases: incidence and diagnosis using fine needle aspiration biopsy. Otolaryngol Head Neck Surg 2002;127(4):294–298
16. Aassar OS, Fischbein NJ, Caputo GR, et al. Metastatic head and neck cancer: role and usefulness of FDG PET in locating occult primary tumors. Radiology 1999;210(1):177–181
17. Safa AA, Tran LM, Rege S, et al. The role of positron emission tomography in occult primary head and neck cancers. Cancer J Sci Am 1999;5(4):214–218
18. Jungehulsing M, Sceidhauer K, Damm M, et al. 2[F]-fluoro-2-deoxy-D-glucose positron emission tomography is a sensitive tool for the detection of occult primary cancer (carcinoma of unknown primary syndrome) with head and neck lymph node manifestation. Otolaryngol Head Neck Surg 2000;123(3):294–301
19. Greven KM, Keyes JW, Williams DW, et al. Occult primary tumors of the head and neck: lack of benefit from positron emission tomography imaging with 2-[F-18]fluoro-2-deoxy-D-glucose. Cancer 1999;86(1):114–118
20. Miller FR, Beeram M, Eng T, et al. Positron emission tomography in the management of unknown primary head and neck carcinoma. Arch Otolaryngol Head Neck Surg 2005;131(7):626–629
21. Lee NK, Byers RM, Abbruzzese JL, et al. Metastatic adenocarcinoma to the neck from an unknown primary source. Am J Surg 1991;162(4):306–309
22. McQuone SJ, Eisele DW, Lee DJ, et al. Occult tonsillar carcinoma in the unknown primary. Laryngoscope 1998;108(11 Pt 1):1605–1610
23. Koch WM, Bhatti N, Williams MF, et al. Oncologic rationale for bilateral tonsillectomy in head and neck squamous cell carcinoma of unknown primary source. Otolaryngol Head Neck Surg 2001;124(3):331–333
24. Alvi A, Johnson JT. Development of distant metastasis after treatment of advanced-stage head and neck cancer. Head Neck 1997;19(6):500–505
25. Grandi C, Alloisio M, Moglia D, et al. Prognostic significance of lymphatic spread in head and neck carcinomas: therapeutic implications. Head Neck Surg 1985;8(2):67–73
26. Leemans CR, Tiwari R, Nauta JJ, et al. Regional lymph node involvement and its significance in the development of distant metastases in head and neck carcinoma. Cancer 1993;71(2):452–456
27. Bernier J, Cooper JS, Pajak TF, et al. Defining risk levels in locally advanced head and neck cancers: a comparative analysis of concurrent postoperative radiation plus chemotherapy trials of the EORTC (#22931) and RTOG (# 9501). Head Neck 2005;27(10):843–850
28. Kowalski LP, Bagietto R, Lara JR, et al. Prognostic significance of the distribution of neck node metastasis from oral carcinoma. Head Neck 2000;22(3):207–214
29. Ellis ER, Mendenhall WM, Rao PV, et al. Does node location affect the incidence of distant metastases in head and neck squamous cell carcinoma? Int J Radiat Oncol Biol Phys 1989;17(2):293–297
30. de Bree R, Deurloo EE, Snow GB, et al. Screening for distant metastases in patients with head and neck cancer. Laryngoscope 2000;110(3 Pt 1):397–401
31. Jesse RH, Perez CA, Fletcher GH. Cervical lymph node metastasis: unknown primary cancer. Cancer 1973;31(4):854–859
32. Marcial-Vega VA, Cardenes H, Perez CA, et al. Cervical metastases from unknown primaries: radiotherapeutic management and appearance of subsequent primaries. Int J Radiat Oncol Biol Phys 1990;19(4):919–928
33. Grau C, Johansen LV, Jakobsen J, et al. Cervical lymph node metastases from unknown primary tumours. Results from a national survey by the Danish Society for Head and Neck Oncology. Radiother Oncol 2000;55(2):121–129
34. Fernandez JA, Suárez C, Martínez JA, et al. Metastatic squamous cell carcinoma in cervical lymph nodes from an unknown primary tumour: prognostic factors. Clin Otolaryngol Allied Sci 1998;23(2):158–163
35. Nieder C, Gregoire V, Ang KK. Cervical lymph node metastases from occult squamous cell carcinoma: cut down a tree to get an apple? Int J Radiat Oncol Biol Phys 2001;50(3):727–733
36. Lonneux M, Lawson G, Ide C, et al. Positron emission tomography with fluorodeoxyglucose for suspected head and neck tumor recurrence in the symptomatic patient. Laryngoscope 2000;110(9):1493–1497
37. Kubota K, Yokoyama J, Yamaguchi K, et al. FDG-PET delayed imaging for the detection of head and neck cancer recurrence after radiochemotherapy: comparison with MRI/CT. Eur J Nucl Med Mol Imaging 2004;31(4):590–595
38. Weir L, Keane T, Cummings B, et al. Radiation treatment of cervical lymph node metastases from an unknown primary: an analysis of outcome by treatment volume and other prognostic factors. Radiother Oncol 1995;35(3):206–211

39. Strojan P, Anicin A. Combined surgery and postoperative radiotherapy for cervical lymph node metastases from an unknown primary tumour. Radiother Oncol 1998;49(1):33–40

40. Friesland S, Lind MG, Lundgren J, et al. Outcome of ipsilateral treatment for patients with metastases to neck nodes of unknown origin. Acta Oncol 2001;40(1):24–28

41. Colletier PJ, Garden AS, Morrison WH, et al. Postoperative radiation for squamous cell carcinoma metastatic to cervical lymph nodes from an unknown primary site: outcomes and patterns of failure. Head Neck 1998;20(8):674–681

42. Coster JR, Foote RL, Olsen KD, et al. Cervical nodal metastasis of squamous cell carcinoma of unknown origin: indications for withholding radiation therapy. Int J Radiat Oncol Biol Phys 1992;23(4):743–749

43. Davidson BJ, Spiro RH, Patel S, et al. Cervical metastases of occult origin: the impact of combined modality therapy. Am J Surg 1994;168(5):395–399

44. Harper CS, Mendenhall WM, Parsons JT, et al. Cancer in neck nodes with unknown primary site: role of mucosal radiotherapy. Head Neck 1990;12(6):463–469

45. Wang RC, Goepfert H, Barber AE, et al. Unknown primary squamous cell carcinoma metastatic to the neck. Arch Otolaryngol Head Neck Surg 1990;116(12):1388–1393

46. Medini E, Medini AM, Lee CK, et al. The management of metastatic squamous cell carcinoma in cervical lymph nodes from an unknown primary. Am J Clin Oncol 1998;21(2):121–125

47. Argiris A, Smith SM, Stenson K, et al. Concurrent chemoradiotherapy for N2 or N3 squamous cell carcinoma of the head and neck from an occult primary. Ann Oncol 2003;14(8):1306–1311

48. Lefebvre JL, Coche Dequeant B, Van JT, et al. Cervical lymph nodes from an unknown primary tumor in 190 patients. Am J Surg 1990;160(4):443–446

49. Andersen PE, Warren F, Spiro J, et al. Results of selective neck dissection in management of the node-positive neck. Arch Otolaryngol Head Neck Surg 2002;128(10):1180–1184

50. Chepeha DB, Hoff PT, Taylor RJ, et al. Selective neck dissection for the treatment of neck metastasis from squamous cell carcinoma of the head and neck. Laryngoscope 2002;112(3):434–438

51. Barkley HT Jr, Fletcher GH, Jesse RH, et al. Management of cervical lymph node metastases in squamous cell carcinoma of the tonsillar fossa, base of tongue, supraglottic larynx, and hypopharynx. Am J Surg 1972;124(4):462–467

52. Mendenhall WM, Millio NRR, Cassisi NJ. Squamous cell carcinoma of the head and neck treated with radiation therapy: the role of neck dissection for clinically positive neck nodes. Int J Radiat Oncol Biol Phys 1986;12(5):733–740

53. Reddy SP, Marks JE. Metastatic carcinoma in the cervical lymph nodes from an unknown primary site: results of bilateral neck plus mucosal irradiation vs. ipsilateral neck irradiation. Int J Radiat Oncol Biol Phys 1997;37(4):797–802

54. Mack Y, Parsons JT, Mendenhall WM, et al. Squamous cell carcinoma of the head and neck: management after excisional biopsy of a solitary metastatic neck node. Int J Radiat Oncol Biol Phys 1993;25(4):619–622

55. McGuirt WF, McCabe BF. Significance of node biopsy before definitive treatment of cervical metastatic carcinoma. Laryngoscope 1978;88(4):594–597

56. Eisbruch A, Dawson LA, Kim HM, et al. Dose, volume, and function relationships in parotid salivary glands following conformal and intensity-modulated irradiation of head and neck cancer. Int J Radiat Oncol Biol Phys 1999;45(3):577–587

57. Chao KS, Majhail N, Huang CJ, et al. Intensity-modulated radiation therapy reduces late salivary toxicity without compromising tumor control in patients with oropharyngeal carcinoma: a comparison with conventional techniques. Radiother Oncol 2001;61(3):275–280

58. Yao M, Dornfeld KJ, Buatti JM, et al. Intensity-modulated radiation treatment for head-and-neck squamous cell carcinoma–the University of Iowa experience. Int J Radiat Oncol Biol Phys 2005;63(2):410–421

59. Chao KS, Ozyigit G, Tran BN, et al. Patterns of failure in patients receiving definitive and postoperative IMRT for head-and-neck cancer. Int J Radiat Oncol Biol Phys 2003;55(2):312–321

60. Peters LJ, Goepfert H, Ang KK, et al. Evaluation of the dose for postoperative radiation therapy of head and neck cancer: first report of a prospective randomized trial. Int J Radiat Oncol Biol Phys 1993;26(1):3–11

61. Erkal HS, Mendenhall WM, Amdur RJ, et al. Squamous cell carcinomas metastatic to cervical lymph nodes from an unknown head and neck mucosal site treated with radiation therapy with palliative intent. Radiother Oncol 2001;59(3):319–321

62. Cohen EEW, Lingen MW, Vokes EE. The expanding role of systemic therapy in head and neck cancer. J Clin Oncol 2004;22:1743–1752

63. Shehadeh NJ, Becker M, Yoo G, et al. Unknown head and neck primary treatment with neck dissection followed by chemoradiotherapy. Proc Am Soc Clin Oncol 2004

64. Bonner JA, Harari PM, Giralt J, et al. Radiotherapy plus cetuximab for squamous-cell carcinoma of the head and neck. N Engl J Med 2006;354:567–578

65. Adelstein DJ, Li Y, Adams GL, et al. An intergroup phase III comparison of standard radiation therapy and two schedules of concurrent chemoradiotherapy in patients with unresectable squamous cell head and neck cancer. J Clin Oncol 2003;21(1):92–98

66. Pignon JP, Bourhis J, Domenge C, et al. Chemotherapy added to locoregional treatment for head and neck squamous-cell carcinoma: three meta-analyses of updated individual data. MACH-NC Collaborative Group. Meta-Analysis of Chemotherapy on Head and Neck Cancer. Lancet 2000;355(9208):949–955

67. Argiris A, Stenson KM, Brockstein BE, et al. Neck dissection in the combined-modality therapy of patients with locoregionally advanced head and neck cancer. Head Neck 2004;26(5):447–455

68. Brizel DM, Prosnitz RG, Hunter S, et al. Necessity for adjuvant neck dissection in setting of concurrent chemoradiation for advanced head-and-neck cancer. Int J Radiat Oncol Biol Phys 2004;58(5):1418–1423

69. Pellitteri PK, Ferlito A, Rinaldo A, et al. Planned neck dissection following chemoradiotherapy for advanced head and neck cancer: is it necessary for all? Head Neck 2006;28(2):166–175

70. Brize lDM, Albers ME, Fisher SR, et al. Hyperfractionated irradiation with or without concurrent chemotherapy for locally advanced head and neck cancer. N Engl J Med 1998;338(25):1798–1804

71. Zuur CL, van Velthuysen ML, Schornagel JH, et al. Diagnosis and treatment of isolated neck metastases of adenocarcinomas. Eur J Surg Oncol 2002;28(2):147–152

72. Nasri S, Namazie A, Dulguerov P, et al. Malignant melanoma of cervical and parotid lymph nodes with an unknown primary site. Laryngoscope 1994;104(10):1194–1198

11

Surveillance of the Patient

Peter M. Som and Eric M. Genden

It is been estimated that each year, more than 400,000 new cases of head and neck cancer will be diagnosed and that these represent 5.4% of all cancers with an overall risk of death of 40%.[1,2] Regardless of the treatment protocol for patients with a primary head and neck cancer, it has been demonstrated that when cancers are diagnosed early, the rate of survival and cure rates are improved.[3–6] Similarly, it has been suggested that the earlier recurrent disease is identified and treated, the better may be the outcome, although this remains somewhat speculative.[7]

In spite of the fact that the majority of treatment initiatives have been directed toward providing a cure, over the past several decades there has been little improvement in the cure rate for most patients with head and neck cancer.[8–15] Although the percentage of patients cured may have changed little, their disease-free survival appears to be improving, and most patients are now dying from distant metastases or from second primary tumors rather than from local or regional recurrences.[9–11] Therefore, although the overall cure rate of patients with a recurrence of a head and neck cancer may be little affected by contemporary combined modality therapy, the opportunity to provide prolonged disease-free survival with an acceptable quality of life is the goal and commitment of a surveillance program.[9]

◆ Considerations for a Surveillance Program

Routine clinical examinations form the basis of any surveillance program, and it is a common practice for clinicians to see patients every 2 months for the first 24 months after therapy. Imaging studies should be coordinated with periodic clinical visits to identify recurrent disease or a second primary tumor prior to clinical presentation.[9,12,13,15] To take advantage of the current state of technology, such imaging should include both morphologic-based computed tomography (CT) or magnetic resonance imaging (MRI) and molecular-based positron emission tomography (PET) im-

aging. The addition of such imaging to the clinical evaluation is especially germane to the posttreatment neck, which is often stiff and "woody" making it difficult to palpate a deeply situated mass. A surveillance program should also take into consideration high-risk patients with a history of advanced disease, low neck metastasis, extracapsular nodal spread, continued smoking and/or alcohol abuse, and the adverse histologic prognosticators such as perineural invasion and limited lymphocytic response.[16–20] These patients will require more vigilant follow-up and more aggressive treatment.

There is sufficient data to support the notion that the majority of recurrences and deaths resulting from head and neck cancers occur within the first 1 to 2 years after initial treatment.[9,21] This implies that any surveillance program should be most diligent during this time period. Additionally, once a patient has one upper aerodigestive tract cancer, there exists the threat of a second primary tumor, be it synchronous or metachronous. The incidence of such a second primary tumor varies from 5 to 36%.[3] This suggests that a surveillance program should be designed to identify not only an early recurrence but also a second primary tumor, and as these second primary tumors may take years to develop, long-term (annual) surveillance should be a part of the program.

Because pulmonary metastasis is the most common site for distant metastasis, pulmonary surveillance should be a part of any head and neck cancer surveillance protocol. This can be best accomplished by periodic CT scans and/or coregistered PET-CT scans. In addition, if PET-CT is utilized as a pretreatment (staging) study, it also offers the possibility of identifying not only a clinically silent metastasis but also a second primary tumor (in the chest, abdomen, or pelvis) prior to initial therapy for the head and neck cancer.[1,2,22,23]

Morphologic Imaging

There are two distinct choices for a morphologically based imaging modality to utilize in a surveillance protocol; CT and

MRI. Each has its unique benefits. CT has been shown to be more accurate than MRI in identifying pathologic cervical adenopathy.[24] Typically, a CT multidetector examination of the neck takes between 10 and 20 seconds of scanner time, with the entire contrast examination taking only ~10 minutes. By comparison, typical MRI scanner times for each sequence are between 4 and 7 minutes, with the entire study taking ~45 minutes. Compared with CT, MRI may be more sensitive to artifacts from body movement, vascular pulsations, rapid respirations, and repeated swallows, all of which may be present in patients with head and neck cancer. Specifically, many of these patients have difficulty lying supine for a prolonged time because of dyspnea, pain, or difficulty handling their secretions. This discomfort is often manifested as restlessness and/or rapid breathing while lying supine, and the markedly shorter CT scanning time favors the use of this modality.

In contrast, if there are numerous surgical clips in the neck that cause significant degradation artifacts on CT, such artifacts tend to be greatly reduced on MRI. Contrast MRI is superior to CT in identifying tumor extension through the skull base and dura, and the closer to the skull base, the more may be the advantage of MRI over CT scanning. Lastly, dental amalgams may cause severe degradation artifacts on CT images through the oral cavity. Such artifacts tend to be less degrading on MRI scans, and MRI may be better for assessing disease in this region.[25] On the average, ~10% of patients reject the MRI study due to claustrophobia, and patients with pacemakers cannot have the study. Patients with metallic body fragments or some implants also may not be able to have the MRI examination. The main rejection-related problem with contrast CT studies is patient allergy to iodine-based contrast agents, a problem that in most cases can be overcome by premedicating these patients with steroids. A consideration of study costs reveals that in general, a contrast CT study is about one third the cost of a contrast MRI study. Finally, access to CT scanners is, in general, easier than it is to MRI scanners. Taking all of these factors into account, we considered CT to be the preferential morphologic imaging study. This is also especially germane if PET-CT examinations are incorporated into the surveillance plan, as the CT portion of the study can be compared with prior CT studies (apples to apples not apples and oranges). As discussed, however, in selected cases an MRI study may be more appropriate and become the modality of choice for those patients.

Positron Emission Tomography

[18F]Fluoro-2-deoxy-D-glucose (FDG)-PET scanning is issuing in a new era of molecular imaging. There is, however, confusing literature on how and when best to utilize this modality. There is little controversy regarding a negative PET study as the negative predictive value (NPV) of PET is between 90% and 95%. This high figure has suggested to many physicians that the best way to utilize PET is for its NPV.[26,27] The current resolution of PET scanners is of the order 3 mm³, and although a negative PET does not completely rule out the presence of tumor, it does strongly suggest that no gross tumor mass is present and that no further immediate treatment may be indicated.

However, when a PET scan shows an area of increased activity in the neck, the exact cause of this increased standard uptake value (SUV) is less clear. The differential diagnosis includes tumor, reaction to surgery, radiation therapy, or chemotherapy, as well as more established causes such as infection, increased muscle activity and/or hypertrophy, the presence of surgical hardware, normal accumulations within the major salivary glands and/or soft palate, brown fat, and benign tumors such as a Warthin's tumors. As many of these circumstances are common to the posttreatment head and neck patient, a false-positive study is a realistic possibility especially within the immediate 4 to 6 months after treatment. PET studies alone have been reported to have a positive predictive value between 65% and 80%[28,29]; however, if PET-CT is performed, many of the more common false-positive causes can be eliminated by anatomic localization of the site of increased activity. For PET-CT studies performed after radiation for head and neck cancers, the sensitivity improved from 55 to 95% and the NPV increased from 90 to 99% when comparing studies done 1 month after treatment with studies performed more than 1 month after treatment[29]; however, some earlier studies have suggested that PET can be reliably utilized within as little as 6 weeks of completing a chemotherapy–radiation therapy treatment.[30]

Although unresolved at present, the general tendency is to wait at least 3 to 4 months after treatment to obtain a more reliable PET-CT study for predicting the presence of cancer. Thus, PET-CT has become the primary imaging modality because it not only offers pretreatment evaluation of the primary tumor, regional disease, distant metastasis, and a silent second primary tumor, but also it can identify morphologically overlooked tumor in the posttreatment neck.[31,32] In addition, recent studies have shown that the SUV value of the primary tumor on an initial pretreatment PET-CT study directly correlates with outcome. This relationship was not shown for nodal SUV.[33] Once a positive PET-CT site is identified, its cause must be clarified, and this is best done by either ultrasound or CT-guided fine-needle aspiration biopsy. To maximize the yield on such procedures, a cytologist should be present at the time of biopsy. This is a critical step, as definitive differentiation of persistent or recurrence tumor from a reactive node may be impossible on the posttreatment FDG-PET–CT study alone.

◆ The Mount Sinai Surveillance Protocol

Pretreatment and Surveillance Protocol

All patients receiving treatment for a head and neck cancer undergo a pretreatment PET-CT, which includes coverage of the neck, chest, abdomen, and pelvis. All of the CT studies in the protocol should be performed as contrast-enhanced examinations unless contrast cannot be administered because of a severe allergy or a contraindicated medical condition. The field of view (FOV) for the neck CT is ~25 cm, with a reconstructed scan thickness of 2.5 mm. To avoid beam hardening artifact, the patient's arms are lowered to their sides for the head and neck portion of the study. When the chest/abdomen/

pelvis portion of the CT examination is performed, the FOV is between 36 and 40 cm and the patient's arms are raised over their head. The FOV for the PET portion of the studies should correspond with the CT FOV values mentioned above.

Posttreatment Assessment

A baseline CT scan is obtained 4 to 6 weeks after initial treatment has ended. This creates a posttreatment CT study to which future examinations can be compared. Taking into account the notion that the greatest surveillance should be in the first two posttreatment years, we recommend that patients have PET-CT studies every 4 months for the first 2 posttreatment years. We start the cycle with a PET-CT scan 4 months after treatment. The surveillance continues with PET-CT studies every 6 months for the third and fourth posttreatment years. Finally, patients should have yearly PET-CT studies ongoing from the fifth posttreatment year or until the physician deems further studies unnecessary.

The PET-CT results are clearly starting to influence further treatment. As just one example, in a recent study patients who had no evidence of disease (NED) for residual lymphadenopathy and who had a negative PET-CT 3 months after radiation therapy did not develop regional disease, and surgery could be withheld. Even if small residual was seen, but it was PET-CT negative, surgery could be withheld.[34] Although this concept is not yet held by all physicians, the PET-CT results are definitely starting to influence future treatment algorithms.

The management of the treated head and neck cancer patient has always been a challenge; however, we believe that the combination of coordinated physical examination and PET-CT has the potential to provide accurate information regarding the preclinical presence of both recurrent tumor and second primary tumors. It is hoped that this information will lead to better treatment decisions and better patient outcomes. The future of PET-CT lies with new agents that will better differentiate between tumor and inflammatory reaction. Many such agents are currently on the horizon, and it is hoped that soon they will be clinically available to help more quickly and definitively identify recurrent disease.

◆ Clinical Cases

The following example cases serve to demonstrate the decision problems encountered by clinicians when they are faced with a positive surveillance PET-CT study.

Case 1 A 56-year-old man had a T1 anterior tongue carcinoma surgically removed. He was treated with radiation therapy after surgery and comes for a PET-CT study 4 months after treatment. Clinically he is NED. His PET-CT study shows diffuse activity within the tongue and two foci of activity in the posterior larynx (**Fig. 11–1**). What is the most likely cause of these findings, and what is the next clinical step in following this patient?

Discussion The PET examination takes from 1 to 2 hours to perform, and during the examination, most patients talk to the physicians and technicians. The PET-CT is sim-

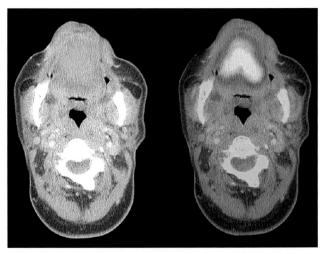

Figure 11–1 PET-CT study from case 1 showing diffuse activity within the tongue and two foci of activity in the posterior larynx.

ply showing normal activity within the tongue muscles and within the cricoarytenoid muscles of the larynx (**Fig. 11–2**). There is no evidence of a focal tumor mass. With an essentially negative PET-CT study, this patient can be watched until the next planned observation point.

Case 2 A 62-year-old woman had a history of oral cavity cancer treated surgically 2 months ago. She then had a left second molar mandibular tooth extracted, and the extraction site did not heal. Shortly after that, she developed left level I adenopathy. Her PET-CT study shows focal uptake in the molar tooth area (**Fig. 11–3**) and mild activity in the level I nodes (**Fig. 11–4**). Sclerosis rather than bone destruction was seen in the mandible on the CT scan. What is the most likely cause of these findings, and what is the next clinical step in following this patient?

Discussion The absence of bone destruction and the presence of sclerosis on the CT scan makes carcinoma invasion

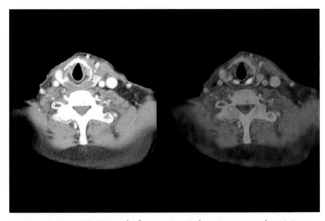

Figure 11–2 PET-CT study from case 1 showing normal activity within the tongue muscles and within the cricoarytenoid muscles of the larynx. No evidence of a focal tumor mass is present.

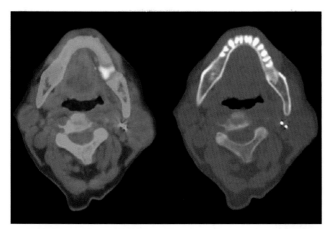

Figure 11–3 PET-CT study from case 2: focal uptake in the molar tooth area.

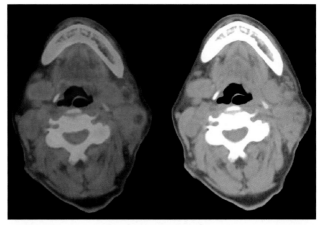

Figure 11–4 PET-CT study from case 2: mild activity in the level I nodes.

of the mandible unlikely and chronic inflammation likely. The level I nodes could be either reactive or metastatic, as they only have a low SUV (2.7). Both the tooth extraction site and a level I node were biopsied, without evidence of tumor. This case demonstrates how inflammatory disease can mimic tumor recurrence. The patient was watched carefully over the next 2 to 3 months with no evidence of tumor recurrence. She has remained disease-free for 1 year after this study.

Case 3 A 68-year-old man had a right stage II tongue cancer and a IIB right neck node. He underwent extirpation of the primary tumor with a flap reconstruction and a right neck dissection. He comes for his 4-month posttreatment PET-CT study, and a focus of increased activity is identified around one of the clusters of surgical clips (**Fig. 11–5**). What is the most likely cause of this finding, and what is the next clinical step in following this patient?

Discussion Nontumorous increased PET activity can occur around surgical clips presumably due to local low-grade inflammation; however, in this clinical setting, a small tumor mass cannot be excluded, especially as the artifact from the clips on the CT scan obscures visualization of any

small soft tissue mass. The site of increased PET activity should be biopsied using either an ultrasound-guided or CT-guided technique to ensure that the correct area was biopsied. At least five needle passes should be made to maximize the chances of getting tumor in the specimen. A cytologist, if possible, should be present to ensure sample quality. Such a CT-guided biopsy was performed, and no tumor was found. This patient was watched carefully over the next 18 months, and his PET-CT studies have remained unchanged. He is clinically disease-free.

Case 4 An 84-year-old woman presents with a left tongue mass and a fixed left tongue. Her initial PET-CT study (**Fig. 11–6**) shows increased activity in the tumor bed. Her tongue carcinoma is treated with brachytherapy. She has been well for 10 months and now returns with pain in the treated area. Her follow-up PET-CT study (**Fig. 11–7**) shows some activity within the tumor bed. What is the most likely cause of this finding, and what is the next clinical step in following this patient?

Discussion This PET-CT study was performed 10 months after the completion of her brachytherapy treatment. It was performed off protocol schedule because the patient

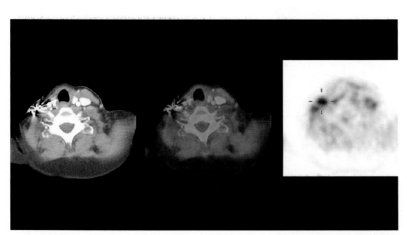

Figure 11–5 Four-month posttreatment PET-CT study from case 3 displaying a focus of increased activity around one of the clusters of surgical clips.

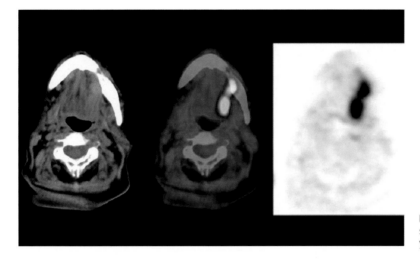

Figure 11–6 The initial PET-CT study from case 4 shows increased activity in the tumor bed of an 84-year-old woman.

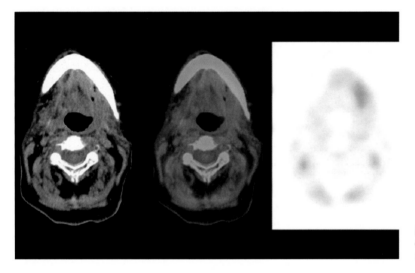

Figure 11–7 Pathway for the development of epithelial malignancy: (**A**) cellular evolution and (**B**) de novo development.

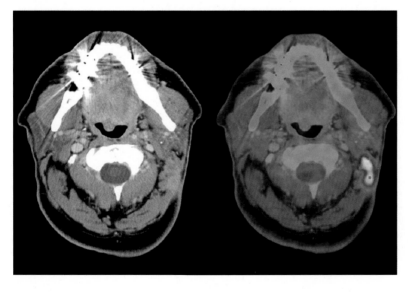

Figure 11–8 The 4-month PET-CT scan of a 47-year-old man (case 4) who had a left tonsillar carcinoma with an N0 neck and was treated with a chemoradiation therapy regimen. The scan shows activity in left level II nodes.

developed pain. The increased activity within the primary tumor site indicates the presence of tumor, as any reactive change from the radiation therapy should have resolved by this time. A biopsy confirmed the presence of tumor. Because of her age and associated health issues, only palliative care was given.

Case 5 A 47-year-old man had a left tonsillar carcinoma with an N0 neck. He was treated with a chemoradiation therapy regimen. He comes for his 4-month PET-CT scan, which shows activity in left level II nodes (**Fig. 11–8**). What is the most likely cause of this finding, and what is the next clinical step in following this patient?

Discussion By 4 months after radiation therapy, any associated reactive changes should have resolved. Thus, the notably increased activity with the left level IIB nodes strongly suggests the presence of tumor. This patient had a neck dissection, and these were the only positive nodes in the specimen.

References

1. Slootweg P, Richardson M. Squamous cell carcinoma of the upper aerodigestive system. In: Gnepp D, ed. Diagnostic Surgical Pathology of the Head and Neck. Philadelphia, PA: W.B. Saunders; 2001:19–78
2. Pisani P, Parkin DM, Bray F, Ferlay J. Erratum: Estimates of the worldwide mortality from 25 cancers in 1990. Int J Cancer 1999;83:870–873
3. Wenig B. General principles of head and neck pathology. In: Harrison LB, Sessions R, Hong WK, eds. Head and Neck Cancer: A Multidisciplinary Approach. Philadelphia, PA: Lippincott-Raven; 1998:253–349
4. Vokes EE, Weichselbaum RR, Lippman SM, Hong WK. Head and neck cancer. N Engl J Med 1993;328:184–194
5. Parker SL, Tong T, Bolden S, Wingo PA. Cancer statistics, 1996. CA Cancer J Clin 1996;46:5–27
6. Parkin DM, Laara E, Muir CS. Estimates of the worldwide frequency of sixteen major cancers in 1980. Int J Cancer 1988;41:184–197
7. Goodwin WJ Jr. Salvage surgery for patients with recurrent squamous cell carcinoma of the upper aerodigestive tract: when do the ends justify the means? Laryngoscope 2000;110:1–18
8. Leon X, Quer M, Orus C, del Prado Venegas M. Can cure be achieved in patients with head and neck carcinomas? The problem of second neoplasm. Expert Rev Anticancer Ther 2001;1:125–133
9. List MA, Rutherford JL, Stracks J, et al. Prioritizing treatment outcomes: head and neck cancer patients versus nonpatients. Head Neck 2004;26:163–170
10. Malone JP, Stephens JA, Grecula JC, Rhoades CA, Ghaheri BA, Schuller DE. Disease control, survival, and functional outcome after multimodal treatment for advanced-stage tongue base cancer. Head Neck 2004;26:561–572
11. Bhatia R, Bahadur S. Distant metastasis in malignancies of the head and neck. J Laryngol Otol 1987;101:925–928
12. Hudgins PA, Burson JG, Gussack GS, Grist WJ. CT and MR appearance of recurrent malignant head and neck neoplasms after resection and flap reconstruction. AJNR Am J Neuroradiol 1994;15:1689–1694
13. Hudgins PA. Flap reconstruction in the head and neck: expected appearance, complications, and recurrent disease. Eur J Radiol 2002;44:130–138
14. Som PM, Biller H. Computed tomography of the neck in the post operative patient: radical neck dissection and myocutaneous flap. Radiology 1983;148:157–160
15. Som PM, Urken ML, Biller H, Lidov M. Imaging the postoperative neck. Radiology 1993;187:593–603
16. Leemans CR, Tiwari R, Nauta JJ, van der Waal I, Snow GB. Recurrence at the primary site in head and neck cancer and the significance of neck lymph node metastases as a prognostic factor. Cancer 1994;73:187–190
17. Shingaki S, Suzuki I, Kobayashi T, Nakajima T. Predicting factors for distant metastases in head and neck carcinomas: an analysis of 103 patients with locoregional control. J Oral Maxillofac Surg 1996;54:853–857
18. de Bree R, Deurloo EE, Snow GB, Leemans CR. Screening for distant metastases in patients with head and neck cancer. Laryngoscope 2000;110:397–401
19. Alvi A, Johnson JT. Development of distant metastasis after treatment of advanced-stage head and neck cancer. Head Neck 1997;19:500–505
20. Brandwein-Gensler M, Teixeira MS, Lewis CM, et al. Oral squamous cell carcinoma: histologic risk assessment, but not margin status, is strongly predictive of local disease-free and overall survival. Am J Surg Pathol 2005;29:167–178
21. Greene F, Page D, Fleming I, et al., eds. Cancer Staging Manual. 6th ed. New York, NY: Springer-Verlag; 2001
22. Schmid DT, Stoeckli SJ, Bandhauer F, et al. Impact of positron emission tomography on the initial staging and therapy in locoregional advanced squamous cell carcinoma of the head and neck. Laryngoscope 2003;113:888–891
23. Schwartz DL, Rajendran J, Yueh B, et al. FDG-PET prediction of head and neck squamous cell cancer outcomes. Arch Otolaryngol Head Neck Surg 2004;130:1361–1367
24. Curtin HD, Ishwaran H, Mancuso A, et al. Comparison of CT and MR imaging in staging of neck metastases. Radiology 1998;207:123–130
25. Dammann F, Horger M, Mueller-Berg M, et al. Rational diagnosis of squamous cell carcinoma of the head and neck region: comparative evaluation of CT, MRI, and 18FDG PET. AJR Am J Roentgenol 2005;184:1326–1331
26. Kubota K, Yokoyama J, Yamaguchi K, et al. FDG-PET delayed imaging for the detection of head and neck cancer recurrence after radiochemotherapy: comparison with MRI/CT. Eur J Nucl Med Mol Imaging 2004;31:590–595
27. Conessa C, Herve S, Foehrenbach H, Poncet JL. FDG-PET scan in local follow-up of irradiated head and neck squamous cell carcinomas. Ann Otol Rhinol Laryngol 2004;113:628–635
28. Stokkel MP, Terhaard CH, Hordijk GJ, van Rijk PP. The detection of local recurrent head and neck cancer with fluorine-18 fluorodeoxyglucose dual-head positron emission tomography. Eur J Nucl Med 1999;26:767–773
29. Fischbein NJ, Aassar OS, Caputo GR, et al. Clinical utility of positron emission tomography with 18F-fluorodeoxyglucose in detecting residual/recurrent squamous cell carcinoma of the head and neck. AJNR Am J Neuroradiol 1998;19:1189–1196
30. Ryan WR, Fee WE Jr, Le QT, et al. Positron-emission tomography surveillance of head and neck cancer. Laryngoscope 2005;115:645–650
31. Goerres GW, Schmid DT, Bandhauer F, et al. Positron emission tomography in the early follow-up of advanced head and neck cancer. Arch Otolaryngol Head Neck Surg 2004;130:105–109; discussion 120–121
32. Schwartz DL, Rajendran J, Yueh B, et al. Staging of head and neck squamous cell cancer with extended-field FDG-PET. Arch Otolaryngol Head Neck Surg 2003;129:1173–1178
33. Schwartz DL, Rajendran J, Yueh B, et al. FDG-PET prediction of head and neck squamous cell cancer outcomes. Arch Otolaryngol Head Neck Surg 2004;130:1361–1367
34. Yao M, Smith RB, Graham MM, et al. The role of FDG PET in management of neck metastasis from head-and-neck cancer after definitive radiation treatment. Int J Radiat Oncol Biol Phys 2005;63:991–999

Index

Note: Page numbers followed by *f* and *t* indicate figures and tables, respectively.